D1550281

REFORMING HEALTH SECTORS

The 1990's have seen a fundamental questioning of the nature, form and content of health systems. Evidence has accumulated that in terms of efficiency and equity, no country can be satisfied with the performance of its health system. Concerns include: the extent to which health systems are responsive to health needs as opposed to professional preferences; the need to ration access to care and how best to do it; how to make services more responsive to users; and how to ensure that the needs of the poorest and most disadvantaged are met. Countries across the world whether rich or poor, are attempting to change how health systems are financed organised, and managed. Proposed reforms are often radical; progress in implementing reforms is often slow; consensus is notably absent. These papers by leading academics and practitioners shed light on reform ideologies, strategies, and experiences.

Anne Mills is a professor of Health Economics and Policy at the London School of Hygiene and Tropical Medicine

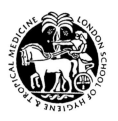

London School of Hygiene & Tropical Medicine
Eighth Annual Public Health Forum

REFORMING HEALTH SECTORS

Edited by
Anne Mills

Series Editor
Alice Dickens

London School of Hygiene & Tropical Medicine, London, UK

KEGAN PAUL INTERNATIONAL
London and New York

First Published in 2000 by
Kegan Paul International Limited
UK: P.O. Box 256, London WC1B 3SW, England
Tel: 020 7580 5511   Fax: 020 7436 0899
E-mail: books@keganpaul.com
Internet: http://www.keganpaul.com
USA: 61 West 62nd Street, New York, NY 10023
Tel: (212) 459 0600   Fax: (212) 259 3678
Internet: http://www.columbia.edu/cu/cup

Distributed by
John Wiley & Sons
Southern Cross Trading Estate
1 Oldlands Way, Bognor Regis
West Sussex, PO22 9SA, England
Tel: (01243) 779 777   Fax: (01243) 820 250
E-mail: cs-books@wiley.co.uk

Columbia University Press
61 West 62nd Street, New York, NY 10023
Tel: (212) 459 0600   Fax: (212) 259 3678
Internet: http://www.columbia.edu/cu/cup

© Kegan Paul International, 2000

Printed in Great Britain, IBT Global London

ISBN: 0-7103-0642-3

British Library Cataloguing in Publication Data
Applied for

Library of Congress Cataloging-in-Publication Data
Applied for

Contents

Contributors

Sara Bennett, Health Policy Unit, London School of Hygiene & Tropical Medicine, Keppel Street, London WC1E 7HT, UK

Somsak Chunharas, Health Systems Research Institute, Building of the Department of Mental Health, Tivanon Road, Nonthaburi, Thailand

Robert G. Evans, Centre for Health Services and Policy Research, University of British Columbia, 429-2194 Health Sciences Mall, Vancouver, BC V6T 1Z3, Canada

Josep Figueras, World Health Organization, European Regional Office, Scherfigsvej 8, DK 2100 Copenhagen Ø, Denmark

Julio Frenk, Executive Vice-President, Mexican Health Foundation, Periferico Sur No 4809, Col. El Arenal Tepepan, Deleg. Talalpan 14610, Mexico DF, Mexico

Declan Gaffney, School of Public Policy, University College London, 29/30 Tavistock Square, London WC1, UK

Lucy Gilson, Centre for Health Policy, University of the Witwatersrand, PO Box 1038, Johannesburg 2000, South Africa

David Harrison, Health Systems Trust, 504 General Building, Cnr Smith and Field Streets, Durban 4001, South Africa

Theodore R, Marmor, Yale University School of Management, Box 208200, 135 Prospect Street, New Haven, CT 06520-8200, USA

Nicholas Mays, Director of Health Services Research, King's Fund Policy Institute, 11-13 Cavendish Square, London W1M 0AN, UK

Barbara McPake, Health Policy Unit, London School of Hygiene & Tropical Medicine, Keppel Street, London WC1E 7HT, UK

Anne Mills, Health Policy Unit, London School of Hygiene & Tropical Medicine, Keppel Street, London WC1E 7HT, UK

Allyson Pollock, School of Public Policy, University College London, 29/30 Tavistock Square, London WC1, UK

Tom Rathwell, Director, School of Health Services Administration, Dalhousie University, 5599 Fenwick Street, Halifax, NS, B3H 1R2, Canada

Richard B. Saltman, Department of Health Policy and Management, The Rollins School of Public Health, Emory University, 1518 Clifton Road NE, Atlanta, GA 30322, USA

Helena Luz Sánchez, Asociación Colombiana de la Salud, Carrera 12# 70-98, Santa Fe de Bogotá, Colombia

Richard Scheffler, School of Public Health, 405 Earl Warren Hall, University of California at Berkeley, Berkeley 94720-7360, USA

Gill Walt, Health Policy Unit, London School of Hygiene & Tropical Medicine, Keppel Street, London WC1E 7HT, UK

Francisco José Yepes, Executive Director, Asociación Colombiana de la Salud, Carrera 12# 70-98, Santa Fe de Bogotá, Colombia

Foreword

David Nabarro

Chief Health and Population Adviser, UK Department for International Development, London, UK

The Eighth Annual Public Health Forum at the London School of Hygiene & Tropical Medicine was a very important event, attended by a healthy mix of senior civil servants, programme managers, representatives of international organizations and academics from the South and the North.

The British Government published its White Paper on International Development in November 1997. Together with colleagues, I have been considering the implications of the material in the Paper for our stance on international health, and on the process of health sector development.

The links between ill-health and poverty are inescapable. However, we question the degree to which they are being adequately addressed by health action taking place throughout the world. What is the reality? High levels of illness and suffering in many communities is a consequence of people's poverty. A poor person affected by serious illness is less likely to be in a position to take advantage of opportunities, and improve well-being, than is one who is wealthy.

The poorest twenty per cent of the world's people—around one thousand million—are: ten times more likely to die young (under 15 years) than the richest 20%; nine times more likely to die of communicable diseases, and twice as likely to die from accidents and injury. Poor women, who are more at risk in general, are at least two hundred times more likely to die of causes related to pregnancy and childbirth. Millions of women and men, particularly adolescents, still cannot access adequate reproductive health care. Serious illness of an adult in a poor household is associated with increased poverty, both now and in future generations.

These inequities, in access to productive resources, to opportunities, to health care and education, are experienced everywhere. They have major implications for health action. The challenge is not just to address absolute poverty, but to establish and maintain equitable approaches to human development everywhere—in countries with higher, as well as lower, Gross National Products.

But was this not what the 'primary health care revolution' was all about? It was designed to address inequity and bring health benefits to poor people. Provision of primary health care was often pursued as a technical issue, increasing the accessibility of low cost health care, redistributing resources to fund inexpensive services and making them available more widely.

The emphasis was on using some public funds to get a minimum package of services to poor people. But a poor people's service is often perceived to be a poor service by those for whom it is designed. Poor people are reported to seek care from providers outside government, or to trek to large hospitals in the hope that they have a chance of accessing services that better-off people take for granted.

The context has changed a lot over the past two decades. Twenty years ago, primary care was sometimes seen as a minimalist requirement for countries to be seen to be tackling the health needs of their poorer people. The situation is different now. Governments increasingly want to prioritize public funds so that they address inequities. As they examine the way in which public funds for health are spent, they are becoming more explicit about the purpose of public finance for health care, the intended consequences, the overall resource availability, the way in which resources are used (i.e. laws, systems, practices), and incentive systems that favour public policies.

In practice, such attempts to change the health sector, so that it addresses inequity, are complex to implement. There are always debates about how scarce resources can best be spent. Different groups use advocacy skills, political links, professional unity and, sometimes, industrial action, to influence both the ways in which resources are allocated and the attention paid by legislators to what is done with them. Changing the ways in which health sectors work is, and always will be, inextricably locked up in political processes: in choices about ways in which resources are allocated and used.

International organizations play their roles in these political processes. They are, to a greater or lesser extent, concerned to address inequities in global health and access to health care. They may also be interested in the efficiency with which resources are used to achieve these outcomes. Their views on optimum patterns of resource use can influence decisions taken by national authorities. The reality of these difficulties at the interface between those who provide external assistance, and those who make use of it, is being more widely accepted.

The sector wide approach to health development is one attempt to establish a process in which all parties can openly debate their concerns, while seeking not to undermine in-country processes. It requires a degree of agreement on policies and priorities for health action, and negotiation is inevitable.

Changing the way in which health sectors work is much more than a technical issue—getting minimal packages of health care to large numbers of people. It is about ways in which pro-poor social policies can be expressed within the health sector, given the range of competing demands for scarce resources. It is vitally important that we learn from the experiences of others, in a way that encourages openness about political realities, the need for negotiation and compromise, and continued efforts to establish milestones for an often unpredictable process. The papers in this volume were commissioned in order to help in this process, by providing an overview of key issues and country experiences in health sector reform

Financial support for the Seventh Annual Public Health Forum *Reforming Health Sectors* was provided by a grant from the UK Department for International Development (DFID), and by the Health Economics and Financing Programme at the London School of Hygiene & Tropical Medicine, which receives a DFID programme grant. We are most grateful for these funds, which facilitated the involvement of many developing country participants. However, the Department for International Development can accept no responsibility for any information or views expressed in this book.

1
Reforming health sectors: fashions, passions and common sense

Anne Mills

London School of Hygiene & Tropical Medicine, UK

I originally thought about the possibility of organizing a Public Health Forum on the subject of health sector reform in 1994, and wrote it into a five-year work plan for the year 1998. I recall colleagues saying that surely by then health sector reform would have given way to some new fashion, and that it was just a passing fad. That is clearly not the case, and while the precise terminology may change, there seems little chance of major reform to health systems disappearing from the policy agenda.

A major reason for this persistence is that reform pressures are not coming merely from within the health sector, but are part of what has been termed a 'public management revolution', which attempts to reshape and improve governance, and change relationships between the State, the market and society (Minogue *et al*, 1997). A key component of this revolution has been new approaches to the management of public sector activities which involve a slimmed down State, reduced levels of public expenditure, increased efficiency in the provision of public services through mechanisms such as contracting and competition, and an extension in the role of the private sector. The social sectors have not been immune from these ideas:

> The conception of social policy as being the professional and/or hierarchical provision of welfare services is being actively replaced by a different image: that of provision by commercial and public interest bodies, with the state playing a regulatory, purchasing and residual providers role (Mackintosh, 1995)

Given the importance of these ideas in recent years in the UK—indeed the UK has been seen as a world leader in putting these ideas into practice—there is a need to be careful not to adopt an unduly anglocentric approach. However, it is generally acknowledged that the new public management is a widespread phenomenon. A number of multilateral agencies, notably the World Bank and the OECD, have been promoting the idea of an emerging consensus on the key characteristics of social sector reform, which would combine a strong role in setting overall policy for the State, with a pluralist approach to service delivery involving a range of different actors.

The World Bank, for example, in the much quoted *World Development Report* of 1993, emphasizes improving the quality and efficiency of government services through decentralization and performance-related incentives, and greater diversity and competition in the supply of health services, including competition between public and private providers (World Bank, 1993).

The OECD, in its 1992 review of the reform of health care in seven OECD countries, identified signs of convergence on an approach to the financing and organization of health care where funding is obtained from taxation or compulsory social insurance contributions, the financial intermediaries are public or quasi public bodies, and they have contractual relationships with providers whether public or private: in other words there is a separation between the funding organizations and providers in contrast to the traditional integrated approach of many publicly funded health systems (OECD, 1992).

A fashionable language is already apparent: terms commonly bandied about include

- purchaser provider split
- quasi markets, internal markets
- competition, contestability
- managed competition/managed care
- contracting
- selectivity and targeting of services to priority groups.

Within this complex field of action and research, the aim of this chapter is to:

- map the terrain of health sector reform
- identify common themes where they exist
- separate out rhetoric from reality.

In doing so, I will draw unashamedly but with due acknowledgement on the writings of some of the key theorists and researchers in health sector reform whose chapters follow in this volume. I will not attempt to analyse experience or draw conclusions on reform strategies since that is the task of the remainder of the book.

There are dangers in this broad approach of analysing overall themes, in particular of discerning patterns where they do not exist. This is especially a danger given the focus of this meeting on the entire world, encompassing countries at very different levels of development, and I will return at the end to issues of the similarity and differences in reform themes and strategies across the world, and the extent to which countries can learn from each other.

In the attempt to cover reforms across the world, I use a diversity of different country groupings, for which I can claim no special virtue. However, since the level of complexity of the health system and particularly of the formal private sector is strongly affected by income level, I most frequently categorize countries by the groupings of low, middle and high income, and formerly socialist.

Health sector reform: what is it?

Health systems have been under recurring scrutiny—for example,with notable reforms to the British National Health Service in 1974 and 1985—but only in recent years has the term 'health sector reform' come to be used (McPake and Machray,1997). The term is used with a distinct connotation that what is occurring is something more than evolutionary, haphazard or marginal change. And since major change is sought, and elements of the health system are inter-related, reform usually implies that a number of changes are occurring at once.

Josep Figueras and colleagues (1997) have provided a list of key elements which help to define when change might be termed reform, and hence help to define the subject matter of this meeting. In terms of the process of change, they suggest key elements are:

- structural rather than incremental or evolutionary change
- change in policy objectives followed by institutional change rather than redefinition of policies alone
- purposive rather than haphazard change
- sustained and long term rather than one-off change
- political and 'top down' process led by national, regional or local governments.

They also suggest that the content of reform is marked by diversity rather than uniformity of measures, and is determined by country-specific characteristics of the health system. The latter may well be true of the European region, their prime concern, but has not been perceived to be always the case outside the developed world where there has been concern about the role of external agencies in influencing reform design (Mogedal *et al*, 1995; Sandiford and Martinez, 1995).

These elements of reform are well summarized in Cassels' definition: 'health sector reform (is) concerned with defining priorities, refining policies and reforming the institutions through which those policies are implemented' (Cassels, 1995). However, such changes are not an end in themselves: it is necessary to state the goals or objectives that reform is intended to serve. This is included in a definition taken as the starting point at a WHO intercountry meeting on health sector reform in sub-Saharan Africa:

> Health sector reform is a sustained process of fundamental change in policy and institutional arrangements, guided by government, designed to improve the functioning and performance of the health sector, and ultimately the health status of the population (Sikosana *et al*,1997).

Health sector reforms are in practice being driven by a number of key problems of health systems.

In the first place, it is thought in many countries that the levels of health produced by the health system are lower than what is believed to be technically possible, and certainly lower than those achieved by the health systems of other countries with access to the same body of knowledge and similar levels of resources. For example, one force for change in the United States has been the recognition that the US has poor life expectancy and high infant mortality despite an expenditure on health care far higher than any other country (Smith, 1997). For Latin America, a recent analysis has compared what levels of health might be expected in the region given its level of income *per capita*, and what is actually achieved (Inter-American Development Bank, 1996) (Table 1.1). Clearly the health system is not the only explanation for these gaps, but it is likely to be an important one.

Table 1.1 The health gap in Latin America and the Caribbean in 1995

Indicator	Observed level	Expected level	Gap (%)
Health services coverage (% of population)	78	89	14
Under-five mortality (per 1000 births)	47	39	17
Life-expectancy at birth (years)	69.5	72	4
Burden of disease and injury (lost DALYs per 1000 people)	231.6	200.1	14

Source: Inter-American Development Bank (1996)

Analyses consistently indicate both a strong relationship between income *per capita* and health indicators such as life expectancy, and certain countries performing worse than others at the same level of income (World Bank, 1993). Over time, increases in knowledge and medical technology, among other things, have permitted countries to achieve higher levels of health with a given income (Figure 1.1). Dean Jamison has termed this 'shifting the curve'. He has also coined the phrase 'joining the curve' to explain the scope for countries with poorer health indicators than might be expected given their level of income to improve health status through improving the performance of their health system (Jamison, 1997).

A second key problem, and one of the explanations for the first problem of poor performance in terms of health status, is that health systems operate with low or very variable levels of efficiency. For example, it is argued that many countries implement programmes of low cost-effectiveness, while not providing enough of the most cost-effective programmes. This has been a key criticism of the spending priorities of low income countries (World Bank, 1993), but the criticism can equally well be levelled at higher income countries (Maynard and

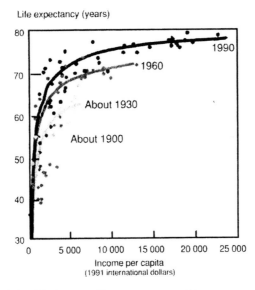

Figure 1.1 The relationship between life expectancy and income per capita for selected countries and periods. Source: World Bank 1993

Bloor, 1995). In terms of technical efficiency, studies of facility costs invariably show great variation in costs across similar types of services, to an extent that is not easily explained by differences in quality but is more likely to be due to problems of managing resources (Mills, 1997). Some countries—particularly those in the developed world—have also experienced high levels of cost inflation to the point where cost containment has been seen as one of the highest priorities (Abel-Smith and Mossialos, 1994).

Quality is a third key problem, especially in the poorer countries where funds are very limited, health service inputs in short supply, and staff poorly paid and hence poorly motivated. Furthermore, where facilities—whether publicly or privately owned—need to generate their own revenue, this can lead to gross o/ver-use of technology. For example China has been experiencing a high technology equipment race since the government regulated pricing structure permits considerable profits to be made from diagnostic equipment such as CT scanners, while maintaining prices of routine hospital services well below costs (World Bank, 1997a).

Another important dimension of quality is that of interpersonal relations between staff and clients. In centralized, integrated public health care systems, in rich and poor countries alike, staff are often criticized for their lack of courtesy to patients and lack of responsiveness to their needs.

The fourth key problem is the mismatch between population expectations for health care, the possibilities for health care interventions created by technological development, and the resources available to finance health care. In the poorest countries this can mean that a significant proportion of the population are without effective access to even basic levels of care. In the richer countries it means that governments have to consider ways of setting priorities and defining limits to what can be provided. In all countries there are difficult issues of how best to ration health care.

This mismatch between needs, demands and resources is being aggravated in all countries by changes in demography and disease patterns. In the middle range of countries, demographic and epidemiological transitions are resulting in changes in the age-structure of the population and a shift in the pattern of disease: from a preponderance of common infections, malnutrition and reproductive events as leading causes of death to a predominance of non-communicable diseases, injuries and new infections (Zwi and Mills, 1995). However, in many countries the 'old' communicable diseases and the 'new' chronic diseases exist side by side, thus imposing what has been termed a double burden (Frenk *et al*, 1989).

The fifth and final key problem is that of equity. Most low and middle income countries fare poorly in terms of both equity of access to care, and equity of payment for care, with a few notable exceptions (Birdsall and Hecht, 1997). Poorer households commonly use health care less frequently, especially in rural areas where access is more difficult and expensive. For example Table 1.2 shows a consistent pattern of the probability of seeking care being higher for higher income quintiles, with the differential by income quintile being less in urban areas.

However, even in urban areas with good access, the poor may end up spending a much higher proportion of their income on health care than higher income groups, partly because public subsidies do not meet their needs well.

Table 1.2 The proportion seeking care in three countries, by income quintile

	1	2	3	4	5
Rural quintiles					
Côte d'Ivoire	23	35	49	39	44
Ghana	26	39	41	46	46
Peru	20	20	30	34	39
Urban quintiles					
Côte d'Ivoire	49	58	63	65	64
Ghana	40	46	55	58	59
Peru	35	44	48	53	57

Source : Baker & van der Gaag (1993)

For example in a city in the north of Thailand, the poorest income quintile spent *per capita* on health care more than three times the amount spent by quintiles 2, 3 and 4 (Pannarunothai and Mills, 1997). One explanation for this, in Thailand and elsewhere, is that the system of public subsidies benefits the rich more than the poor. For example in Kenya, the richest 20% of the rural population capture a much higher proportion of subsidies than the poorest 20%, largely because they are more frequent users of the hospitals that absorb the bulk of public subsidies (Figure 1.2).

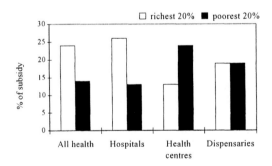

Figure 1.2 The share of public health expenditure received by the poor, rural Kenya, 1993. Source: Birdsall and Hecht (1998)

Such degrees of inequity are not seen in developed world countries where the coverage of publicly funded health care is universal. However, concerns about equity still remain, notably with respect to the incidence of payment for health care and the access to care of particular disadvantaged groups (van Doorslaer *et al*, 1993).

The goals of health sector reform follow from this list of key problems. Common to all sets of objectives are the short hand terms of efficiency, equity of access, and consumer satisfaction. However, there are some notable differences in definitions:

- the prime concern may be the overall share of GNP consumed by health care (OECD 1992) or the share of public revenue (Cassels, 1995): the latter has been a concern of those governments wishing to downsize and to shift the balance of responsibility to private pockets
- consumer preferences are not always mentioned: the OECD explicitly mentions maximizing both health outcomes and consumer satisfaction (OECD, 1992), while objectives specified for low income countries often emphasize health outcomes alone, as measured by indicators such as DALYs;[1]
- financial sustainability may be a key objective for low income countries (McPake and Kutzin, 1997)
- equity of access may be qualified in terms of access to a minimum package of care
- equity in financing health care may be replaced by the more limited objective of income protection (OECD,1992) or protection from catastrophic payments (Cassels, 1995)
- freedom of choice for consumers may be specified as an objective in its own right (OECD, 1992).

The above objectives are driven largely by the values of economics. However, there are likely to be other objectives that health systems—particularly that part funded by governments—seek to meet, if not always defined explicitly. These may include meeting the demands of key influential groups (Reich, 1995; Birdsall and Hecht, 1997), and providing employment (Busse and Wismar, 1997). If this is not taken into account, there is a danger of misinterpreting the reasons why governments embark on health sector reforms, and what they aim to achieve from them.

---

[1] It can be argued that objectives such as consumer satisfaction can be subsumed under the broad term of social preferences, which should be taken into account in any measure of population health status (Murray, 1995) and certainly are part of the assessment of allocative efficiency (Maynard and Bloor, 1995). However, in practice the measures of health status that we have are weak in their reflection of social preferences.

The terrain of health sector reform: fashions and passions

Before embarking on an analysis of key reform themes, it is necessary to map out the field of action: or in other words define the health system that is the target of reform efforts. A number of frameworks are available of differing degrees of complexity (e.g. Frenk and Donabedian,1987; Roemer, 1991; Frenk, 1994; Hoffmeyer and McCarthy,1994). I have chosen one of the simplest frameworks (Figure 1.3). This is less all-encompassing than some, in that it focuses primarily on the health care system, but it is adequate for exploring the key reforms that countries are putting in place. It identifies four key actors:

- the government, which structures and regulates the system;
- the patients/population who as individuals and households ultimately pay for the health system and receive services
- financial intermediaries who collect funds and pay providers, and may operate at national or lower levels
- the providers of services, who themselves can be categorized in various ways such as by level (primary, secondary, tertiary), ownership (public, private for profit, private not for profit), degree of organization (formal, informal), or medical system (allopathic, ayurvedic etc.).

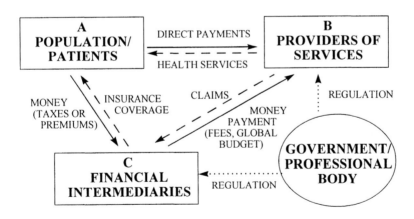

Figure 1.3 The terrain of health sector reform. Source: Reinhardt 1989

These actors perform the four key functions of health systems, namely those of:

- regulation
- financing

- purchasing
- providing.

While this looks quite simple and straightforward, a key difficulty with this structure and categorization, and indeed with any structure, is that in both 'unreformed' and 'reformed' systems, these roles may be divided up in different ways between different actors, and one actor may perform several functions. For example in public integrated systems the government is also the financial intermediary; and in health maintenance organizations, the same organization may manage the raising of funds, purchasing services and providing services, thus collapsing the roles of financial intermediary and provider.

Nonetheless, this structure does provide a basis for considering reform approaches. These, together with key reform topics, are considered in subsequent sections as follows:

The government (overall role, regulation, specifying benefit packages, safeguarding and promoting public health)

The population (role in health care system, financing mechanisms e.g. user fees, insurance)

Financial intermediaries (purchasing, contracts, payment mechanisms)

Providers (decentralization, competition, diversity of ownership, reform to levels of care, evidence-based medicine, quality improvement).

The government

A noted feature of health reforms in many countries has been an increased emphasis on regulation, and a clarification of the key roles of government. These are accepted to include:

- setting and enforcing standards including minimum quality standards
- monitoring the behaviour and performance of providers and insurers (where they exist), including ensuring information is available to do so
- defining an appropriate package of services and/or benefits
- regulations to encourage efficient and equitable financing and delivery of services and to constrain cost inflation (Saltman, 1995).

These roles are not necessarily the functions of the government alone, but may be shared with a range of professional bodies.

In the poorest countries, the emphasis of reforms has been on amending out-of-date legislation and ensuring that new private sector activities are brought within the scope of the law (Russell and Attanayake, 1997; Smithson *et al*, 1997; Bennett and Muraleedharan, 1998; Kumaranayake, 1997). Countries have also introduced legislation that is more permissive with respect to private medical practice (Ngalande-Banda and Walt,1995).

Middle-income countries and those experiencing rapid economic growth have had to cope with a much more diverse range of actors in the private sector, many of them with powerful influence. Updating legislation has been important, but so have been more sophisticated ways to influence behaviour such as reforming payment systems, using the media to educate consumers, and encouraging the development of accreditation schemes now being actively pursued in countries in all regions of the world, for example Thailand (Supachutikul, 1996), Estonia, Georgia (Saltman and Figueras, 1997) and Mexico. Countries with extensive private insurance such as South Africa have in addition been struggling with the dilemmas of how best to regulate the insurance industry (van den Heever, 1997).

In some of these countries, along with some of the most wealthy set of countries, a key feature of new approaches to regulation is the attempts to encourage a competitive market which it is hoped will encourage efficient behaviour without the need for strict command and control regulatory mechanisms. In effect this approach seeks to encourage self-regulation. This has also been proposed for countries with very limited capacity for government regulation (World Bank, 1993).

Beyond regulation, the role that the government adopts in the health system depends crucially on past and present social perceptions of its role in health (Maynard and Bloor, 1995; Saltman and Figueras, 1996). At its crudest, the opposing views can be characterized as firstly a view of health care as a social good, where access to health care is regarded as a citizens' right and should not be affected by income or wealth. At the other extreme, health care can be regarded as just another market commodity, which is rationed by price. These tend to define two ends of a spectrum, with countries falling between according to the extent to which the state intervenes in the health care market.

The belief that the government should assume responsibility for ensuring all citizens get care, regardless of their level of income, has been a feature of many health systems across the world, even though many did not deliver this in practice. A key feature of reform trends in low- and middle-income countries is that this belief is currently being severely questioned. In particular it is argued that aside from their regulatory role, governments in low- and middle-income countries should confine themselves to ensuring the provision of a cost-effective package of basic services for the poor, preferably leaving it to other actors to finance and provide health care for other income groups (World Bank, 1993). Even for services for the poor, the possibility is left open that many of these may be funded by the state but provided by others.

The most radical reforms seem to have taken place in countries in Central and Eastern Europe and the Former Soviet Union, where formerly centrally-run services have been transferred to local government or private ownership (Saltman and Figueras,1997). Some privatization of specific facilities has taken place in other regions of the world, though in general the pace of change has been slow (Mills, 1997). More marked has been an uncontrolled and unplanned process of privatization of facilities, where government's inability to finance services adequately, and/or encouragement of facilities to generate a substantial proportion of their revenue, have led to public facilities in practice operating as private enterprises (for example: China (World Bank, 1997a) and Uganda (Asiimwe *et al*, 1997)).

Selective targeting of a basic package of services to the poor is a reform theme only in poorer countries but the issue of the definition of a package has been universal, as has been the application of cost-effectiveness or cost-utility analysis as part of the process of defining the package. The developed world has been experimenting with a diversity of approaches to setting priorities, and public debate has been seen as an important component of priority setting (Maynard and Bloor, 1995; Saltman and Figueras, 1997; Smee, 1997). In contrast in low-income countries, the setting of priorities has been top down and recommended on the basis of technical analysis (World Bank, 1993).

The one area where there seems to be general agreement over the state's role is that of promoting and protecting public health. Yet despite this, reform efforts appear to concentrate on the medical care system, leaving unanswered the crucial questions of how best to pursue public health more broadly defined.

The population

The people at large can be involved in health reform and are affected by it in three key ways:

- as part of reformed managing and policy-making structures
- as patients
- as payers.

Europe demonstrates a variety of approaches to involving citizens at both collective and individual levels, and in recent years has seen the strengthening of mechanisms to protect patients' rights (Saltman and Figueras, 1997). Outside Europe, efforts seem more muted, successes less common. Some mechanisms are similar, for example the introduction of health or hospital boards with citizen representation (Mogedal *et al*, 1995), though there has been little evaluation of experience. In many of the poorest countries, local government structures are weak, ruling them out as an immediate means for ensuring local representation (Mills *et al*, 1990). Often community involvement is seen to occur via NGOs rather than government health services (Mackintosh,1995). Similarly, little attention has been paid to patient rights, and patients tend to appear as the object of reforms, rather than as the subject.

In contrast, people as payers appear prominently in reforms in low-income countries. Indeed, a universal component of health reforms appears to be changes in financing arrangements. User fees have been a very common component of reform packages, especially in Africa but also in central and eastern Europe (Gilson and Mills, 1995; Saltman and Figueras, 1997). Their prime motivation has usually been to raise revenue, unlike in high-income countries where if they are promoted, this is on the grounds of restraining demand.

The other key reforms concerning financing have involved risk-pooling mechanisms. A virtually universal feature of reform approaches has been the notable absence of proposals to place increased reliance on tax finance, except in a few countries where the alternative of insurance is clearly not feasible. In contrast, the introduction or reform of insurance has been a common component of reform across the world. Approaches to health insurance considered include

- compulsory social insurance
- medical savings accounts
- community-based voluntary insurance
- voluntary private insurance, especially as supplementary to basic compulsory social insurance.

In general, where a sufficient proportion of the population is in formal employment, compulsory social insurance has been the preferred option. A key issue, however, has been the organizational arrangements for insurance, considered further below.

Financial intermediaries

In both countries introducing compulsory insurance, and those engaged in reforming existing systems, a key and controversial issue has been whether or not to encourage competition between insurance funds and to encourage choice of insurer. In Western Europe, countries have proceeded very cautiously. In contrast, there is very active exploration of arrangements that would permit competitive pressures to be felt by financial intermediaries in some countries in Latin America, and central and eastern Europe. Londoño and Frenk (1997), for example, propose a model of reform for Latin America which involves organizations competing to enroll individuals, and being compensated by a risk-adjusted capitation payment. This approach is, for example, being implemented in Colombia (see Yepes and Sánchez, this volume), and Argentina (World Bank, 1997b).

As part of the reconsideration of the roles of both financial intermediaries and providers, there has been increased specification of the purchaser role. The purchasing role is one of defining needs, specifying tasks, arranging for service provision, and monitoring spending and performance. Traditionally, financial intermediaries, whether part of a government bureaucracy or a public or quasi-public insurance fund or agency, have taken a passive approach to providers, reimbursing whatever they spend and undertaking little analysis of efficiency or quality. The reform programmes of a number of countries now include emphasis on a more active purchaser, which may be a patient (Saltman, 1995), but is more usually an institutional purchaser such as a health authority, an insurance agency or a provider. Perhaps the best known introduction of the purchaser role is the UK, but there are many other examples. Management reforms being discussed in South Africa, planned in Zimbabwe (Russell *et al*, 1997) and implemented in Zambia specify a purchasing role for district authorities. In the US, managed care organizations are actively engaged in controlling the provision of care (Scheffler, this volume). In the UK, some Swedish counties, and New Zealand, general practitioners have taken on budgets to purchase services not previously part of their responsibilities (Malcolm 1997; Saltman and Figueras 1997). In Thailand the social security office accredits and monitors hospitals which are eligible to provide care to the compulsorily insured (Tangcharoensathien and Supachutikul, 1997).

Along with the specification of the purchaser's role has come an emphasis on contractual arrangements between purchasers and providers. At one extreme these arrangements may be seen as no more that the formalization of a management relationship, as where annual contracts are agreed between a national ministry of health and an executive agency (Zambia) or a regional health authority (Trinidad), or between a province and a district (South Africa, Zambia, Zimbabwe). At the other extreme the contracts may be awarded on a competitive basis, and may be legally binding (as in New Zealand: Ashton, 1998).

Also linked to the relationship between purchaser and provider is the payment mechanism: the basis on which funds are transferred from purchasers to providers. Health sector reforms commonly involve changes to traditional modes of payment, though the nature of the reforms depends on the starting point and is severely constrained by powerful interest groups, hence a great variety of reforms are apparent in practice. In general, fee-for-service methods of payment are seen to be undesirable, and there is also now a history of countries introducing fee-for-service payment in new compulsory insurance schemes and suffering the consequences of cost inflation (for example: Korea: Yang, 1997; Czech Republic: Saltman and Figueras, 1997). Yet fee-for-service payment systems are very difficult to change where they already exist except by capping total expenditure and allowing the point value of services to decrease if the volume of services provided is greater than allowed for.

Conversely, countries such as those in eastern and central Europe which provided salaries to primary care providers have sought to raise remuneration levels and encourage greater productivity by using a mix of salary, fee-for-service and capitation. Indeed, capitation appears to be one of the areas where there is most experimentation worldwide. Traditionally an approach for paying primary care providers, it is being extended to pay for hospital care as well in Thailand for example (Tangcharoensathien and Supachutikul, 1997), and is the basis for payment in many managed care arrangements.

Global budgets for hospitals have been a feature in Europe under very different funding regimes. Concern that they do not provide incentives to efficiency has led to introduction of measures of hospital activity such as bed days or cases, or even service-specific payments (Saltman and Figueras, 1997). Some similar reform trends can be seen elsewhere: Thailand, Taiwan, Korea and Mexico are all considering case-based payments to hospitals. In general, whatever the precise nature of reforms to payment mechanisms, the concern is that the payment method should transmit the right incentives to encourage good performance.

Providers

Key reform themes concerning providers have been decentralization, competition, diversity of ownership, reform to levels of care, evidence-based medicine, and quality improvement.

Even in health systems which maintain a strong public role in provision, decentralization has been a common and almost universal theme. Indeed, the extent to which it is being adopted throughout the world raises expectations of a pendulum swing in the opposite direction in the not too distant future. At the national level, decentralization has taken the form of restructuring the role and functions of ministries of health (Kutzin, 1995), with some countries creating executive agencies to take over management responsibility at national level (e.g. Zambia, Ghana), leaving the ministry to concentrate on regulation, policy and monitoring. Some form of decentralization to intermediate and local levels is also a common theme, with most countries choosing to decentralize services within a hierarchical structure with the MOH at the top, though there are a few notable examples of devolution of health to local government (e.g. Philippines). Finally, decentralization even further, to hospital level, is a common trend in countries with centrally funded, public systems of health care provision. In the poorest countries, because of limits on management capacity, this reform may be confined to teaching hospitals, but in some countries such as Indonesia a wider range of hospitals are being made 'autonomous' (Bossert et al, 1997).

Competition between providers is similarly being widely promoted as a means to encourage efficiency, though with rather more caution and doubts about its effects than in the case of decentralization. However, the doubts are rather more evident with respect to developed country health systems (e.g. Smee, 1997) than in developing countries where the desirability of using competition as a stimulus to efficiency is widely emphasized.

Diversity of ownership is similarly being promoted as a means to increase competitive pressures, especially on poorly performing public systems of provision. Some African countries formerly known for their opposition to private medical practice have liberalized laws and allowed new cadres (e.g. paramedical staff) to practise privately (Ngalande-Banda and Walt, 1995; Bennett et al, 1994). African governments have also been urged to give greater emphasis to NGOs. In a number of South East Asian countries tax incentives have been provided for the construction of private hospitals (e.g. India: Bennett and Muraleedharan, 1998; Philippines: Herrin,1997; Thailand: Bennett and Tangcharoensathien, 1994).

Strengthening the role of primary care has long been a theme in reforms in many countries, though often without substantial changes in resource allocation patterns. In Europe it has been said that although reform documents typically emphasize PHC, in practice it has often been treated as a marginal player (Saltman and Figueras, 1997). The same might be said throughout the world, with few exceptions. However, experiments with giving primary care doctors funds to purchase other services have aroused a lot of interest though the primary level itself may require substantial strengthening before this is possible. Many low- and middle-income countries have poorly developed public primary care centres, and in urban areas substantial numbers of private clinics which are heavily patronized as well as public and private hospitals which have large, open access out-patient departments. Efforts to create high quality primary care services, with a gatekeeper role for the primary care doctor, do not as yet appear to feature strongly in reforms.

Finally, part of many reform packages has been measures to improve the quality of the care provided. In rich countries a range of approaches is being used, including evidence-based medicine, technology assessment, clinical guidelines, medical audit, and quality assurance methods. These are beginning to feature in less wealthy countries, but in the poorest countries more basic problems have been addressed, such as availability of drugs and supplies, improvement of staff skills, and maintenance of equipment.

Common sense

Following this broad review of reform themes, common sense might react and say that order is being imposed where there is none; and that in practice countries are adopting very different approaches to reform, and moving at very different speeds. Certainly what I have said should not be taken to imply that all countries are adopting a similar package of reforms and producing similarly structured health systems. Rhetoric may appear similar due to the spread of ideas around the world and the activities of agencies involved in both transferring knowledge and recommending reforms. However, in practice, reforms are shaped by the particular forces operating in the local setting, and influenced by their starting point. So the fact that we currently see clear differences in the arrangements and funding of health systems throughout the world itself will dictate that many differences will remain.

Moreover, the current craze for reform and urge to effect major change leads to a rhetoric of reform that often masks the truth that fundamental change has not occurred. Paradoxically, it is appearing that new public management ideas are making greatest inroads where existing state structures and bureaucracies are weak, creating the danger that weak state provision may be replaced by unregulated non-state provision. Precisely those countries where state bureaucracies are strongest and most need reform, are those which are amongst the hardest to change. In addition, societies with a number of strong institutional interest groups and no effective mechanism to agree change often face major barriers to reform. A review of a large number of largely rich countries comments that

> the patterns that emerge—in country after country—are largely comprised of promises and pronouncements rather than ample evidence of firm implementation (Björkman and Altenstetter, 1997).

One of the areas of greatest disagreement in reform policies has been whether or not competition should be a key strategy in improving efficiency. In terms of competition between insurers, it is notable that European reforms have been much more cautious than at least the language of reform elsewhere. For Europe, it has recently been concluded that

> efforts to create more market orientated behaviour among third party insurers by introducing competitive incentives among them have met ...economic and social obstacles

and that

> It remains to be demonstrated whether competition between insurers leads to more efficient and effective health care, and whether newly implemented mechanisms that combine solidarity with competition will be successful in sustaining both policy objectives (Saltman and Figueras, 1997).

On the provider side there appears to be less argument over the beneficial effects of some degree of competition, though there is concern that there will be a lack of effective competition in many areas and that regulation may be ineffective in ensuring that competition has positive results (Bennett, 1997).

Given the tendency to promote similar reforms in different contexts, it is vital to emphasize that the same reforms implemented in different contexts can have very different effects. This point can be illustrated by taking the example of capitation. In the UK, it has been used for many decades to pay primary care physicians. While there have undoubtedly been some concerns that capitation may encourage more referrals than necessary, and some degree of under-provision of care, these concerns have not been major ones. In contrast, since capitation was introduced in Thailand to pay for the compulsorily insured, there have been major concerns that hospitals, especially private hospitals, have sought to minimize the amount of care provided (Tangcharoensathien *et al*, 1999). Key to the actual results of a specific reform is likely to be the institutional context in the country, including an informed patient body, formal monitoring systems, quality assurance procedures, and especially professional ethics. As Abel-Smith and Mossialos (1994) commented,

> Under any system of payment it is the ethics and social commitment of the doctor which matter most of all. Where standards are low in these respects no financial structure can induce doctors to be what they are not.

Similar concerns have been raised about the effect of making public hospitals autonomous and requiring them to raise a substantial proportion of their income: in the absence of constraining influences both internal and external, they may simply turn themselves into private enterprises serving those who can pay. There is already evidence from China on the dangers (Jie, 1997; World Bank 1997a), and evidence from Indonesia that hospitals given greater autonomy have restricted the access to services of poorer groups (Bossert *et al*, 1997).

An important dimension of the context is the state's capacity to monitor and regulate. As stated earlier, reforms place great emphasis on the regulatory role of the state. However, given the prevailing view that the state has failed in the direct provision of health care, it is not clear why there is greater faith in its ability to regulate, especially the more sophisticated forms of regulating that seek to avoid the 'command and control' mode. For the richer countries, it has been said that

> the current state must have even more strengths and abilities than its archaic predecessors if it is going to capitalise on the virtuous efficiencies of the market place without suffering the latter's side effects which in humanitarian terms are unacceptable (Björkman and Altenstetter, 1997).

This is a tall order for the poorest countries.

There are two other areas where common sense must intrude on reform fashions. The first is the tendency to argue that the objectives of efficiency and equity can be satisfied at the same time. However, there are increasing suggestions that they may demand a trade off. For example, increased autonomy has tended to increase rather than decrease government allocations to hospitals, and hence has worsened the inequity of public funding patterns (Govindaraj and Chawla, 1996), and employing competitive pressures to improve efficiency may lead providers and insurers to discriminate against those with greater health risks.

The second is the argument that equity objectives are best met by strictly targeting public support to needy groups. In contrast, there are clear dangers of targeting which result in segmented systems. A service only for the poor is likely to remain a poor service (Mackintosh, 1995; 1997; Reddy and Vandemoortele,1996; Burgess, 1997).

Conclusions

I began by noting the emphases of a number of agencies on an emerging consensus. The IADB's agenda, for example, contains many of the reforms I have reviewed:

> Public finance and regulation, provider autonomy and consumer empowerment are the cornerstones of improved functioning....Public sources are better allocated according to outcomes and with increased autonomy by providers. Payment methods based on capitation are preferred. Equity can be improved when access to services is guaranteed by the public funding that individuals bring with them to the ..clinic, rather than by proximity to a centrally planned facility. Consumer decision making powers can be strengthened with greater information regarding the quality of diverse providers, with greater voice in the functioning of purchasing agencies and providers and with greater options for choosing amongst numerous providers (Inter-American Development Bank, 1996).

Not dissimilar conclusions have emerged from European experience, though with less emphasis on the consumer as a purchaser.

In contrast, an alternative view is beginning to be heard, that 'reform needs to be tightly embedded in the diverse institutional structures of individual countries and areas' (Mackintosh, 1995), and that approaches based on principles of strict regulation, competition and contracts are doomed to fail because those regulated will always find ways to manipulate the situation to benefit themselves. Instead, it may be better to encourage the development of co-operation and socially oriented values and motives (Zuckerman and de Kadt, 1997).

It is remarkable how the so-called emerging consensus is not backed by adequate evidence that the proposed models will in fact achieve what they are intended to. Perhaps this is not surprising: many reforms are driven more by ideological motivations than objective analysis. However, given that the language of reforms is that of rational analysis, and that the improvements they are intended to bring are vital, it is important that more attention be paid to monitoring and evaluating the achievements of reform, and to researching the effects of specific reform strategies.

Indeed, the remarkable absence of good-quality research is increasingly being noted (Janovsky, 1996; World Health Organization, 1996; Smee, 1997). Two key areas require emphasis. The first is research closely tailored to the needs of country decision makers, and done in such a way that its results can readily be used. The second is research that by comparing the experiences of a number of countries, is able to generalize beyond the very specific circumstances of each country study. It is usually the case in the area of health system research that we rarely have gold standards by which we can say that a result is good or bad and that the same result will be obtained regardless of the context. Instead, we need comparative research to study the relative effectiveness of similar strategies in different country contexts. An important aim of this book is to contribute to the exchange between researchers and decision-makers that is required if we are to be able collectively to identify and implement effective reforms.

References

Abel-Smith B, Mossialos E. *Cost Containment and Health Care Reform. A Study of the European Union.* London: London School of Economics and Political Science, 1994
Ashton T. Contracting for health services in New Zealand: a transaction cost analysis. *Social Science and Medicine*, 1998; **46**: 357–367
Asiimwe D, McPake B., Mwesigye F *et al.* The private-sector activities of public-sector health workers in Uganda. In: Bennett S, McPake B, Mills A (eds) *Private Health Providers in Developing Countries: Serving the Public Interest?* London: Zed Books, 1997: 141–157
Baker JL, van der Gaag J. Equity in health care and health care financing: evidence from five developing countries. In: van Doorslaer E, Wagstaff A, Rutten F (eds) *Equity in the Finance and Delivery of Health Care. An International Perspective.* Oxford: Oxford University Press, 1993, pp 356–394
Bennett S. *The Mystique of Markets: Public and Private Health Care in Developing Countries.* London: London School of Hygiene & Tropical Medicine, PHP Departmental Publication No. 4, 1991
Bennett S. Health-care markets: defining characteristics. In: Bennett S, McPake B, Mills A (eds) *Private Health Providers in Developing Countries: Serving the Public Interest?* London: Zed Books, 1997, pp 85–101

Bennett S, Muraleedharan VR. *Reforming the Role of Government in Tamil Nadu Health Sector*. Birmingham: Development Administration Group, University of Birmingham, 1998. The role of Government in Adjusting Economies, Paper no. 28

Bennett S, Ngalande-Banda E, Teglgaard O. *Public and Private Roles in Health. A Review and Analysis of Experience in sub-Saharan Africa*. Geneva: World Health Organization, 1994 (WHO/ARA/CC.97.6)

Bennett S, Tangcharoensathien V. A shrinking state? Politics, economics and private health care in Thailand. *Public Administration and Development*, 1994; **14**: 1–17

Birdsall N, Hecht, R. Swimming against the tide: strategies for improving equity in health. In: Colclough C (ed) *Marketizing Education and Health in Developing Countries - Miracle or Mirage?* Oxford: Clarendon Press, 1997: 347–366

Björkman JW, Altenstetter C. Globalised concepts and local practice: convergence and divergence in national health policy reforms. In: Altenstetter C, Björkman JW (eds) *Health Policy Reform, National Variations and Globalisation*. Basingstoke: Macmillan Press, 1997

Bossert T, Kosen S, Harsono B, Gani A. *Hospital Autonomy in Indonesia*. Data for Decision Making Project. Boston: Harvard School of Public Health, 1997

Burgess RSL. Fiscal reform and the extension of basic health and education coverage. In: Colclough C (ed) *Marketizing Education and Health in Developing Countries - Miracle or Mirage?* Oxford: Clarendon Press, 1997

Busse R, Wismar M. Health care reform in Germany: the end of cost containment? *Eurohealth*, 1997; **3**: 32–34

Cassels A. Health sector reform: key issues in less developed countries. *Journal of International Development*, 1995; **7**: 329–348

Figueras J, Saltman, R, Mossialos E. *Challenges in Evaluating Health Sector Reform: an Overview*. London: London School of Economics and Political Science, 1997

Frenk J. Dimensions of health system reform. *Health Policy*,1994; **27**: 19–34

Frenk J, Bobadilla JL, Sepulveda J, Lopez Cervantes M. Health transition in middle-income countries: new challenges for health. *Health Policy and Planning*, 1989; **4**: 29–39

Frenk J, Donabedian A. State Intervention in medical care: types, trends and variables. *Health Policy and Planning*, 1987; **2**: 17–31

Gilson L, Mills A. Health sector reforms in sub-Saharan Africa: lessons of the last 10 years. In: Berman P (ed) *Health Sector Reform in Developing Countries. Making Health Development Sustainable*. Boston, Harvard University Press, 1995, pp 277–316

Govindaraj R, Chawla, M. *Recent Experiences with Hospital Autonomy in Developing Countries - What can we learn?* Data for Decision Making Project. Boston: Harvard School of Public Health, 1996

Herrin A. Private health sector performance and regulation in the Philippines. In: Newbrander W (ed) *Private Health Sector Growth in Asia. Issues and Implications*. Chichester: John Wiley & Sons, 1997, pp 157–173

Hoffmeyer UK, McCarthy TR. *Financing Health Care*. Volume I. Dordrecht: Kluwer Academic Publishing, 1994

Inter-American Development Bank. *Economic and Social Progress in Latin America*. Special section 'Making Social Services Work'. Washington DC: Johns Hopkins University Press for the Inter-American Development Bank, 1996

Jamison D. Presentation to Health Policy/Systems Research Initiative. An informal consultation. 10–12 April 1997, Lejondal, Sweden (unpublished)

Janovsky K (ed) Health Policy and systems development. An agenda for research. Geneva: World Health Organization, 1996 (WHO/SHS/NHP/96.1)

Jie C. The impact of health sector reform on county hospitals. *IDS Bulletin*, 1997; **28**: 48–52

Kumaranayake L. The role of regulation: influencing private sector activity within health sector reform. *Journal of International Development*, 1997; **9**: 641–649

Kutzin J. Experience with organizational and financing reform of the health sector. Geneva: World Health Organization, 1995 (WHO/SHS/CC 94.3)

Londoño J-L, Frenk J. Structured pluralism: towards an innovative model for health system reform in Latin America. *Health Policy*, 1997; **41**: 1–36

Mackintosh M. Competition and contracting in selective social provisioning. *European Journal of Development Research*, 1995;7: 26–52

Mackintosh M. Informal regulation: a conceptual framework and application to decentralised mixed finance in health care. Paper prepared for the conference on Public Sector Management for the Next Century, Institute of Development Policy and Management, Manchester, 29 June–2 July, 1997

Malcolm L. New Zealand's experience of radical health reform: from market competition to managed collaboration. *Eurohealth*, 1997; **3**: 29–31

Maynard A, Bloor K. Health care reform: informing difficult choices. *International Journal of Health Planning and Management*, 1995;10: 247–264

McPake B, Kutzin J. *Methods for Evaluating Effects of Health Reforms.* Geneva: World Health Organization, 1997. Current Concerns series, ARA Paper number 13. (WHO/ARA/CC/97.3)

McPake B, Machray, C. International comparisons of health sector reform: towards a comparative framework for developing countries. *Journal of International Development*, 1997; **9**: 621–629

Mills A, Vaughan JP, Smith DL, Tabibzadeh I. *Health System Decentralization. Concepts,1 issues and Country Experience.* Geneva: World Health Organization, 1990

Mills A. Improving the efficiency of public sector health services in developing countries: bureaucratic versus market Approaches. In: Colclough C (ed) *Marketizing Education and Health in Developing Countries. Miracle or Mirage?* Oxford: Clarendon Press, 1997 pp 245–274

Minogue M, Polidano C, Hulme D. Re-organising the State towards more inclusive governance. *Insights*, 1997; **23**: 1–2

Mogedal S, Steen SH, Mpelumbe G. Health sector reform and organizational issues at the local level: lessons from selected African countries. *Journal of International Development*, 1995; 7: 349–367

Murray CJL. Towards an analytical approach to health sector reform. In: Berman P (ed) *Health Sector Reform in Developing Countries. Making Health Development Sustainable.* Boston, Harvard University Press, 1995, pp 121–142

Ngalande-Banda E, Walt G. The private health sector in Malawi: opening Pandora's Box? *Journal of International Development*,1995; 7: 403–22

OECD. The Reform of Health Care: a Comparative Analysis of Seven OECD Countries. Health Policy Studies No. 2. Paris: OECD, 1992

Pannarunothai S, Mills A. The poor pay more: health-related inequality in Thailand. *Social Science and Medicine*, 1997; **44**: 1781–1790

Reddy S, Vandermoortele J. *User Financing of Basic Social Services.* New York: United Nations Children's Fund (UNICEF), 1996

Reich MR. The politics of health sector reform in developing countries: three cases of pharmaceutical policy. In: Berman P (ed) *Health Sector Reform in Developing Countries: Making Health Development Sustainable*. Boston: Harvard University Press, 1995, pp 59–99

Roemer MI. National Health Systems of the World. Volume 1: The Countries. New York: Oxford University Press, 1991

Russell S, Attanayake N. *Sri Lanka—Reforming the Health Sector: Does Government have the Capacity?* Birmingham: Development Administration Group, University of Birmingham, 1997. Role of Government in Adjusting Economies. Paper No. 14

Russell S, Kwaramba P, Hongoro C, Chikandi S. *Zimbabwe: Reforming the Health Sector: Does Government have the Capacity?* Birmingham: Development Administration Group, University of Birmingham, 1997. Role of Government in Adjusting Economies. Paper No. 20

Saltman R. *Applying Planned Market Logic to Developing Countries' Health Systems: an Initial Exploration.* Geneva: World Health Organization, 1995. Forum on health sector reform; Discussion paper no 4.

Saltman R, Figueras J. On solidarity and competition: an evidence-based perspective. *Eurohealth*, 1996; **2**: 19–20

Saltman RB, Figueras J (eds) *European Health Care Reform. Analysis of Current Strategies.* Copenhagen: World Health Organization, 1997. WHO Regional Publications, European Series no.72

Sandiford P, Martinez J. *Health Sector Reforms in Central America.* Liverpool: Liverpool School of Tropical Medicine, 1995

Sikosana PLN, Dlamini QQD, Issakov A. Health sector reform in sub-Saharan Africa: a review of experiences, information gaps and research needs. Geneva: World Health Organization, 1997 (WHO/ARA/CC/97.2)

Smee CH. Bridging the gap between public expectations and public willingness to pay. *Health Economics*, 1997; **6**: 1–9

Smith R. The future of healthcare systems. *British Medical Journal*, 1997; **314**: 1495–1496

Smithson P, Asamoa-Baah A, Mills A. *The Case of the Health Sector in Ghana.* Birmingham: Development Administration Group, University of Birmingham, 1997. Role of Government in Adjusting Economies. Paper No. 26

Supachutikul A. *Situation Analysis on Health Insurance and Future Development.* Bangkok: Health Systems Research Institute, 1996

Tangcharoensathien V, Supachutikul A. Compulsory health insurance development in Thailand. Bangkok: Health Systems Research Institute, 1997

Tangcharoensathien V, Supachutikul A, Lertiendumrong J. The social security scheme in Thailand: what lessons can be drawn? *Social Science and Medicine*, 1999; **48**: 913–923

van Doorslaer E, Wagstaff A, Rutten F (eds) *Equity in the Finance and Delivery of Health Care. An International Perspective.* Oxford: Oxford University Press, 1993

van den Heever A. Regulating the funding of private health care: the South African experience. In: Bennett S, McPake B, Mills A (eds) *Private Health Providers in Developing Countries: Serving the Public Interest?* London: Zed Books, 1997, pp158-173

World Bank. *Investing in Health: World Development Report 1993.* New York: World Bank, 1993

World Bank. *Financing Health Care: Issues and Options for China*. Washington DC: World Bank, 1997a. (China 2020 Series, Volume 4)

World Bank. Argentina: facing the challenge of health insurance reform. Washington DC: World Bank, 1997b

World Health Organization. *Investing in Health Research and Development. Report of the Ad Hoc Committee on Health Research Relating to Future Intervention Options*. Geneva: World Health Organization, 1996

Yang B-M. The role of health insurance in the growth of the private health sector in Korea. In: Newbrander W (ed) *Private Health Sector Growth in Asia: Issues and Implications*. Chichester: John Wiley & Sons, 1997, pp 61–81

Zukerman E, de Kadt E (eds) *The Public-Private Mix in Social Services—Health Care and Education in Chile, Costa Rica and Venezuela*. Washington DC: Inter-American Development Bank, 1997

Zwi A, Mills A. Health policy in less developed countries: past trends and future directions. *Journal of International Development*, 1995; 7: 299–328

2
Health for all or wealth for some? Conflicting goals in health care reform

Robert G. Evans

Department of Economics and Centre for Health Services and Policy Research, University of British Columbia, and Canadian Institute for Advanced Research

Death of a steersman: the myth of shared goals

All proponents of health reform seek to improve the health of the populations served. Or so they say. Yet the policies and strategies offered are extraordinarily diverse, and to a considerable degree inconsistent or in direct conflict with each other. And they arise from radically different visions of the 'good' —i.e. healthy— society. The health promoters' fit, well fed, socially well adjusted and depressingly well-behaved citizenry are worlds apart from the compliant pill-poppers implicit in the approach of NERA and the PPBHC[1]; the professionally guided, scientifically-tuned health care of the Cochrane Collaboration is not on the same planet as the consumers' paradise of Friedman-esque fantasy[2]. If all share a common goal, some at least are holding the map upside down.

A popular reconciliation is offered by the 'steersman' metaphor. We are all in the same boat, trying to reach the same destination, but navigation is complex and

---

[1] The PPBHC (Pharmaceutical Partners for Better Health Care) supported the NERA study (Hoffmeyer and McCarthy, 1994) which purported to show that the underfunding of health care is universal and large—outside Switzerland!— and that the only remedy is more private financing (Towse, 1995).

[2] Friedman (1962) offered a vision of a health care system organized entirely through private competitive markets. He asked: 'Why are there not [private] department stores of medicine?' but has been unable to hear the answers.

difficult. We therefore debate how best to advise the steersman in choosing a route – disagreeing over means, not ends. In particular the determinants of health are far from well understood, and there is room for considerable difference of opinion over how 'we' should proceed. On this interpretation, progress in understanding should lead to convergence of policy recommendations. More research is needed.

This picture, while containing elements of truth, is fundamentally in error. Two features of the current reform debate are of particular significance.   First, it is striking that in discussions of reform, so small a role is played by the growing literature on, and understanding of, the determinants of health itself. That dog rarely barks. There is in particular a growing interest in the sources and significance of 'inequalities in health' within populations, and in possible policy responses. But these discussions are carried on largely in isolation from those about the reform of the health care system. Indeed some of the more radical proposals for system change would appear on current understanding to pose a significant threat to population health.[3]

Second, although they may be re-phrased in a new and often rather impenetrable language imported from the worlds of insurance and management consulting, most of the ideas are in fact quite old. We are watching re-runs of the debates that took place at the origins of our public funding systems, and before. Old ideas have found their way back onto the agenda, at least for discussion, in complete disregard not only of the evolving evidence on the determinants of health, but of the working experience of health care systems over the last fifty years. That history, and accompanying progress in research, have provided a number of important lessons on the implications and consequences of different ways of organizing and funding care. A number of 'reformers' appear, however, to have missed those classes (or dropped the course entirely).

These observations cannot be reconciled with the presumption of a population united in the goal of improving health, and disagreeing only over the best means to achieve it.   In fact the most persistent and intractable conflicts over the proper direction for health care reform arise from disagreements over ends, not means. These in turn are rooted in fundamental conflicts of economic interest in every society.   'More research' can certainly clarify, but can never resolve, these conflicts.   In this context the steersman metaphor serves only to divert attention (sometimes deliberately) from the real forces at work.

'A Wedge for Understanding': recognizing heterogeneity in populations

A more enlightening perspective arises from the observation and interpretation of 'heterogeneity', through a process that has been basic to understanding the

---

[3] A particularly retrograde 'reform' argument is that governments should concern themselves with improving the broader social and environmental determinants of health... and get out of the business of funding and regulating health care! The second half of the recommendation appears to be the real objective.

determinants of health of populations. Populations can be partitioned into sub-groups on a variety of different measures—age, sex, occupation, income, education, region of residence.... If one finds unambiguous and systematic differences in health status across such partitions, then they presumably contain information about the determinants of health. The direction of causality may not be clear—indeed each may be correlated with some other unobserved variable(s)—but there is *some* systematic relationship between the partitioning variable and the health measure.

Particular attention has been given to the universally observed relationship between measures of social class—income, education, occupational status—and various measures of health outcome, particularly mortality. The exploration of such 'inequalities', however, easily becomes politically polarized, for obvious reasons. The more general observation is that such heterogeneities, whatever their normative significance, represent a 'wedge for greater understanding' of the determinants of health.[4]

The 'Representative Agent'—representing whose interests?

Most economic theory, by contrast, rests on the assumption (normally implicit) that populations consist of identical individuals. Of course 'people are different'; and for some purposes—the analysis of insurance markets, for example—these differences become critical. But they can be captured in a probability distribution (of health outcomes, for example) that is identical across individuals. People are different, but in a random way; there will be no systematic differences among sub-populations. (Empirical studies must, of course, take account of some, at least, of the characteristics of their individual observations.)

One can then represent the behaviour of an entire population by that of a single, 'representative agent'—typically rational, informed, and self-interested. That agent's behaviour is predicated upon a particular structure of objectives and constraints, and its responses to changes in that structure become theoretically predictable. The (average) behaviour of the entire population is then predicted by scaling up that of the representative agent. In this conceptual framework, conflicts of interest are not merely impossible, but inconceivable. How can identical individuals—much less a single representative individual—have conflicting objectives?

To the extent that discussions of health care reform are carried on by economists, or more generally in terms of economic concepts and modes of thinking, the representative agent sneaks in with the intellectual baggage. It provides a natural basis for the steersman metaphor—how do we identify and carry out those reforms that are best for all of us?—and 'distributional problems are

---

[4] ...[T]here is a tremendous potential to exploit heterogeneity in populations as a wedge for greater understanding.' (Sapolsky, 1993).

ignored'.[5] But distributional problems do not disappear just because the analyst ignores them. Important in themselves, they also have significant effects on the economist's chosen concern of resource allocation.

A focus on heterogeneities, by contrast, leads one to look for ways of partitioning the population. Can we identify sub-groups with differing economic interests, for whom alternative reform strategies are likely to lead to very different distributions of both economic and health burdens and benefits? Is there a systematic relationship between the 'reforms' advocated by different groups, and their differing economic interests? Such an approach permits one to express the pretty obvious notion that people—not just individuals but rather well-defined and more or less self-aware sub-groups within the population—are pursuing very different objectives in any reform process. The persistence of ancient debates in new language, and the extraordinary resistance to evidence of some of the traditional positions, reflect these persisting conflicts of interest.

Such an observation would be rather banal and obvious in an elementary course in politics or public policy. Conventional economic modes of thinking, however, with the 'representative agent' solidly embedded in the foundations, can make the obvious unthinkable. The reality of conflicting goals cannot be grasped by 'models' of a society as a single big (rational, informed) individual. (Translating such models into less accessible mathematical language, however, can make the inadequacy less transparent.)

The clash of competing interests, however, does not take place in a 'zero-sum' world. How a health system is organized and financed has an important influence on the distribution of burdens and benefits in the society it serves; but some systems do 'work' better than others, in terms meaningful to an external observer. Some are overall and on average more efficient, effective, humane, and acceptable to their publics, and others less so. It is possible to evaluate reform proposals in terms of their probability of improving or making worse the overall functioning of a health care system (so long as one does not insist on too much precision). Some reforms, on the other hand, clearly offer 'partial gain for general pain', and their proponents go to some lengths to hide that fact.

More fundamentally, our advancing understanding of the determinants of health of populations suggests that different choices in health care reform may have effects on those determinants, above and beyond their influence on the nature, quantity and distribution of health services themselves. The scale of health care systems in modern economies, as well as their significance at critical and vulnerable points in the lives of individuals, give them an especial salience. Health care reforms may be helpful or hazardous to health, in ways separate from and additional to their effects on the use of health care *per se*.

---

[5] Arrow (1976) p. 3; see also Reinhardt (1992) and esp. (1998).

Expenditures, incomes, and revenues: the fundamental accounting identity in all health care systems

Partitioning a population into relevant categories is an accounting rather than an economic exercise, though the categories are motivated by economic considerations. In any population (society, economy) there are three distinct roles that an individual may play with respect to the health care system. S/he may use health care goods or services; s/he may provide resources for their production (including administration and management); and s/he may contribute to the revenues that finance them. In a modern health care system everyone contributes to some degree, most will in the course of a year use some services, but only a minority (though more than is usually realized) will provide resources for their production.[6]

Each of these activities can be represented by a financial flow. Individuals contribute revenues, primarily through various forms of taxation and to a lesser extent through direct payments for services or premiums to private insurers. These revenues then become the expenditures on health care that are received by the various forms of provider organizations—hospitals, clinics, professional practices, pharmacies. (Payments may be made as prices or fees per unit of service, or be implicit in budgetary allocations.)

But all the receipts of these provider organizations—the 'firms' of economic theory—are then attributable to the various individuals that supply resources to them—those who work there, or own or manage them, or invest capital in them, or sell them various forms of supporting goods and services.[7] All the funds that come from individuals, thus return to individuals. This circular flow is depicted in Figure 2.1.[8]

---

[6] There is an inherently arbitrary element (and some interested controversy) in decisions on where to place the boundaries of a health care system, though the central activities that engage most of the people and account for most of the funding are readily identified. Clearly health care cannot include all activities that have an influence upon health. The three-part identity begins from a list of types of commodities that have, by whatever process, been agreed to be 'health care' (the elements of the Q vector). Their prices can then be observed or estimated, and one can (in principle) identify all the different resources that were used up in producing these—and only these—and the payments made for those resources. These total costs can then be partitioned exhaustively among the three sources of revenue.

[7] Provider organizations will typically buy goods and services from other firms —the pharmacist, for example buys drugs from a wholesaler, who buys from a manufacturer. But all of these payments in turn flow through to individuals working or investing in those firms. Revenues remaining in a particular firm can all be attributed either to the firm's creditors, or to its owners—'no land without a lord'.

[8] A number of simplifications have been imposed for the sake of clarity, without loss of generality. More detail is provided in Evans et al (1994b).

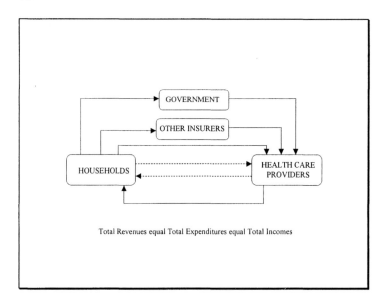

Figure 2.1 Alternative ways of paying for health care

Summing over all the individuals in the society, the total value of the resources supplied—labour, effort and skills, capital, raw materials—must equal the total value of the services produced, and that in turn must equal the total amount of revenue raised for their reimbursement. There is a fundamental accounting identity (a sub-component of the general national income identity) linking total expenditure on health goods and services, total revenues raised to pay for those services, and total incomes earned from the provision of services.

TOTAL REVENUE ≡ TOTAL EXPENDITURE ≡ TOTAL INCOME

This identity, however, is a relation among financial magnitudes, and money *per se* produces neither health care nor health. At best it provides access to the things that do. So we expand the relationship:

$$T + C + R \equiv P \times Q \equiv W \times Z$$

Revenues are raised via taxation (T), direct charges (C), and private insurance premiums (R). Total expenditure can be factored into the unit prices of the various health care commodities, and the quantities of each. P and Q are thus vectors whose elements list all the different types of commodities provided/used. These in turn are produced by combining various inputs or resources, Z, that are paid at a rate per unit, W. An element of the vector W might be a wage rate, for example; the corresponding element of Z would be a type of labour input measured in hours.

This framework makes obvious the distinction between the levels of health expenditure in a system, $P \times Q$, and the levels and types of services actually provided—Q. It is the latter that contribute to health. Their production requires not money but the use of real resources Z. An increase (decrease) in W, the rate of remuneration of resource suppliers, will pass through in higher (lower) prices and require the assembly of greater (lesser) financial contributions through T, C, and/or R. But it will have no necessary direct effect on service provision or on health.[9]

Gainers and losers: who sits (and stands) where in the flow of funds?

Such a change will, however, very definitely re-distribute incomes among the different individuals in the society. An increase in nurses' wages W, for example, paid from government revenues, will (if the elements of Z and Q do not change) shift money from the pockets of taxpayers to those of nurses. P, the implicit price of hospital care, and T, the amount of tax revenue needed to pay for it, both increase.[10] Alternatively an increase in drug prices P, funded by an increase in user charges C, flows into higher rates of return on capital invested in drug companies (a component of Z). W rises, and money is transferred from patients to shareholders.

Although the three-part identity above holds for the entire society, it does not hold for each individual, and probably not for any.[11] The total amount of money paid out by individuals, returns to individuals, as noted above, but the amount each receives will not be equal to the amount s/he contributed, and the discrepancies may be very large. We can partition the population on the basis of the relationship between their contributions to, use of, and income from the health care system.

The first partition isolates those individuals for whom $W \times Z$, their total income from supplying resources, exceeds either the amount they contribute, or the total cost of the services they use. (This will typically be true of doctors, nurses, and others who are clearly health care workers, but will also include suppliers of specialized supporting goods and services—drug or equipment sellers, but also health insurers and benefits managers.) For this group, health expenditures are (primarily) income, and their perspectives on proposals for reform are shaped accordingly.

---

[9] It may affect the willingness of resource owners to offer them for the production of health care, e.g. the supply of workers, but that is another story.

[10] Governments could, of course, borrow or cut other spending instead of raising taxes. But borrowing implies a cost to future taxpayers, while cuts in other spending still constitute an increase in T, the amount of tax revenue spent on health. The losers will be, not taxpayers in general, but those who would have received that other spending as income.

[11] In order to 'ignore distributional considerations' Arrow (1976) did assume that the identity holds for every individual, with the addition of an expectations operator on C and Q. This is empirical nonsense, however convenient theoretically.

The rest of us are primarily users of, and payers for, health care services (though we may also, for example, belong to a pension plan that invests in a mutual fund that holds shares in a drug company or private laboratory). But we can be further partitioned according to whether our contributions to the system, T+C+R, exceed or fall short of the expenditures generated on our behalf, P × Q.

Such a partition could not be made in a health care system that was fully funded by out-of-pocket payments. User charges C would equal P × Q, in total and for each individual.[12] But no such system exists. In all developed societies, revenues for health care are primarily raised from (various forms of) taxation. Since these are more or less proportionate to income, and use of care is more or less proportionate to illness, the relatively healthy and/or wealthy contribute more than they spend, and the unhealthy and/or unwealthy contribute less. Public financing for health care transfers income from the former to the latter. Any reform that affects the proportion of revenues flowing through the different channels will redistribute income between (and of course within) these groups.

The differing economic interests of these three sets of individuals—providers, the healthy and wealthy payers, and the unhealthy and unwealthy users—go far to explain the pattern of intellectual debate and political conflict over health care reform. They distort, and sometimes crowd out entirely, what one might naively hope would be a collective search for 'the best'—or at least better ways of organizing, providing and funding care.

Disagreements over how to advise the steersman are not randomly distributed across the population, a result of incomplete information and imperfect reasoning power. Rather they are rooted in clear conflicts of economic interest, in which those who disagree may, and often do, have very similar (albeit unacknowledged) understandings of the likely impacts of different policies. It is the goals that are in dispute.

Reform proposals and their implications: tracing the links to health and wealth

Interested advocates of particular 'reforms' may of course make claims of general health benefits (among others) as part of their attempt to recruit wider public support. The actual impact of any change in policy may be more difficult to predict, and is likely to be conditional on a number of particular factors—God and the devil are both in the details. Nonetheless the rapidly accumulating understanding of the determinants of health, and the considerable international experience with the behaviour of health care systems, should make possible at least a rough assessment of the probable impacts of particular policies.[13]

---

[12] Assuming also that the unit prices of all services equalled their costs, so that no buyer/user was subsidized by any other.

[13] It must be recognized however that any such attempt, if it receives wider attention, will itself become part of the advocacy process.

Changes to health care systems may influence the health of populations through three broad channels. They may affect:

1. The level, mix, and allocation of the services provided by that system: Who gets how much of what kind of care?
2. The balance of resources between health care and other public or private goods: How much does the production of health care draw away from other economic activities, with potential effects on health? and
3. The distribution of income among the members of society: What (relative) incomes do providers earn, and how is the bill for their services divided up?

The probable impact of any given proposal can then be assessed under each of these heads.

To impose some order on a 'zoo' of reform proposals, note that the three-part identity offers a classification. Some focus primarily on the levels and patterns of expenditure, the $P \times Q$, others on the use and payment of resources, or the incomes generated by the health care system. Still others would change the sources of revenue for health care—the endless 'public-private' wrangles, for example. But as the identity reminds us, all will have effects across the whole equation. And all will have (more or less) identifiable patterns of winners and losers.

Evidence-based medicine: toward effectiveness and efficiency in health care?

Consider first the movement for evidence-based medicine, which seeks to influence directly the mix and volume of services provided. It is hard to disagree in principle with proposals to reform health care by generating more reliable evidence on 'what works—for whom—and what does not', and then using this evidence to modify patterns of service. The classic description in the Book of Common Prayer still holds good today, and it is clear that by changing the values of the elements of the vector Q, stopping things that do more harm than good (or doing nothing in particular, whether or not they do it very well) and doing more of the rest, we could either save money, or be healthier, or both.

It is not so much the totally useless services that are at issue—though those exist—but the services that are ineffective or harmful for some or most of the patients to whom, or in the amounts that, they are currently provided. No one questions the value of antibiotics. But if one third of all antibiotic prescriptions written in the United States, or 50 million scrips a year, are unnecessary, this is both an economic absurdity and a major public health hazard (Levy, 1998). Nor are the Americans unique.

So is the Cochrane Collaboration a clear contributor to improved population health? Probably, but there are several sources of potential slippage. All are traceable to the link between service provision and incomes – $P \times Q \equiv W \times Z$. Users of services may have an unambiguous interest in more effective health care, but providers do not.

The determination that a particular product or service has no value, either at all or in a significant proportion of its current uses, is a direct threat to the incomes of those who supply (and are paid for) it. If an element of Q falls, the associated Z falls too.[14] 'Money is saved' because the owners of certain resources are now paid less—perhaps not at all. Conversely the finding that an intervention is of value in a wider range of applications is in effect a call to increase its use—and associated incomes.

Recall also that the Z represent not only the services of clinicians and others 'at the coal face.'   They include (owners of and workers in) commercial firms supplying products and services to be used under their direction, or directly to the public—drug and equipment manufacturers, for example. Their advertising—a normal commercial practice—produces a continual barrage of combined information and 'dis-information'—partial truths, deceptive implications, and outright misrepresentations—with the sole purpose (as with any commercial advertising) of expanding sales. Such advertising includes but goes far beyond the use of the traditional media, to include very sophisticated approaches to clinicians disguised as various forms of 'scientific' communications.

This leads to an obvious bias in the uptake of evidence. Clinicians have always been much more reluctant to give up an activity than to take on a new one. They appear to operate on the principle of 'When in doubt, do', requiring a higher standard of proof before accepting that something should not be done (e.g. Banta *et al*, 1981; Wennberg, 1990).   If the evidence is clear that a procedure is unambiguously harmful, it is pretty certain to be stopped.   But if, as is more common, there is no evidence of harm, only lack of clear evidence of benefit, clinical practice will change much more slowly if at all.

Commercial advertisers powerfully strengthen this bias. Findings of effectiveness, real or apparent, become part of marketing campaigns. Findings of lack of effect, or of risk, are given much less prominence, distorted, or simply ignored.[15] Nor could it be otherwise, given the incredibly powerful economic incentives bearing on the commercial sector—there is just too much money at stake. Regulatory agencies try to offset this inevitable bias, but are always overloaded, under-resourced, and out-gunned.

---

[14] If payment continues to be made for idle resources, there is an implicit increase in W. More likely, resource owners (typically professional workers) will attempt to introduce or expand some other element of Q—'to meet new needs' —and so keep themselves employed and paid. If they are successful, expenditures do not fall.

[15] In a few notorious cases, (unsuccessful) attempts have been made to suppress negative findings. The incidence of successful suppression is, of course, unknown.

In this context the generation of better evidence alone may simply provide more arguments for system expansion. Indeed, since research resources are scarce, clinical epidemiologists who want their work to have impact might be well advised preferentially to investigate those interventions they suspect *will* turn out to be of (possibly wider) benefit. Who needs the hassle?

In what way, however, would this be a bad thing? Such a selection bias would disappoint those who hope that better evidence will, by reducing ineffective care, lead to lower cost (Wennberg, 1990). But if the effectiveness of the health services is on average improving, even though their cost is rising, then surely this is a contribution to the health of the population. It would be even better if one could phase out ineffective (and particularly harmful) care with equal speed. But even if this were possible, it is not obvious a priori that a system that provided all and only effective health care would be less expensive, even in the United States.[16]

And that, of course, is the problem. It may well be that there is a virtually infinite supply of services with very low but non-zero benefit. To the extent that better evidence identifies these services more precisely, it provides support for expanding the scope of care. Explicit rationing is tougher than implicit. But resources, as economists repeat by rote, are scarce and have opportunity costs. If any service with a positive health pay-off—no matter how small—is to be provided, this must eventually divert resources from other activities, public or private, that also have positive effects on health. 'Partial strength produces general weakness.' (Sir Robert Seppings, quoted in Gordon, 1978). It is possible to have too much of a good thing (Lavis and Stoddart, 1994); too much (low-value) health care can be hazardous to population health.

Reforms that improve the evidence base underlying health care practice seem unambiguously to advance population health through channel one above. But they carry a risk through channel two, hypertrophy of the health care system itself. Moreover the considerable methodological advances that have supported the evidence-based care movement impart their own biases to the choice of routes to health. It is quite simple—in principle anyway—to conduct a randomized controlled trial (RCT) of a drug or well-defined clinical manoeuvre. Many of the other factors that appear to contribute to health cannot be tested in this way. How does one conduct an RCT of more or less egalitarian income distributions?

That is not an argument for 'justification by faith alone', as one might infer from some of the more woolly-minded (or economically motivated) proponents of 'alternative medicine'. But if the RCT is treated not only as a 'gold standard' – which for some purposes (not all) it clearly is – but as the only mode of evaluation with any validity, all evaluations will be rigged in advance. Only health care interventions (and those paid for providing them) will be demonstrably effective.

---

[16] There is certainly some expert opinion that it would be, at least in the United States, but no one really knows.

Other supposed contributors to health, however plausible, will not be supported by 'valid scientific evidence'.[17]

Finally, the evidence-based approach to reform can be diverted into quite different channels by the advocates of 'core services' or 'basic benefits'. Implicit in the efforts to evaluate effectiveness is the understanding that ineffective (and *a fortiori* harmful) services should not be provided at all. And certainly no one should pay for them. But if no one pays, then no one is paid. An obvious alternative for suppliers of such services, if they are removed from public payment programmes, is to sell them in the private market-place.

By shifting attention from what is done (and why) to who pays, the core services 'reformers' blunt the threat to jobs and incomes, to W × Z. Any cost containment potential can be converted into cost shifting—lowering T while raising C and possibly R. Indeed total incomes can actually be raised, not merely maintained. Once a health service has been moved into the private sector the absence of public controls permits higher prices, while the opportunities for advertising (overt and covert) and more liberal case selection lead to higher volumes as well.[18] (This of course requires an appropriate match of service and clientele: no one wants to offer expensive services for low-income people in a private market.)

This particular application appears to be far from the intent of the advocates of evidence-based medicine. But steady improvement in the science base underlying medical practice could lead to the identification of an ever-increasing range of low-benefit, high-cost services that no universal public system ever could, let alone should, cover. If so, this is certain to feed into arguments for private markets in health care, and may thus influence population health through channel three (see below). The advocates of 'reform' will be those who hope to sell these services, unencumbered by evidence of minimal effect.

Who pays, and how much? Rearranging the sources of revenue

They will, moreover, have allies. Shifting attention to the sources of revenue for health care, from the level and mix of the Q to the balance among the T, C, and R, opens up another whole class of reform proposals, and their associated interests. Here the focus is not on what is done, but on who pays. 'Reform' is primarily about getting someone else to pay.

Imposing (or raising) direct charges on users of care, with or without supplementary private insurance, lowers the proportion of revenue from taxes.

---

[17] This is a slight over-statement; there are well-known RCTs of non-medical interventions. But they tend to be very expensive, very long term, and very few.

[18] The pharmaceutical industry's growing interest in and commitment to 'Direct To Consumer Advertising' (DTCA) reflects their understanding of the profit potential in private markets with weaker restrictions on communications strategies.

There are many variants on this theme. Traditional approaches charge each user so much per visit, hospital day, or prescription, or a proportion of total expenditures, or for all expenditures up to some fixed amount per time period. More complex schemes involve integration of patient liability with the income tax: a currently fashionable version, medical savings accounts, adds a longitudinal dimension. Introducing or expanding a 'private tier' of care alongside a public system has similar effects.[19]

The Sheriff of Nottingham rides again

Such proposals link financial liability more closely with health care use, and less with ability to pay. More complex forms may make the linkage less transparent; but all, at the end of the day, raise C and lower T. They may also raise R; increased user charges provide something for private insurance to cover. Since, as noted above, tax funding transfers income from the healthy and wealthy to the unhealthy and unwealthy, all these policies shift it back again.[20]   They are regressive income transfers, in Lomas' words the policies not of Robin Hood but of the Sheriff of Nottingham (Lomas and Contandriopoulos, 1994). The more heavily a national system relies on private financing, the larger the proportion of overall health care costs that will be borne by those with lower incomes. The international evidence is most comprehensively assembled and analysed by van Doorslaer *et al* (1993).[21] But the central point emerges most strikingly from the United States data in Figure 2.2, drawn from Rasell *et al* (1993) and Rasell and Tang (1994).

---

[19] A private tier of care for the better-off may appear to link financial liability with ability to pay. But those who pay for care privately would also have to pay a higher proportion of the taxes necessary to support such a standard of care for themselves—and everyone else. What is lost on the roundabouts is made up on the swings.

[20] But suppose the state itself collects user fees and places them in general revenue, with no direct flow through to providers of care? These then represent, quite literally, 'taxes on the sick'. T, C, and R are unchanged in the accounting identity but the tax base has become more regressive, linking liability more closely with illness, and less closely with ability to pay.

[21] '...[O]ut-of-pocket payments tend to be a highly regressive means of financing health care but the impact of private insurance is more nuanced ...' (van Doorslaer *et al*, 1993). Private insurance supplementary to a more or less universal public system is a 'luxury' primarily bought by people with higher incomes. But if private insurance is purchased by a large proportion of the population because public coverage is restricted or non-existent, the distribution of its costs is highly regressive. In general the larger the user charges and the more people who must pay them, the more regressive are the costs of private insurance to cover them.

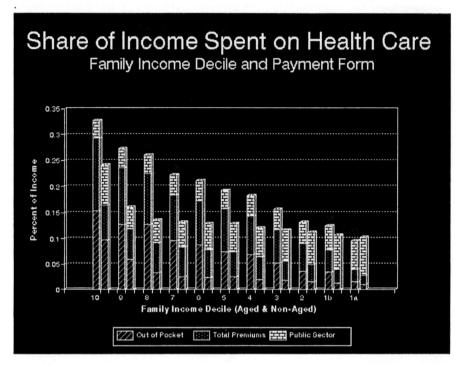

Figure 2.2

Family expenditure data were analysed to identify how much was spent on health care by families in each income decile, through each of taxation, private insurance premiums, and out-of-pocket payments. Higher income families spent more, on average, in each category. But they spent a much lower *proportion* of their incomes, on either direct charges or private insurance. Only taxation was (mildly) progressively distributed. Moreover, this was true of families with aged heads, even though the United States has a universal public insurance programme for the elderly. But that programme requires its beneficiaries to pay large user fees; those that can afford it have private 'Medigap' insurance.

This point seems to be well enough understood by the advocates of private payment. Such proposals have a long history of support from the wealthy and healthy. More recently these have been seeking to broaden their constituency to include the healthy and unwealthy—younger people—by focusing attention on a supposed 'inter-generational conflict'. (The strategy is fundamentally deceptive, because most of the currently young will get old but few will get rich. They may, however, get old too soon and smart too late.)[22]

---

[22] Why, after all, should they be different from their predecessors?

The traditional arguments for such reforms do not, of course, emphasize redistributive effects. Rather they allege benefits in improved efficiency and effectiveness in health care—and implicitly in population health. Faced with direct charges, patients will be more selective in their use of care, and less likely to use ineffective or harmful services. The level and mix of Q will change, and on average the effectiveness of care will improve.

Moreover, informed consumers faced with prices will shop more carefully for services, forcing suppliers to be more competitive. Prices will fall, and more efficient suppliers will capture a larger share of the market. 'More efficient' means using fewer resource inputs per unit of output, a lower ratio of Z to Q, thus permitting lower P for given W. Total expenditures may rise or fall. But since they will (by hypothesis) reflect the preferences of informed consumers expressed through competitive markets, whatever level they attain must be right.

All this is simply elementary economic theory, describing the market for 'widgets'.[23] In fact experiment and common observation both show that, faced with direct charges, patients are not able to discriminate between effective and ineffective services. (The whole history of quackery should have told us that.) Reforms that increase the costs to users do deter the use of care that, in the judgement of experts anyway, is appropriate. Not surprisingly, these deterrent effects are strongest among those with lowest incomes.[24]

Moreover, whatever the behaviour of providers might be in the hypothetical world of the economics textbooks, in reality they are quite capable of suppressing 'perfect competition' so as to protect their incomes. Professional organizations, in particular, have been the most persistent advocates of private funding over the decades (Barer et al, 1994) because they anticipate that their income opportunities are greater in a mixed funding environment. International experience bears out this expectation.

Indeed, professional spokesmen often explicitly advocate increased user charges to increase total costs—raising C and/or R while holding T constant—arguing that this will support health-enhancing increases in Q. It will also, however, support income-enhancing increases in P, and in any case must inevitably increase $W \times Z$.[25]

Reforms focusing on the sources of revenue appear therefore to have two potential channels of effect on population health. By increasing (or decreasing)

[23] Rice (1998) provides an extended and up-to-date critique of efforts to apply 'off-the-shelf' economic theory to health care systems.

[24] A number of papers on this point emerged from the RAND Health Insurance Experiment: Brook et al (1983); Lohr et al (1986); Shapiro et al (1986); Siu et al (1986); Lurie et al (1989). But the basic point was demonstrated earlier by Enterline et al (1973a, 1973b), and the differential impact by income class was shown by Beck and Horne (1980).

[25] As noted above, private markets tend to be less resistant to price increases than are public payers. They also provide more opportunities for expanding sales volumes—Q—through various forms of promotion, because no countervailing agency has a direct incentive to restrain them. The health benefits of such promotion are at best open to question.

financial barriers they redistribute access to and use of care services within the population. But they also redistribute among individuals the burden of paying for whatever care is provided, as well as influencing the overall size of that burden.

The effect on population health of redistributing access and use of care is pretty obvious, though the magnitude may be questioned in particular cases.   Financial deterrents do not differentially discourage inappropriate or 'unnecessary' care-seeking, and do have a greater impact on use by people with lower incomes. So they re-allocate care away from lower income people—who tend to be less healthy—and towards those with greater ability to pay.[26] The healthy and wealthy get more, the unhealthy and unwealthy get less.   Insofar as care is effective, this presumably reduces population health.[27]

But changes in health care financing also affect the distribution of income both among individuals and across income classes. The less users respond to prices (and empirical estimates suggest that the price elasticity of demand is quite low), the closer user charges approach to pure income transfers. Substituting private for public finance raises disposable incomes at the upper end of the income scale (after taxes, transfers, and direct payments for health care), and lower them at the lower end.

Inequality and ill-health: a pathogenic reform agenda?

There is a strong relationship, within every population studied, between income distribution and health status. Income is associated with health, and greater inequality of income with greater inequality of health. There is increasing evidence that greater inequality is also associated with lower average health status.[28] From a population perspective, therefore, 'Sheriff of Nottingham' reforms pose threats to health quite independent of their influence on the levels and patterns of health care use.

The potential significance of this channel increases if we consider the pathways through which income inequality might have their effects on health. Those pathways, in high (average) income populations, go far beyond sheer material

---

[26] In a supply-constrained environment, user charges can push lower-income people out of the market, improving the access of those with higher incomes such that their use actually increases. This is an important aspect of the appeal of private funding to the wealthy and unhealthy—they can be more sure of getting the care that they (think they) need.

[27] Gorey *et al* (1997), for example, compared cancer survival rates in Toronto with those in Detroit. They found that survival rates are significantly correlated with socio-economic status in Detroit, where access to care depends upon income, but not in Toronto, where it does not. But upper income Torontonians fared no worse; the overall results favoured Canada.

[28] Wilkinson has been a particular champion of the latter view, though he has not been alone—see his (1995) exchange with Judge (1995). More recent evidence has come from US research (Kaplan *et al*, 1996; Kennedy *et al*, 1996; Davey Smith, 1996).

deprivation and biological insufficiency. A health gradient is observed across the entire income distribution. In general, hierarchical position is associated with the availability of internal or external resources (e.g. education, income, social support) to cope with external threats—'stress' in the broadest sense (e.g. Evans *et al*, 1994a). Conversely vulnerability—inability to cope with challenges—appears to be in itself a source of illness. Animal studies offer powerful support for this view (e.g. Sapolsky, 1993; Evans *et al*, 1994a; Evans, 1996).

The relationship between the health status of individuals and their level of 'coping resources' (including income) has been shown in population-based studies (Mustard *et al*, 1997). But equally important, as discussed by Lynch and Kaplan (1997) in a recent survey, are the effects on individual health of characteristics of the social environment—and in particular the degree of inequality of income—that have no meaning as individual-level measures. They also note that the relevant measure of inequality should be based on the distribution of income (ideally wealth) after the redistributive activities of governments—taxes, transfers, and 'income in kind' such as publicly provided health care or education.

Reforms to health care funding that transfer costs from public to private budgets clearly increase inequality of income on this measure, and will therefore— at least on these findings—increase the dispersion and probably lower the overall level of health in the population. The magnitude of the effect may be open to question, but the direction seems pretty clear[29].

More specifically, however, illness and injury are themselves a major source of stress: they present threats and challenges on a number of levels. The sense of vulnerability of the individual is linked with perceptions of both the probability and severity of such threats, and the availability of resources to cope with them—access to and effectiveness of health care. Matters of health are thus always news, and health care is never far from the top of the political agenda. And the tighter (looser) the link between personal resources and access to high-quality health care, the greater (less) the sense of vulnerability associated with lower income.

In short, if the answer to the question 'Can I get care when I need it?' is 'Only if you have the money', then lower income means greater vulnerability. And vulnerability, in humans and other animals, predisposes to illness.

Provider organization and payment: the many modes of 'managed care'

---

[29] But by shifting financial responsibility for health care, might not governments release public funds to address broader determinants of health? This would require that the level of public revenues be maintained after health costs and responsibilities were shifted. The advocates of privatization also tend to be the advocates of government downsizing, 'rolling back the frontiers of the state'. Health care funding is in most countries one of the most popular of public programmes, legitimizing the role of the state more generally. It seems unlikely that in transferring this activity, governments could find support for expanding their roles in other areas.

But an alternative answer, 'No, because the care you need is not available (or not approved in your case)' is hardly more comforting.[30] The third and most complex area of health care reform involves changing the ways in which providing organizations are structured and paid, with the intent of changing both the types and amounts of services offered to patients, and the processes of their production. The focus here is on the $W \times Z$, in the hope of increasing efficiency (Q/Z) or effectiveness ('better' mix of Q). Possibilities range from American visions of private, for-profit 'integrated delivery systems' in hot competition for profitable 'portfolios of insured lives'; through variants on the theme of capitated groups of providers, budget-holding or commissioned; to the more mundane and very crude 'macro-management' that is implicit in the process of negotiating fee schedules, budgets, or global cost caps.[31]

These reform efforts have their origins in cost control pure and simple. Public and private payers focused initially on P and W, trying to hold down fees and wage rates. But it was quite quickly discovered that 'demand' can be driven by income aspirations and the availability of capacity—people and facilities. If fees are held down, service volumes rise; if wages are held down, services are withdrawn in various ways. Payers were thus forced to broaden their range of targets.

Direct controls on capacity and budgets, on Z and $P \times Q$, have had significant effects on cost escalation, but these are always politically vulnerable to variations on the charge of 'under-funding'. Providers claim that the overall level of care provided is simply inadequate to meet patients' needs, putting their health at risk ('people are dying'), and can produce 'waiting lists' (and sometimes deaths) to prove it. Questions as to the effectiveness and efficiency of the system itself, the appropriateness of the level and mix of Q and the ratio of Q to Z, are side-stepped—unless payers raise them directly.

To do so could imply a much-expanded role for payers in the management of the care services. The difficulty of direct management has led, however, to widespread interest in more indirect approaches—in changing the information, organization and particularly the modes of payment of providers so that they will manage themselves differently. With different incentives, they might be more willing to take up information on effectiveness, and to seek ways of lowering costs. This is the attraction of the broad range of reforms under the general heading of 'managed care'.

---

[30] It is an interesting question as to whether the latter response might be more or less stressful than the former. Is the knowledge that others are getting what they need (through money or connections) more troubling than a sense of solidarity and shared sacrifice? The answer may turn on perceptions of the reasons for shortage (external catastrophe vs. administrative stupidity and waste) or of the relative deservingness of others (they need/earned/inherited/stole their preferred status).

[31] 'Managed care' as defined by Rosenbaum and Richards (1996) includes universal public systems of health insurance, at least to the extent that they 'manage the health care practices of participating providers'.

This approach leads into variants of capitation—paying people or organizations a fixed sum to provide 'all necessary care' (perhaps of a specific type) to a defined population. To encourage effective care, however, one might also want to 'reimburse by results' linking the capitation payment at least in part to the health outcomes achieved. But then, why restrict such organizations to providing only health care? It is but a step to the truly intriguing idea of contracting for health itself, not merely health care. Provider organizations might then attempt to influence the whole spectrum of health determinants, being paid according to their success (Kindig, 1997). One can imagine this creating powerful commercial incentives not only to extend our understanding of the determinants of health, but also to apply that knowledge as broadly as possible.

Paradox in private markets: can you get here from there?

This is leading edge stuff, attempting to harness the forces of the competitive market-place to the promotion of health. But there are a couple (at least) of fundamental paradoxes in this programme. One is perhaps the central problem in managed care; the other is a quiet embarrassment for health promoters. Neither is approaching resolution.

The most powerful incentives to overcome barriers to efficiency and effectiveness, and to address determinants of health that lie beyond health care, are generated by profit-driven competition among private commercial organizations. But such an environment also creates the most powerful incentives for patient selection—managing the care of people who are not sick, or not sick in complex and ambiguous ways—and for under-serving those who are. (Death, after all, is very cost-effective.)

If managed care organizations are to be rewarded or penalized for the long-term consequences of their interventions, or lack thereof, this will require not only an extraordinary data base to identify such consequences, but also long-term (possibly lifetime) enrolment contracts. These may be acceptable neither to managers nor to the managed. But spot market trading of 'insured lives' yields maximum returns to the clever selector of the healthy and the hard-nosed withholder of care, not the expert producer of health.[32]

The second paradox is implicit in the expression: 'empowering people to make healthy choices'. But empowered people do not always make the choices you believe they should.[33] That you ignore my good advice is bad enough, but if my firm is going to lose money when you are unhealthy then I will try to control your

---

[32] Of course efforts would be made to regulate such behaviour, but one should not be optimistic about the outcome.

[33] As Luther found out after translating the Bible. Anabaptists have been persecuted ever since.

behaviour, through financial penalties or the 'health police'. There will be endless wrangles about who is responsible for bad outcomes.

Nor does management come free. Some forms of 'managed care' introduce large numbers of new managers, marketers, and other income claimants— increasing the Z term in the basic identity. This translates into higher prices, as each clinical service must now include in its (explicit or implicit) price an increased burden of administrative overhead (Woolhandler and Himmelstein, 1991; Himmelstein *et al*, 1996). P goes up—unless the incomes of clinical personnel can be pushed down.

'Managed care', though supposedly focused on efficiency and effectiveness, can also slide into another form of 'Sheriff of Nottingham' policy. Suppose competitive private integrated delivery systems (or a National Health Service) offer a basic level of care. But a 'point of service' option (or a private tier) is also made available, whereby those who can afford it can buy more convenient (or better quality?) services when they feel the need.

Advocates describe this alternative as 'taking the pressure off the public system' which translates as taking the pressure off taxpayers to fund the same level of care for all. Those with higher incomes can assure themselves (what they believe to be) a higher standard without having to contribute to the same for others. Meanwhile providers can feed those perceptions, to increase their own marketing opportunities and prices. 'Managed care', if it takes the form of competition among delivery systems, may well lead down this road. Since a two-track ('deux vitesses') system is both more accessible and less costly for upper-income people, there will always be a market.

Better information for better management: 'PSPB' data systems

So 'managed care' has its problems and risks. Yet health care is *always* 'managed' by someone, and all decisions are based on some sort of information. 'Managed care' reforms address: 'Who manages, under what incentives, and with what information available?' The problems indicated above arise from the particular and very powerful incentives generated by profit-driven competition in a commercial market-place. They are not inherent in management *per se*. Changing the location of managerial decisions, increasing the accountability of those making them, and particularly extending information on which they are based, can lead to 'better management' without the two-edged spur of commercial competition.

Perhaps the clearest link between health care management and the determinants of population health is provided by the newly developing 'person-specific, population-based' data systems (Wolfson, 1994; Roos and Shapiro, 1995). Administrative data from universal, comprehensive programmes of health care reimbursement permit the construction of person-specific trajectories of care. These show, in the words of the old limerick, 'who did what and with which and to whom,' not merely for certain individuals or classes of patients but for whole populations.[34]

These 'PSPB' data systems are beginning to generate more detailed and open information on patterns of care. Linked with other sources of information on health status, they point forwards to much more powerful methods of identifying patterns of practice and assessing outcomes; linked with information on personal and community characteristics they point backwards to the underlying determinants of health itself. The longitudinal structure is of particular importance, because these determinants appear to include certain factors that operate over the whole of the life cycle, becoming embedded at a very young age.

Creatively used, such databases permit both more precise analysis of the social correlates of morbidity and mortality (e.g. Mustard *et al*, 1997) and better targeting of possible interventions. Wider dissemination of their contents could also raise general public understanding and mobilize support. Improved health care management can thus support the more broadly based promotion of health.

The trick now is to develop the organizations—regional boards, commissioning groups, integrated delivery systems?— that will be capable of, and accountable for, translating that information into more efficient and effective patterns of intervention, in and out of the health care system. Some of the tools developed in the American competitive environment may turn out to be useful for this purpose, even if that environment itself looks like another blind alley.

Most importantly, the juxtaposition of data on population health with that on care use can be a way of informing the general public, as well as those responsible for health policy, about the significance of determinants of health beyond the health care system (British Columbia, 1997). If strategies for promoting health are to be developed and to find support as alternatives to health system expansion, they will probably have to be based on information at an equivalent level of specificity—not 'How can we all be healthier?' but 'What to do about condition X?'[35]

Keeping the hyena on a diet

---

[34] Large linked (or more accurately, linkable) data systems containing sensitive personal information about individuals raise obvious issues of privacy and confidentiality. These issues, however, can be and are being dealt with, apparently effectively, by establishing clear criteria and lines of accountability for data access. Much of the agitation over privacy issues appears to come not from individual citizens, but from those who fear, quite correctly, that better data systems might make their own activities more transparent, and accountable.

[35] Again a paradox emerges if care managers are in profit-driven competition. This environment creates powerful incentives to generate information on both the health status of different populations and the relative effectiveness of various interventions. But the information so generated is inevitably proprietary. If it is exposed to external evaluation, it can be copied by competitors. Just because the idea of patenting care protocols or health promotion strategies is absurd, this does not mean that it could not happen.

More generally, if health care delivery is not to crowd out policies to address the broader determinants of health, its global scope and costs must be contained. 'It's hard to advance while there's a hyaena chewing on your foot.' Wildavsky (1977) summarized the fundamental growth dynamic of modern health care systems in his *Law of Medical Money:* 'Costs will increase to the level of available funds . . . that level must be limited to keep costs down.' Failure to limit the demands of health care will make it difficult to find (public or private) resources to improve other aspects of the social and physical environment that contribute to health.[36] Better management of health care may be essential to population health.[37]

The forces arrayed against cost containment are formidable, all driven by the fundamental fact that expenditures equal incomes. Efforts to limit expenditure elicit a standard cry from providers to the public:

> The system is underfunded and your health is at risk! Make the politicians give us more money, or protect yourself privately!

The containment of health care systems will fail unless it is—and is seen to be— consistent with preserving access to effective high-quality health care, at need. Is this possible?

This is really a double question. First, is it technically feasible to maintain and improve the effectiveness of modern health care systems while containing and perhaps even reducing current expenditures? The answer appears to be very clearly yes—in principle. Health care systems throughout the developed world continue to provide inappropriate and ineffective services, in ways that are unnecessarily costly.[38] Wide variations exist, within and between regions, in patterns of care for apparently similar populations and problems. These variations are linked to the availability and aspirations of providers, not the needs of the populations served. The cheerleaders of technology, for whom no (amount of)

---

[36] It is also likely to lead to more private financing, with effects such as those described above.

[37] Attention should not be wasted on an idle dream that improvements in population health could be 'self-financing' by lowering the need for and hence the cost of health care. Apart from the extreme disjunction of time scales, such a hope would be based on a complete misreading of the determinants of health care use and cost.

[38] For example, in-patient hospital use has been falling dramatically in a number of countries. But a pair of recent studies in British Columbia has found that, although acute care use (*per capita*) has fallen roughly 70% since 1969 (McGrail et al, 1998), it would still be possible to halve current use by medical patients if adequate alternative facilities (mostly outpatient) were available (Wright et al, 1997). On the other hand, reductions in in-patient use do not necessarily save costs. Costs and incomes may simply be transferred to other venues and earners (Reinhardt, 1996). More generally, there is a huge literature on both the appropriateness of current care patterns, and the possibilities for resource substitution.

expenditure is without benefit, draw their inspiration from the marketing department.

The second question, however, is more difficult, being primarily one of administrative and ultimately political feasibility. Can knowledge about effectiveness and efficiency be translated into changed behaviour? Restraining costs, whether by brute budget or persuasive protocol, always comes back to restraining incomes. Health care is managed within a 'capacity' environment set by public and private investment policies that determine the long-run path of the Z—in a sense the demand for incomes.[39] Investments in training of highly 'human capital intensive' people such as physicians are especially critical. Once trained, they will expect one way or another to make a living. That means they will have to be paid—by someone. And training places are politically much easier to open than to close.

Similarly, when more generous patent privileges are conferred on drug manufacturers, their prices and profits, P and W, are raised. These privileges both encourage and support increased investment in pharmaceutical innovation—increases in Z—and these too will have to be paid for. There may be more effective ways to advance population health than by developing and consuming ever more, and more expensive, drugs. But once the (very large) investments have been made, their owners will fight tooth and nail to get their return—with a profit.

Short-sighted decisions to encourage particular private investments can thus impose very long-run constraints on management choices. They put in place a level and mix of personnel or products that powerfully influence the pattern of services produced and their overall cost. If the scale and structure of Z is pre-committed, it is hard to change the mix of Q—or reduce P—whatever the form of management.

Efficiency at whose expense: was there someone in that bathwater?

But managed care may also have implications for population health on another level, that go to the core of the belief that the health care services need 'More management, not more money.'   Along with the extensive evidence of inappropriate and simply unevaluated servicing, there is also considerable evidence that (at least in the absence of financial barriers) the sickest people do receive the most care. Since health is correlated with socio-economic status (SES), on average people at lower SES are the heavier users. The SES gradient in use is not, however, uniform across all services. It is found in those forms of care for which outcomes are less well defined, and the boundaries between medical and social needs less clear especially in hospital care for patients with medical and psychological diagnoses and relatively long stays (Roos, 1997).

Yet in-patient care is precisely where cost containment pressures have had the greatest effects. Surgical and diagnostic procedures—which display less of an SES

---

[39] Or in Reinhardt's (1987) terms, the allocation of life-styles to providers.

gradient—are migrating out to ambulatory or short-stay facilities. Lengths of stay are down because people are simply going home—as many of them wish to, and should. But what happens to those with real but ill-defined needs, who are in hospital because the hospital is there?[40]   And by the time they get there, such people are in fact quite sick (Roos, 1997).   Some of the resources released by 'downsizing' might be re-deployed to support them in other ways. But if not? The SES gradient is at least a warning that 'better management' on medical criteria might have adverse implications for the health of vulnerable sub-populations.

Conclusions—and a few suggestions

The relation between health determinants and health care reform is thus a complex one.   Reform of health systems to improve effectiveness and efficiency in the provision of care may be essential if resources are to be made available to address other determinants of health. You have to get the hyena off your foot. On the other hand powerful economic forces tend to distort all reform efforts, trying to blunt or reverse cost containment while inserting regressive cost shifting.   Such distortions are most likely to have negative effects on population health.   But they will never lack for advocates.   There is simply no way around the fact that more expenditures equal more incomes for providers, or that tax-financed health care transfers resources from the healthy and wealthy to the unhealthy and unwealthy.   The economic interests are well-defined, and a permanent feature of every national debate on health care.

'Re-forms' that would substitute private for public funding sources are more or less overt efforts to redistribute access and costs. Their effects on population health seem unambiguously negative. Common sense suggests, and empirical evidence confirms, that linking access more closely to ability to pay results in more care for those with more resources, and less for those with less, and overall a worse match between care use and needs.

But privatizing revenue sources also redistributes access to other goods and services. Paying less (more) in total—taxes plus private charges or premiums—to support the health care system, the healthy and wealthy (unhealthy and unwealthy) have more (less) to spend on other things. Health care finance is part of the general pattern of taxes and transfers in each society that mitigate (more or less) the inequality emerging from the market-place. Privatizing health care funding weakens that mitigating effect, leading to greater economic inequality and probable negative consequences for health.

More private funding would, however, raise total expenditures on health care. Advocates now seem almost unanimous on this point. But these increases are likely to be primarily in incomes, not in services provided, and *a fortiori* not in the most

---

[40] Hertzman suggests that we have in our societies two types of institutions for people who have simply 'given up' and can no longer cope with their lives—hospitals and prisons.

effective services. And the significance of emerging evidence on the broader determinants of health is precisely that further expanding the health care system may NOT be the best route to population health.

'Re-forms' of funding sources deserve particular attention, because these are 'degenerate forms' of virtually every other approach to health care reform. When proposals to improve the functioning of health care systems run into opposition from those whose incomes would be threatened, sooner or later someone will suggest 'more private funding'—cost shifting—as a compromise. But even apart from the distorting effects of economic interest, harnessing health care reform to the improvement of health remains a significant challenge with much still unknown.

Improving the evidence base for health care interventions seems to be making the most rapid progress. But that area also shows clearly the need for organizational structures to ensure both that new knowledge is used appropriately in health care delivery, and that the process of information generation is not itself subject to systematic biases rooted in economic interest. Changing the organization and management of health care systems may improve the uptake of evaluative information, and ideally encourage attention to a broader range of health determinants. A good deal of experimentation is going on with different forms of 'managed care', but settled results are still scarce.

There seems to be a widespread interest in 'primary care reform' based on some form of capitation, and agreement that fee-for-service, as the predominant mode of reimbursing care, has outlived its usefulness. Nor do profit-motivated competitive managed care systems in the United States appear to be overcoming their inherent paradoxes (though Americans have low expectations and a high ideological commitment to the market). But the ball is still very much in play. Whatever the organizational framework, however, controlling the costs of health care in the face of intense provider pressure and public anxiety and scepticism seems certain to require progressively more sophisticated and detailed management, whether by payers or by providers themselves.

The data systems that this will require are, however, now coming into being. Comprehensive population-based data systems assembled from health care utilization data are providing a framework on which to assemble a wide range of other forms of information on personal and community characteristics. Integration of these different sources of information promises to provide support for both better management of health care delivery, and more effective approaches to the determinants of health. (The effective use of such information, however, will still depend upon the development of organizations with the capability and the incentive to do so.)

It would be ridiculous to conclude by offering a 'blueprint' for managing health care services so as best to promote population health. Certain points do, however, seem to emerge from the above discussion.

First, if we are to take advantage of our growing understanding of the determinants of health, it is essential to contain the enormously powerful growth dynamic in the health care system. The hyena must be kept on a diet. Second, better information on 'what works and what does not' in the clinical setting is necessary, but far from sufficient for this purpose. The more difficult challenge is that of institutional design, of developing the organizations that will do the job instead of doing something else. Third, no such reform is likely to have a chance if short-sighted decisions expand the numbers of long term (public or private) income claimants—vesting future interests in health care spending. Fourth, since there are permanent economic interests at stake, any effort to redirect health policy will inevitably be a political struggle. Much better—both detailed and reliable—information on system performance is now needed not only to ensure the integrity of the containment process but also to demonstrate this to a concerned public. The competitive clamour of 'too little' versus 'too much' at a global level is uninformative and distracting. Fifth, the 'person-specific, population-based' data that are necessary for the effective management of a health care system is also a major resource for generating public information. It should be used. Sixth, more detailed information on where, how, and why health differences emerge is required if appropriate policy responses are to be introduced. From an observed mortality gradient by socio-economic status to a more progressive tax system, for example, would be a rather long leap; the connection between symptom and underlying cause is still far from clear. Seventh, for this purpose also an information base assembled from the activities of the health care system can be augmented with individual and community-level data to become a significant source of knowledge about both the broader determinants of health and the effectiveness of interventions—and a source of public information. Eighth, never forget that the Sheriff of Nottingham is always out there, and that he is hazardous to health!

Acknowledgements

This paper draws on my own and others' work supported by the Program in Population Health, Canadian Institute for Advanced Research.

References

Arrow KJ. Welfare analysis of changes in health coinsurance rates. In: Rosett RN (ed) *The Role of Health Insurance in the Health Services Sector*. New York: National Bureau of Economic Research, 1976, Conference Series no. 27

Banta HD, Behney C, Willems JS. *Toward Rational Technology in Medicine: Considerations for Health Policy*. New York: Springer Publishing Company, 1981

Barer ML, Bhatia V, Stoddart GL, Evans RG. The Remarkable Tenacity of User Charges. Ontario: The Premier's Council on Health, Well-Being, and Social Justice, 1994

Beck RG, Horne JM. Utilization of publicly insured health services in Saskatchewan before, during and after copayment. *Medical Care*, 1980; **18**: 787–806

British Columbia Report on the Health of British Columbians: Provincial Health Officer's Annual Report, 1996 Victoria, British Columbia: Office of the Provincial Health Officer, 1997

Brook RH, Ware Jr JE, Rogers WH, *et al*. Does free care improve adults' health? *New England Journal of Medicine*, 1983; **309**: 1426–1434

Davey Smith G. Income inequality and mortality: why are they related? *British Medical Journal*, 1996; **312:** 987–988

Enterline PE, McDonald JC, McDonald AD, Davignon L, Salter V. Effects of free medical care on medical practice—the Quebec experience. *New England Journal of Medicine*, 1973a; **288**: 1152–1155

Enterline PE, Salter V, McDonald AV, McDonald JC. The distribution of medical services before and after 'free' medical care—the Quebec Experience. *New England Journal of Medicine*, 1973b; **289**: 1174–1178

Evans RG, Barer ML, Marmor TR (eds) *Why Are Some People Healthy and Others Not? The Determinants of Health of Populations*. New York: Aldine-de Gruyter, 1994a

Evans RG, Barer ML, Stoddart GL. *Charging Peter to Pay Paul: Accounting for the Financial Effects of User Charges*. Ontario: Premier's Council on Health, Well-Being, and Social Justice, 1994b

Evans RG. Health, Hierarchy, and Hominids: biological correlates of the socioeconomic gradient in health. In: Culyer AJ, Wagstaff A (eds) *Reforming Health Care Systems: Experiments with the NHS*. Aldershot: Edward Elgar, 1996, pp 35–64

Friedman M. *Capitalism and Freedom*. Chicago: University of Chicago Press, 1962

Gordon JE. *Structures, or Why Things Don't Fall Down*. London: Plenum, 1978

Gorey KM, Holowaty EJ, Fehringer G *et al*. An international comparison of cancer survival: Toronto, Ontario, and Detroit, Michigan, metropolitan areas. *American Journal of Public Health*, 1997; **87**: 1156–1163

Himmelstein DU, Lewontin JP, Woolhandler S. Who Administers? Who Cares? Medical administrative and clinical employment in the United States and Canada. *American Journal of Public Health*, 1996; **86**: 172–178

Hoffmeyer UK, McCarthy TR. *Financing Health Care* (two vols.) Dordrecht: Kluwer Academic Publishing, 1994

Judge K. Income distribution and life expectancy: a critical appraisal. *British Medical Journal*, 1995; **311**: 1282-1285

Kaplan GA, Pamuk ER, Lynch JW, Cohen RD, Balfour JL. Inequality in income and mortality in the United States: analysis of mortality and potential pathways. *British Medical Journal*, 1996; **312**: 999–1003

Kennedy BP, Kawachi I, Prothrow-Stith D. Income distribution and mortality: cross section ecological study of the Robin Hood index in the United States. *British Medical Journal*,1996; **312**: 1004–1007

Kindig DA. *Purchasing Population Health: Paying for Results.* Ann Arbor: University of Michigan Press, 1997

Lavis JN, Stoddart GL. Can we have too much health care? *Daedalus*, 1994; **123**: 43–60

Levy SB. The challenge of antibiotic resistance. *Scientific American*, 1998; **278**: 32–39

Lohr KN, Brook RH, Kamberg CJ *et al.* Effect of cost-sharing on use of medically effective and less effective care. *Medical Care*, 1986; **24**: Supplement

Lomas J, Contandriopoulos A-P. Regulating limits to medicine: towards harmony in public and self-regulation. In: Evans RG, Barer ML, Marmor TR (eds) *Why Are Some People Healthy and Others Not? The Determinants of Health of Populations.* New York: Aldine-De Gruyter, 1994, pp 253–283

Lurie N, Kamberg CJ, Brook RH, Keeler EB, Newhouse JP. How free care improved vision in the Health Insurance Experiment. *American Journal of Public Health,* 1989; **79**:640–642

Lynch J, Kaplan GA. Understanding how inequality in the distribution of income affects health. *Journal of Health Psychology*, 1997; **2**: 297–314

McGrail KM, Evans RG, Barer ML, Sheps SB, Hertzman C, Kazanjian A. *The Quick and the Dead: The Utilization of Hospital Services In British Columbia, 1969–1995/96.* Discussion Paper HPRU 98-3D. Vancouver: Centre for Health Services and Policy Research, University of British Columbia, 1998

Mustard CA, Derksen S, Berthelot J-M, Wolfson M, Roos LL. Age-specific education and income gradients in morbidity and mortality in a Canadian province. *Social Science & Medicine*,1997; **45**: 383–397

Rasell E, Bernstein J, Tang K. *The Impact of Health Care Financing on Family Budgets.* Briefing Paper 39. Washington DC: Economic Policy Institute, 1993

Rasell E, Tang K. *Paying for Health Care: Affordability and Equity in Health Care Reform.* Working Paper No. 111. Washington DC: Economic Policy Institute, 1994

Reinhardt UE. Resource allocation in health care: the allocation of lifestyles to providers. *The Milbank Quarterly*, 1987; **65**: 153–176

Reinhardt UE. Reflections on the meaning of efficiency: can efficiency be separated from equity? *Yale Law and Policy Review*, 1992; **10**: 302–315

Reinhardt UE. Spending more through 'Cost Control': Our obsessive quest to gut the hospital. *Health Affairs*, 1996; **15**:145–154

Reinhardt U. Abstracting from distributional effects, this policy is efficient. In: Barer ML, Getzen T, Stoddart G (eds) *Health, Health Care and Health Economics: Perspectives on Distribution* New York: John Wiley, 1998, pp 1–53

Rice T. *The Economics of Health Care Reconsidered.* Chicago: Health Administration Press, 1998, p 194

Roos NP, Shapiro E (eds) Health and health care: experience with a population-based health information system. *Medical Care*, 1995; **33**: supplement

Roos NP. Preserving and Improving the Delivery of Needs-Based Health Care to Populations: Targets for Reform, or What Do the Determinants Have to Do With It? Winnipeg: Manitoba Centre for Health Policy and Evaluation, 1997 (unpublished)

Rosenbaum S, Richards TB. Medicaid managed care and public health policy. *Journal of Public Health Management and Practice*, 1996; **2**: 76–82

Sapolsky RM. Endocrinology alfresco: psychoendocrine studies of wild baboons. *Recent Progress in Hormone Research*, 1993; **48**: 437–468

Shapiro MF, Ware JE, Sherbourne CD. Effects of cost sharing on seeking care for serious and minor symptoms. *Annals of Internal Medicine,* 1986; **104**: 246–251

Siu AL, Sonnenberg FA, Manning WG *et al.* Inappropriate use of hospitals in a randomized trial of health insurance plans. *New England Journal of Medicine,* 1986; **315**: 1259–1266

Towse A (ed) Financing Health Care in the U.K.: A Discussion of NERA's Prototype Model to Replace the NHS. London: Office of Health Economics, 1995

van Doorslaer E, Wagstaff A, Rutten F (eds) *Equity in the Finance and Delivery of Health Care: An International Perspective.* Oxford: Oxford University Press, 1993

Wennberg JE. Outcomes research, cost containment, and the fear of health care rationing. *New England Journal of Medicine,* 1990; **323**:1202–1204

Wildavsky A. Doing better and feeling worse: the political pathology of health policy. *Daedalus,* 1977; **106**:105–124

Wilkinson RG. Commentary. A reply to Ken Judge: mistaken criticisms ignore overwhelming evidence. *British Medical Journal,* 1995; **311**: 1285-1287

Wolfson MC. Social Proprioception: measurement, data, and information from a population health perspective. In: Evans RG, Barer ML, Marmor TR (eds) *Why Are Some People Healthy and Others Not? The Determinants of Health of Populations* New York: Aldine-De Gruyter, 1994, pp 287–334

Woolhandler S, Himmelstein DU. The deteriorating administrative efficiency of the U.S. health care system. *New England Journal of Medicine,* 1991; **324**:1253–1258

Wright CJ, Bigelow D, Cardiff K *et al.* Acute medical beds: how are they used in British Columbia? Discussion Paper HPRU 97-7D. Vancouver: Centre for Health Services and Policy Research, University of British Columbia, 1997

3
Changing the role of the state

Julio Frenk

Mexican Health Foundation, Mexico DF, Mexico

The role of the state is the key issue in the contemporary debate about health systems. Since health care became an organized matter, interaction between the population and the providers of services has not been direct, but has rather been mediated through a collective agent. Although in the past different social institutions performed such a mediating role, in most countries the state has become the main collective mediator.

Indeed, the development of modern health systems has been characterized by the broad involvement of the state. Undoubtedly, this process has been a motor for progress, as reflected in expanded coverage to the poor, intense institution building, training of a specialized work-force, recognition of health care as a social right and, ultimately, health improvement. Unfortunately, this bright side of progress has been often obscured by the dark side of bureaucratic inefficiency, authoritarianism, social exclusion and corruption. It is not uncommon to find public organizations whose main beneficiaries are their own employees and political clients, rather than the population they are supposed to serve.

Faced with these realities, the reform of the state has become one of the central topics in our turn-of-the-century transition. The rapid pace of change that has characterized the last decades of the 20th century is forcing a rethinking of the social arrangements to regulate, finance and deliver health services. There is no doubt that the vast transformation of the organized response to health problems will count as one of the major achievements of a century that, according to Yehudi Menuhin, '... raised the greatest hopes ever conceived by humanity...' (cited in Hobsbawm, 1994).

Especially after World War II, health systems have emerged everywhere as a prominent social endeavour. The scope of health-care activities has expanded to growing numbers of people and spheres of human life. As the problem-solving capacity of medicine has increased, most societies have constructed an order of discourse that regards health as a basic human need and medical care as a social right. At the same time, there has been a widespread adoption of rationalizing rules and procedures which constrain the direct relationship between patient and provider. A conspicuous change has been the concentration of the production of both knowledge and services in increasingly complex organizations. There is today an expansive and expensive health-care industry operating on a global scale. As costs escalate, pressure has mounted to demonstrate the effectiveness of interventions. Adding another critical dimension are the wide inequalities among and within countries, both in levels of health and in access to services. Such inequalities persist despite the almost universal growth in the supply of health workers, a large proportion of whom have become civil servants. On the political side, both providers and users have become increasingly organized into formal associations struggling to influence the allocation of scarce resources (Frenk and Durán-Arenas, 1993). In all these dimensions of change, the state appears as a main actor occupying the centre stage of health systems.

Whereas the health-care arrangements that became institutionalized during the post-war period generated important benefits, there is a growing sense that they have largely exhausted their usefulness. For this reason, a worldwide search for new arrangements has been launched in recent years. At the heart of this wave of health system reform initiatives lies the issue of the role of the state along with its practical consequences for the public/private mix. Clearly, this issue involves many ethical, political and technical questions (Reich, 1997). Rather than addressing all of them, we will deal mostly with the conceptual aspects of the role of the state, although we will attempt to derive the policy implications for the design of improved health systems.

In order to provide a context for our discussion, the first part will briefly examine the broader question of the recent evolution of the nation-state. This general analysis will allow us then to focus on the specific health arena. To this effect, we will propose a conceptual framework about health systems in terms of a set of structured relationships between populations and service providers, which are mediated by the state. In the last part of the chapter we will develop a functional perspective that will make it possible to visualize the changing roles of the state in health care. As societies strive to redefine these roles, they will be shaping the health systems of the future.

Rethinking the state

The rise of the nation-state as the major political form in the world and the concentration of power in its hands are relatively recent processes, which began in Europe around the middle of the 17th century (Mathews, 1997), continued through the 18th and 19th centuries (Tilly, 1975), and expanded to the entire globe during the 20th century with the end of colonialism and the constitution of a world polity (Meyer, 1980) based on the concept of national sovereignty. The same developmental forces that were unleashed by the increasing intervention of the state laid the foundations for the expansion of the other major organizing institution in the modern world: the market (Lindblom,1977). Alongside these two institutions, recent years have witnessed the emergence of the so-called 'third sector': the heterogeneous constellation of non-governmental organizations (NGOs).[1]

Since at least the end of the Cold War, the triangular relationship among states, markets and civil society has been experiencing what Mathews (1997) calls a 'power shift'. Its main thrust is paraphrased by Slaughter (1977) as a redistribution of power 'away from the state—up, down, and sideways—to supra-state, sub-state, and ... nonstate actors', and by Reich (1997) as a reshaping of the state by the simultaneous operation of forces 'from above, from within, and from below'.

While these changes have no doubt been dramatic, their impact on the vigour of the state has probably been overestimated. There is a swelling literature proclaiming the 'end of the nation-state', with a number of books and articles that have this prophecy as their title (see, for example, Omae, 1995 and Guéhenno,1995). 'New medievalism' is what Slaughter (1977) calls this vision of a future where the nation-state has withered away or has been reduced to a weak actor struggling to find its place in a world order dominated by global markets, transnational corporations, multilateral agencies and networks of NGOs–all of them coexisting with a revival of regionalism and even tribalism (Barber, 1996).

One need not subscribe to this extreme view in order to recognize that the character of the state is indeed changing (World Bank, 1997). Even as their numbers have grown, the notion that nation-states constitute autonomous political entities exercising full sovereignty over strictly-delimited territories is rapidly becoming obsolete. To begin with, the nation-state construct has been applied to a very heterogeneous set of political entities. Only by recourse to abstract attributes is it possible to find a common thread between, on the one hand, the old, stable, powerful and culturally homogeneous nation-states of

---

[1] The dominant position traditionally enjoyed by the state is reflected even in this term, which specifies a negative identity referring back to government. As power becomes more evenly distributed, we should seek a positive name for these organizations. If we accept the definition of 'civil society' as 'the space of uncoerced human association and also the set of relational networks—formed for the sake of family, faith, interest, and ideology—that fill that space' (Walzer, 1991), then we could adopt the term 'civil society organizations' (CSOs), instead of the conventional 'NGOs'.

Western Europe, and on the other hand, the unstable configurations that emerged out of the arbitrary post-colonial division of Africa. An analysis of the development prospects of countries (Reyes-Heroles, 1998) gives a clear picture of the heterogeneity of the international community. Out of the 184 countries that currently form this community, only 30, with less than a quarter of the world's population, are considered developed. There is a second tier of approximately another 30 countries that exhibit viable prospects for development. And then there are 120 countries, four-fifths of the total number of nations, that simply lack the institutional stability to offer a glimpse of hope for sovereign and sustainable development.

In recent years, even the most stable nation-states have begun to face new challenges deriving from the changing character of relationships in the world arena. New global forces are eroding the potency of national borders, facilitating the transfer of goods, services, people, ideas, values and lifestyles from one country to another. This process has led to what Abba Ebban (1995) has called the central paradox of our times: the existence of multiple nations in a world where sovereignty has lost a lot of its traditional meaning. In this world, a number of economic, technological, political and cultural forces are accelerating the integration of the global village (Frenk et al, 1997).

The dual health agenda

The health field is being reshaped by the emerging world order. Indeed, the complexity of an increasingly integrated world whose basic political unit nonetheless continues to be the nation-state confronts national decision-makers with a series of dilemmas. Clearly, national governments retain responsibility for the health of their populations. Yet, these same governments have only limited control over many determinants of health status that arise from interactions at the global level. All countries are exposed to the international transfer of health risks resulting from the rise of global environmental threats, the expanded movement of people and goods that facilitates the spread of pathogens across national borders, the transfer of unhealthy lifestyles, the cross-national variation in environmental and occupational health standards, the trade in legal and illegal hazardous substances, and the improper use of medical technology including prescription practices that give rise to antibiotic-resistant strains.

Governments have not only lost control over many of these determinants. In addition, the technologies to satisfy health needs are increasingly being produced and traded through global processes that transcend the regulatory capacity of individual governments. As mentioned earlier, there is a global medical industry that has become a key component of the world economy. In turn, many of the transnational corporations that form this global industry must face a bewildering array of regulatory practices in different countries.

Apart from fast technological change, our times are also characterized by political and cultural developments with important impact on health. Among other trends, the aspirations of peoples all over the world are being enriched by a universalistic view of human rights, where the equitable access to good-quality health services plays a growing role. As health care is assimilated into the global human rights movement, governments can expect more active demands on the part of their respective populations for better services (Frenk *et al*, 1997).

The problem for low- and middle-income countries is that these global challenges come on top of an already complex picture of national challenges. Complexity stems from the juxtaposition of an epidemiological backlog (represented by common infections, malnutrition and reproductive health problems) with a series of emerging problems (noncommunicable diseases, new infections such as AIDS and injury). The nonlinear, overlapping and polarized character of the epidemiological transition (Frenk *et al*, 1989) is placing major pressures on the health systems of low- and middle-income countries.

The dual nature of global and national challenges leads to what is also a dual agenda for all states: on the one hand, to improve their individual effectiveness in their respective societies; on the other, to enhance their collective action in the world arena. The first item in this agenda has to do with the reform of national health systems, which is extended by the second item to the reform of the world health system.

Both reforms are linked. Improving health conditions within each country is more dependent than ever on effective international organizations that serve as the vehicle for states to share sovereignty in order to deal with global health challenges. In addition, some international agencies have provided a consensus-building forum with major impact on national health policies, as exemplified by the almost universal adoption of the primary health strategy following the Alma Ata Declaration.

In turn, international organizations can only be effective to the extent that their constituent members succeed in putting their respective health houses in order. As we will argue later, an effective national reform would shift the fulcrum of responsibility of the ministry of health from directly operational programmes to strategic activities, including a renewed focus on interactions with other states.

In sum, an effective state must rethink its role both in the domestic management of health affairs and in the mechanisms for international collective action. Space limitations preclude us from further analysing the reform of international health organizations—a topic that we have addressed in detail elsewhere (Frenk *et al*, 1997; Jamison *et al*, 1998). Instead, the remainder of this paper will focus on the renewal of state participation in national health systems.

A conceptual framework

The formulation of policies regarding the public/private mix must start with a clear understanding of the characteristics of state intervention in health care. A fully developed theory would encompass the determinants, modalities, typologies, historical trends and consequences of such intervention (Frenk and Donabedian, 1987). Here we will restrict the analysis to one of the most critical issues in the current debate over health systems reform: the functions of the state.

Goals and means of the state

In attempting to elucidate this issue, it is necessary to address an apparent contradiction in the intrinsic character of the state. On the one hand, there is a high degree of heterogeneity in the state apparatus. Indeed, the state includes a number of quite different organizations, some involved in functions of social control and order maintenance, others in the direct production of goods and services. Yet, on the other hand, it is reasonable to assume that the state apparatus has an organic unity that allows us to identify it as an object of analysis.

In this respect, Weber (1946) made a fundamental contribution when he defined the state as a type of organization whose essential characteristic is its 'monopoly of the legitimate use of physical force'. As such, the state differs in a radical way from other organizations because it is structured not around the attainment of a goal but, instead, around its monopoly over the means of legitimate violence. Thus Weber (1946) argued (and in this he differs both from classical economists and from Marxists) that there is no goal that states have not assumed and, conversely, that there is no state which has assumed all possible goals. The crucial point is that, by being structured around specific means rather than specific goals, the state as an organization has the plasticity to mobilize its resources so as to accomplish a changing set of goals.

The notion of the relative autonomy of the state, which is consistent with the Weberian tradition, emerges as a necessary result of the way that the state is structured around its specificity of means and its goal plasticity. Such a conception attempts to avoid both the normative definitions of what the goals of the state ought to be, as proposed by Neoclassical economic theory, and the material determinism by which certain schools of Marxist thought reduce the state to an instrument of the ruling class (Frenk and Durán-Arenas, 1993).

The implications of this conceptualization for health systems are profound. Because of its goal plasticity, the state has historically assumed different functions. Underneath the concrete proposals found in the current wave of health reforms, there is a deeper core involving a potential paradigm shift in the definition of state functions. We must therefore specify what those functions are.

A functional view of the health system[2]

All too often, health systems are seen as a simple collection of organizations. Instead, we would like to propose a dynamic view of health systems (Cassels, 1995) as a set of *structured relationships* among two major components: populations and institutions (Figure 3.1). The various population groups present a series of conditions which constitute health needs requiring an organized social response from institutions. In every health system this response is structured through a number of basic functions which institutions have to perform in order to address the health needs of populations. As a collective mediator (Johnson, 1972), the state forms part of the institutional constellation of health systems. One of the key issues in health system reform refers to the distribution of functions between public and private institutions.[3]

In specifying the functions of the health system, it is useful to bear in mind the conventional distinction between personal and non-personal health services, a point that will be discussed later in greater detail. Most of the discussion that follows will concentrate on personal health services, i.e. the set of preventive, diagnostic, therapeutic and rehabilitative actions that are applied directly to individuals. This emphasis is justified by the fact that personal health services absorb the vast majority of resources and that most of the debates on health system reform refer centrally to them.

Modern health systems are not limited to the set of institutions that provide services, but also include a diversified group of organizations that generate the resources required to produce those services (Roemer, 1991). Salient among these are universities and similar institutions, which often have the dual role

---

[2] Parts of this section are based, with modifications, on concepts that have been developed in two previous papers (Frenk, 1994; Londoño and Frenk, 1997).
[3] For the purposes of this discussion, we follow the common practice of adopting the narrow definition of the state as the institutions of government providing the administrative, legislative and judicial vehicles for the actual exercise of public authority and power, rather than the broad definition of the state as the total political organization of a society, including its citizens. Similarly, we identify the adjective 'public' with governmental, even though we are well aware that these are not strict synonyms.

of developing human resources and providing health services. Another group of important resource generators are research centres producing knowledge and developing new technologies, as well as the large group of firms forming the 'medical-industrial complex', such as pharmaceutical and medical equipment companies.

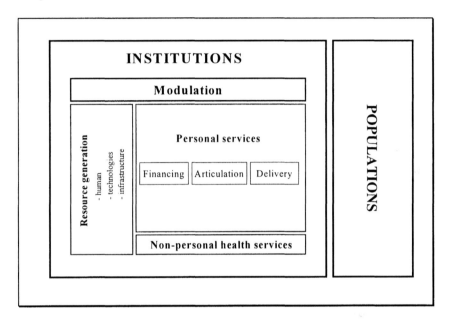

Figure 3.1 Components of health systems. Source: Londoño and Frenk (1997)

Although parts of the discussion that follow will also be relevant to resource generation, the remainder of this chapter will focus on the four core functions of health systems presented in Figure 3.1: modulation, financing, articulation and delivery.

The functions of financing and delivery are the most familiar. In its strict sense, financing refers to the mobilization of money from primary sources (households and firms), as well as from secondary sources (government at all levels and international donors), and its accumulation in real or virtual funds (e.g. social insurance funds, public budgets for health care, family savings) that can then be allocated through a variety of institutional arrangements to produce services. In turn, the delivery function refers to the combination of inputs into a production process that takes place in a particular organizational structure and that leads to a set of outputs (i.e. health services) which generate an outcome (i.e. changes in health status).

Alongside the two traditional functions, every health system has to perform a series of key functions, which can be encompassed under the term 'modulation'.[4] This is a broader concept than regulation. It involves setting, implementing and monitoring the rules of the game for the health system, as well as providing it with strategic direction. Setting rules of the game is a delicate process where the interests of the various actors have to be balanced. Too often, this function has been neglected, particularly in those health systems where the ministry of health devotes most of its human, financial and political resources to the direct delivery of services. Later on, we shall argue that strengthening modulation should be a major element of health system reform. At that point, we will analyse in greater detail the various elements of this key function.

The last function of the health system, as shown in Figure 3.1, can be termed 'articulation'. This function lies between financing and delivery. In most current health systems it has been collapsed into either of those two other functions and has therefore remained implicit. One of the important innovations in many reform proposals has been to make this function explicit and to assign responsibility for performing it to distinct entities. Thus, 'articulation' corresponds to what Chernichovsky (1995) calls 'organization and management of care consumption'. It also encompasses the functions of demand aggregation and consumer representation that are assigned to what the managed competition model calls the 'sponsor' (Enthoven, 1988; Starr, 1994). The term 'articulation' is meant to convey the notion that this function pulls together and gives coherence to various components of health care. As in the case of modulation, we will explain articulation in greater detail later on. At this point it is sufficient to note that articulation encompasses key activities that allow financial resources to flow to the production and consumption of health care. Examples include the enrolment of populations into health plans, the specification of explicit packages of benefits or interventions, the organization of networks of providers so as to structure consumer choices, the design and implementation of incentives to providers through payment mechanisms, and the management of quality of care.

The configuration of the four major health system functions—modulation, financing, articulation and delivery—provides the basis to identify the main institutional models. In this paper we will not spell out the implications of the functional approach to the classification of health systems.[5] It should be stressed, nevertheless, that in some models one or more of the functions may not be explicitly assigned. This is the case of vertically integrated systems, where some functions may be performed only implicitly or may be absent altogether because they conflict with other functions. These omissions are

---

[4] We are indebted to Professor Avedis Donabedian, from the University of Michigan, for having suggested this term.

[5] A typology of health-care modalities throughout the world is proposed in Frenk (1994) and an adaptation to the case of Latin America in Londoño and Frenk (1997).

particularly common for modulation and articulation. Even the implicit nature or the outright absence of a function reveal important aspects of the character of a health system.

The mix of functions lies at the heart of the discussion regarding the changing role of the state. Before we can sketch some of the proposals in this respect, it is necessary to take account of a factor that has often been neglected in such discussion, but which makes it complex and rich.

The heterogeneity of health services

Very often, the academic literature and the policy debate about the role of the state seem to assume that health services constitute a homogeneous good. In fact, they encompass a wide variety of human activities, from pure public goods to items of individual consumption, from life-saving procedures to superfluous interventions.

The category 'health service' represents a social construct that is historically bound. Since about the 18th century, there has been a trend towards expanding the set of activities that fall under that rubric (Foucault, 1973). This trend has been due, among other factors, to the differentiation of medical care as a specialized social institution, to the expansion of technology and to a cultural shift towards explanations of human experience based on scientific reason. State intervention has been a major force in the development of these social forces, since the modern nation-state is usually conceived of as a legitimate agent of rational progress (Meyer, 1980).

The expansion of the domain of health services means that they have become increasingly heterogeneous. It is difficult to find another sector of the economy that encompasses such a variety of outputs. Failing to recognize this heterogeneity limits the usefulness of both research findings and policy prescriptions. In particular, the definition of the role of the state must be grounded on a firm understanding of the intrinsic character of health services. As Bennett and colleagues (1997) cogently argue: 'Any analysis of appropriate roles for public and private sectors in health care is ... inevitably country-specific and moreover should be fairly *product- or service-specific*' [emphasis added].

The picture is further complicated by the fact that health status is influenced by a variety of services other than health care, such as general education. For this reason, Figure 3.2 proposes a classification that begins with the broad category of services for health. An important aspect of the political dynamics of the health system lies in defining the boundaries between health services strictly defined and other services with health effects. (Witness the political feuds in many countries as to whether environmental protection should be the

responsibility of the ministry of health or of an independent agency.)
Intersectoral coordination has to do with the management of this interface.

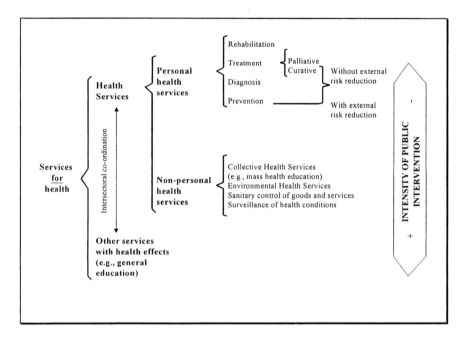

Figure 3.2 Classification of services with health effects

Health services proper are further subdivided into personal and non-personal, as
mentioned earlier. The criterion for this conventional distinction refers to the
exclusivity of consumption. Use of personal health services by one individual
precludes simultaneous utilization by others, whereas non-personal services
constitute public goods since their consumption cannot be appropriated
exclusively by one individual. In turn, personal health services encompass the
usual categories of prevention, diagnosis, treatment and rehabilitation. An
important distinction with respect to prevention and treatment is whether they
entail the positive externality of reducing risks to others, as when they deal with
contagious diseases. The non-personal category includes actions that are
applied by health sector agencies to collectivities (e.g. mass health education)
or to the non-human components of the environment (e.g. basic sanitation), as
well as the sanitary regulation of general goods and services and the
surveillance of health conditions in the population.

As shown on the right-hand side of Figure 3.2, there is a gradient of
intensity of public intervention spanning the different categories of health
services. Non-personal services and personal services with external risk
reduction have traditionally represented the least controversial arenas for public

involvement. Compared to them, the medical care end of the spectrum of health services has offered greater room for debating the legitimacy of state participation, for playing out conflicting interests and for adopting varying forms of intervention.

Part of these controversies stem from the fact that even personal health services without externalities exhibit important differences that must be taken into account when examining the role of the state. While the literature correctly points to market imperfections as a reason for state intervention (Bennett,1997), there are additional criteria to determine the extent of those imperfections. Musgrove (1996) uses the criterion of cost to differentiate private goods, since (apart from public goods) market failure occurs in the case of catastrophically costly services that are financed through insurance. Figure 3.3 proposes two other analytical dimensions that can be useful to distinguish different types of services calling for alternative strategies of state intervention.

The first dimension refers to the degree of discretion to utilize services, which determines the potential for demand to be price-elastic. Many health events are not very serious or do not lead to a felt need, thus allowing for a high degree of discretion in the decision to utilize the corresponding services. Under

DEGREE OF REPEATED UTILIZATION (Potential for consumer sovereignty)	DEGREE OF DISCRETION TO UTILIZE (Potential to be price-elastic)	
	HIGH	**LOW**
HIGH	- Early detection and screening procedures - Health maintenance services	- Treatment of chronic diseases - Treatment of acute repetitive diseases
LOW	- Elective surgery	- Treatment of acute non-repetitive diseases - Medical emergencies

Figure 3.3 Typology of personal health services. (Examples include personal health services without external risk reduction.)

these circumstances, consumers are likely to be more responsive to prices. (The exact extent to which this potential for price elasticity will be realized depends on other attributes of the health care market and of consumers themselves.) In sharp contrast, there are many situations where the consumer has no choice but to use services lest there be serious health consequences. An extreme example is represented by life-threatening emergencies. In this type of situation, it is unrealistic to expect that there will be much room for price competition or shopping around.

The second dimension has to do with the degree of repetition in the utilization of a certain service. It is well known that one of the major ways in which consumers acquire information about the qualities of goods is through repeated consumption. However, there are certain health services that do not lend themselves to such repetition, due to the very nature of the underlying need they are meant to address. Under these circumstances, information asymmetries will become magnified (Pauly, 1978), and the potential for consumer sovereignty will be sharply curtailed. (Again, we are referring here only to a potential, the realization of which will depend on other market variables.)

Combining these two dimensions yields a four-fold typology of personal health services (Figure 3.3). Each of the resulting categories has different implications for market imperfections and therefore for the role of the state. Imperfections are least severe for services in the upper left-hand quadrant, which correspond to Musgrove's (1996) category of low-cost private interventions. These activities exhibit the opposite attributes to what classical insurance theory prescribes as requisites for making an event insurable: they are frequent, the losses in each episode are relatively small and they are highly influenced by individual decisions. In particular, dependence on individual discretion would make these interventions prone to 'moral hazard' if they were to be insured (Pauly, 1974). As a result, traditional insurance products exclude them, leading to gaps in coverage (Barr, 1992).

In the opposite quadrant we find those personal health services for which market imperfections are most marked. These services address health needs that arise too infrequently or are too life-threatening to make it feasible to obtain information in order to guide purchasing decisions (Hsiao, 1990). This situation calls for the kind of regulatory and consumer-protection actions that will be discussed in the next section. Since this type of service is often associated with catastrophic expenditures, public intervention may take the form of mandating or providing insurance. Extreme market failure in services such as medical emergencies might even lead to direct delivery by the state, depending upon country-specific circumstances.

The two remaining quadrants illustrate market imperfections that have been frequently analysed in the literature. When services do not lend themselves to repeated utilization and there is a high degree of discretion (as in elective surgery), information asymmetries can lead to provider-induced demand. When consumers acquire information through repeated utilization of services but have low discretion (as in the treatment of chronic diseases), there is a particularly high potential for adverse selection, with its corresponding response of risk selection by insurers (Musgrove, 1996). This last situation demonstrates the fact that information asymmetries affect not only consumers but also insurers.

Until now, the conventional view has restricted state intervention in the medical care market to extreme market failures usually involving catastrophic expenditures. Yet three new rationales for such intervention are emerging. The first refers to the cost-effectiveness of interventions. Many of the interventions that traditional insurance excludes from coverage count among the most cost-effective. As will be discussed later on, an emerging role of the state is to set explicit priorities in order to assure that those interventions are indeed produced (World Bank, 1993). The second rationale stems from the fact that, despite their heterogeneity, personal health services are often linked to each other. Specifically, failure to cover preventive services often translates into higher costs for curative activities and breaks the continuity of care. For these reasons, the state may create incentives (including direct finance) for comprehensive plans that cover the whole gamut of health services, albeit through schemes that are meant to reduce the potential for moral hazard, such as having providers bear part of the financial risk. The third rationale is grounded on the pervasiveness of information asymmetries, noted above. Such pervasiveness has led Barr (1992) to write: 'Information failures provide both a theoretical justification of and an explanation for a welfare state which is much more than a safety net.'

In summary, the health field must face the complexities arising from the heterogeneity of its products. Both the extent of discretion and the propensity for repetition in the use of services are influenced by cultural norms and economic incentives. Yet they also reflect certain intrinsic attributes of health services, which go beyond cultural and institutional specificities. Faced with this heterogeneity, the state has a repertory of intervention strategies, depending on the combination of functions that it performs. In many countries, however, the choice of strategy has not been guided by the intrinsic attributes of services and the ensuing mix of functions. Instead, the state has adopted differential intervention strategies for different social groups. This has led to segmented health systems, which are marred by inefficiency and inequity. The segmented model is the dominant one in Latin America, and it is increasingly common in other parts of the developing world. (Indeed, certain reform proposals would actually lead to segmentation, as we will see later on.) It is therefore useful to examine in greater detail the logic of such a model. This will set the stage for proposing a paradigm shift in the role of the state, based on the functional conception of the health system.

Segmented health systems[6]

One of the most common solutions to the problem of specifying the role of the state in developing countries has been to divide the health system into several segments, each designed to serve a social group. The structure of such a segmented model can be depicted in a simplified way with the matrix shown in Figure 3.4a. This matrix relates the health system functions of modulation, financing, articulation and delivery to the various social groups.

An initial fundamental distinction has been made between the poor and the non-poor. The non-poor comprises two groups. The first is made up of those working in the formal sector of the economy (and often their relatives as well), who are covered by one or several social security schemes. The second group consists of the middle and upper classes, mostly urban, who are not protected by social security.[7] The health needs of this group are mostly catered for by the formal private for-profit sector, with financing coming principally from out-of-pocket payments. Increasingly, some middle- and upper-class families get coverage from private insurance or prepaid plans, whether purchased directly or offered through employers.

Finally, there are the poor, both rural and urban, who are excluded from social security because they do not have formal employment. In the design of the segmented model, ministries of health are charged with providing personal services to the poor (in addition to producing non-personal health services that benefit the whole population). In many countries, this group also receives care from private non-profit providers, who often resemble their counterparts in government more than those in the for-profit sector.

As can be seen in Figure 3.4a, the segmented model segregates the three population groups into their respective institutional niches. Indeed, this model can be described as a system of vertical integration but horizontal segregation. Each institutional segment—the ministry of health, the social security schemes and the private sector—performs the functions of modulation, financing, articulation (when present) and delivery of services (totally or partially), but does so only for a specific group. Such a configuration of the health system has many problems. First, it makes for duplication and waste of resources, especially in high-technology services. Second, it usually leads to major quality differentials among the various segments. In particular, services reserved for the poor suffer from a chronic shortage of resources (Musgrove, 1996). Third,

---

[6] Parts of this section and the following one are based, with modifications, on concepts that have been developed in two previous papers (Frenk, 1995; Londoño and Frenk, 1997).

[7] Strictly speaking, many members of these classes, especially those with higher incomes, do contribute to social security, but they never use its services. They see their contributions to social security as one more tax rather than as an insurance premium.

segmentation creates incentives for many health professionals (mostly physicians) to seek employment in more than one institution, typically by combining a salaried job in a public organization with private practice. Such a combination often creates conflicts of interest (e.g. referring patients from the public organization to the private practice) and leads to differentials in the quality standards applied by the same physician, which are very problematic from the point of view of professional ethics and of social justice.

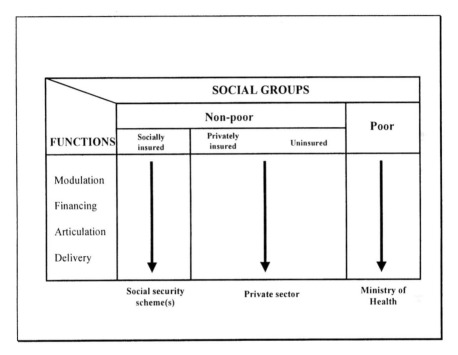

Figure 3.4a Present design of the segmented model. Source: Londoño and Frenk (1997)

While all these limitations are serious, the most important problem with the design of the segmented model is that it does not reflect actual population behaviour. Indeed, people do not necessarily respect the artificial divisions among the three segments. At least in Latin America, there is empirical evidence of a considerable overlap of demand, with a very high proportion of social-security beneficiaries using services provided by the private sector or the ministry of health (González-Block, 1994). The problem is that the burden of such a decision is borne by the consumer, for he or she is forced to pay for the care received elsewhere, despite already having paid an insurance premium. This leads to an important source of inequity: multiple payments, which impose on many families and businesses a disproportionate financial burden.

Another source of inequity is that the overlap in demand is unilateral, since uninsured families cannot use social-security facilities (except in emergencies and for a few high-priority services). Furthermore, many ministries of health have failed in their intended targeting of services for the poor. The notion that private services are reserved for the middle and upper classes, thereby liberating public resources to care for the poor, is not supported by utilization data. In most countries with such data, it turns out that the private sector is an important source of care for poor households, which may spend a higher proportion of their income on out-of-pocket payments than richer households (Frenk, 1995). In addition, the poorest groups often obtain their care in an informal private sector (McPake, 1997), which by definition is unregulated. While the tendency in policy analysis is to emphasize market failures, these are all instances of government failure—in this case, the failure to protect the most vulnerable groups.

There have been several efforts to correct the failures of segmented systems. So far, these efforts have gone in two opposite directions. Some countries have attempted to break the segmentation of the population by nationalizing the health services and unifying all institutions in a single public system. This was probably the most popular reform strategy up until the 1980s and still has many proponents. The search for equity under this strategy has proved to be incompatible with the requirements of efficiency and responsiveness to population needs and preferences.

Either because of ideological preferences or public finance restrictions, other countries have sought to hand over the organization of health services to agencies outside central government. There have been two major variants of this type of reform. The first has been the privatization strategy: Chile provides one of the earliest examples of this policy. The second variant has been the decentralization strategy, with devolution of previously centralized responsibilities to local authorities. A major problem with both variants has been the weakness of the modulatory effort needed to set clear rules of the game for the transfer of responsibilities. Instead, central decision-makers have acted under the implicit assumption that local or private initiative will somehow solve the major constraints in health care delivery. Under these conditions, many privatization and decentralization initiatives have proved to be incompatible with the requirements of equity and, paradoxically, have not yielded the expected gains in efficiency.

Because of this, a growing number of countries have started to look for truly innovative alternatives. In this context, several proposed and implemented reform initiatives have started to develop an option that seeks to achieve an optimal balance among equity, efficiency and quality. While the existing proposals and experiences show important differences, this emerging model is well captured by the term 'structured pluralism' (Londoño and Frenk, 1997).

Structured pluralism: towards a paradigm shift

The concept of 'structured pluralism' tries to convey the search for a middle ground in the public–private polarization that has so hampered the performance of health systems. 'Pluralism' avoids the extremes of monopoly in the public sector and fragmentation in the private sector. 'Structured' avoids the extremes of authoritarian command-and-control procedures in government and the anarchic absence of transparent rules of the game to correct market failures. In this respect, it is interesting to note that opposite extremes can end up having the same deleterious effect. For example, subordination of consumers to providers and insurers is a common outcome of both public monopoly— through lack of choice—and of fragmented private markets—through information asymmetry. Very often the real dilemma is not choice of public or private ownership of facilities, but of provider, insurer or consumer sovereignty. Structured pluralism fosters a more balanced distribution of power than existing models have achieved.

Organizing the system by functions

The solution proposed by structured pluralism can be visualized by referring back to the matrix of functions and social groups. As shown in Figure 3.4b, the proposal is to turn the matrix around. Instead of the present vertical integration with segregation of social groups, there would be explicit and specialized assignment of functions. In other words, the health system would no longer be organized by social groups, but by functions (Frenk, 1995). Indeed, a key feature of this model is that it identifies explicitly each of the four functions. In this way, it promotes a specialization of actors in the health system. This is why structured pluralism involves a new institutional configuration for the health system. In this scheme, modulation would become the main mission of the ministry of health, as the entity in charge of giving strategic direction to the whole system. Instead of being one more provider of services—usually the weakest—the ministry of health would assure a balanced, efficient and equitable interaction among all actors by structuring the appropriate rules and incentives. As we will argue later, this emphasis on modulation should not lead to bureaucratic concentration of power. On the contrary, having set transparent and fair rules of the game, ministries of health could increasingly delegate the actual operation of many modulatory functions to participatory organizations of civil society that are not captured by special interests.

The next function, financing, would become the major responsibility of social security, which would be gradually extended in order to achieve universal protection under principles of public finance. Compared with current financial arrangements, there would be a greater emphasis on demand-side than on supply-side subsidies. Instead of allocating a historical budget to each facility regardless of performance, each insured person would represent a potential payment contingent on the choice of insurer and provider by the consumer.

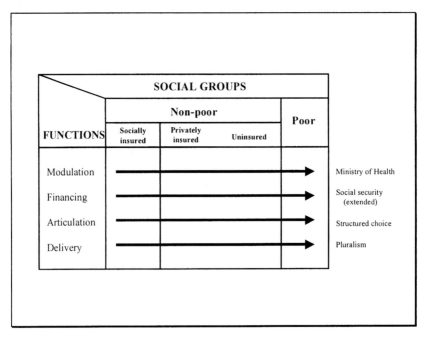

Figure 3.4b Proposed design of structured pluralism. Source: Londoño and Frenk (1997)

Managing that payment would be a key element of the articulation function, which would now become explicit and would be carried out by specialized institutions. These could generically be called 'organizations for health services articulation' (OHSAs). There are several options for the specific development of these organizations, depending on the conditions of each country. In urban areas, OHSAs would compete to enrol individuals and families. In rural areas, conditions are usually not ready for this kind of open competition. Nevertheless, even there it is possible to foster pluralism that is responsive to population needs. Indeed, in order to stimulate choice and efficiency it is not necessary to have all the conditions for full-blown competition. Often, it suffices to have 'market contestability', which refers to the potential participation of alternative agencies in the organization of services, in a situation where block grants or annual contracts can only be arranged with one such agency. For rural areas in many developing countries, market contestability would obtain if several agencies would compete annually for broad contracts to serve specific populations. Finally, as a consequence of greater choice in the articulation function, the direct delivery of services would be opened up to a pluralist array of institutions, both public and private.

In sum, the challenge for structured pluralism is to increase the options both for consumers and for providers, while having explicit rules of the game that will minimize the potential conflicts between equity and efficiency. Increasing the options for consumers is accompanied by an extension of prepayment in a context of public finance to assure and redistribute resources. Increasing the options for providers is accompanied by their integration into efficient networks, which are clearly articulated and modulated. Alongside the traditional functions of financing and delivery, it is the emphasis on modulation and articulation that gives the 'structured' character to this kind of pluralism.

In examining the organization of health systems by functions, it is useful to return to our previous discussion about the goals and means of the state. Out of the entire constellation of goals that governments can pursue in health care, only modulation requires the means that are exclusive to the state. Given the centrality of this function to the changing role of the state, it is necessary to explain it in greater detail.

Modulation: the core public function

There seems to be a growing awareness that the modulation function has been insufficiently specified and implemented in most health systems. As these systems become more open and diverse through decentralization and increased competition, modulation will have to be strengthened. This is a key feature for present and future reforms.

Increasingly, discussions about reform options are focusing on the need to establish fair and transparent rules in order to foster a harmonious development of the system. Such rules are the essence of institutions, as they make it possible to reduce uncertainty by providing stability to interactions (North, 1990). This is a specialized function that must be differentiated from both financing and delivery, so as to avoid conflicts of interest and assure the transparency of the myriad transactions occurring in modern health systems. Hence, modulation must be carried out by neutral agents who can rise above any special interest.

While there is still much to be debated and decided concerning the specifics of modulation, in practically all health systems this function is a public responsibility. This does not mean that the actual operation of all modulatory functions must be carried out by the government. In fact, there is cross-national variation in the extent to which other actors participate in the operation of some of those functions (like certification or accreditation). Nonetheless, there is widespread consensus that the ultimate responsibility is public, meaning that a politically legitimate agent must be responsive and accountable to the interests of the entire collectivity. As explained below, in almost all countries modulation encompasses a core of public functions.

In contrast, there is wide variation in the degree of state intervention concerning the other three functions of the health system, i.e. financing, articulation and delivery. The real debate no longer concerns a Manichæan choice between nationalization or privatization, but the best distribution of functions between public and private institutions so as to optimize population well-being. In this public/private mix, the importance of modulation as an essential public responsibility is underscored precisely by the growing pluralism in the other functions.

In fact, the emphasis on modulation represents a shift in conception of the central mission of ministries of health. It is therefore part of the broader discussion about the reform of the state. This reform has proposed that public organizations should stop being owners of facilities and producers of goods and services. Instead, government should channel its energy into promoting public interest, proposing strategic directions, providing comprehensive security, mobilizing resources, setting standards, catalysing private activity, giving transparency to markets, protecting consumers, evaluating performance and assuring justice.

When translated to the specific realm of health care, the reform of the state means that ministries of health should gradually move away from the direct provision of services, into the strategic modulation of the system. Of course, government retains a direct responsibility for the financing and delivery of those health services that have the characteristics of public goods, as discussed earlier. Even in this case, however, there are many possible innovatory ways for governments to fulfil their responsibility through efficient, responsive, participatory and autonomous modes of organization.

Shifting their central mission towards modulation would actually strengthen ministries of health. It is the concern with the details of direct operation of services that weakens them. Their true strength lies in their capacity to mobilize social energy for a common purpose. Such a catalytic role is the essence of modulation. In order to perform it, modulation includes five more specific functions:

1. System development. It encompasses the following elements:
- policy formulation;
- strategic planning;
- priority setting for resource allocation, including the process of building consensus around those priorities;

- intersectoral advocacy, so as to promote 'healthy policies' that will act on the social, economic, environmental and cultural determinants of health status;
- social mobilization for health, including community participation;
- development of criteria and standards for the assessment of performance of financing agencies, articulating organizations, and individual and institutional providers of services;
- capacity strengthening through promotion of investments in physical infrastructure, human resources, scientific research, technological development and information systems.

2. Co-ordination. There are many situations in health care that require concerted action in order to achieve objectives efficiently. This is the case, for example, with complex and costly tertiary technologies where it may be desirable to limit the number of providers in order to achieve economies of scale. Another case is represented by massive public health campaigns, which commonly involve the collaboration of many organizations. In general, co-ordination may be required among territorial units, levels of government, or public and private organizations. There must be an agent in the health system with the authority to convene these multiple actors in the pursuit of common objectives.

This does not mean, however, that co-ordination must be carried out in an authoritarian manner. On the contrary, one of the challenges for new institutional development under structured pluralism involves the promotion of efficient and equitable transaction modalities among public and private agents. The task of co-ordination becomes then one of strategic design that will give transparency and consistency to those transactions. Hence, co-ordination should not be carried out through discretionary interventions by bureaucracies, but through clear rules of the game that facilitate interactions in a pluralist environment. Once those rules are set as a part of modulation, the actual activities leading to co-ordination of health care can then be performed as part of the articulation function. For example, contracts and information represent valuable tools to achieve transparent co-ordination in health care. A system increasingly based on explicit contracts for the performance of functions can produce a more efficient and less authoritarian control of compliance (Mills, 1997; Perrot et al, 1997). The provision of information so that every actor can make rational decisions and the others can know about them is another essential element of this new institutional development.

3. Financial design. In order to increase coverage and quality, modern health systems must face two key financial challenges: mobilize the required resources and contain costs. Often, progress on one of these fronts can place obstacles to the other; hence it is necessary to strike a balance between them. Such a balance

can only be achieved through a careful design of the financial scheme. This design of financing, as distinct from its operation, is an important part of modulation. Without a careful design, the system can suffer either from shortage of resources or from cost explosion. Setting clear financial rules is essential to achieve sustainable reform. In particular, this part of modulation aims to provide global consistency to the resources in the system.

The function of financial design involves key decisions that will determine the structure of incentives in the system, such as the use of public funds for the benefit packages (especially if they are mandated); the amounts of capitation payments and the possible risk adjustments for them; the budget cap for the system as a whole; the formulae for resource allocation among territorial units, levels of government or non-governmental institutions; and the use of policy instruments, such as taxes and subsidies, that are aimed at changing population behaviour.

4. Regulation strictly defined. This includes two main types: sanitary regulation of goods and services, and health-care regulation. The former refers to the conventional efforts by sanitary authorities to minimize the health hazards that might be generated by the goods and services provided throughout the economy, especially those are directly consumed by human beings, such as foodstuffs. Even more crucial for our present discussion is the second kind of regulation, which is applied to the specific sectors of the economy dealing directly with health care. Thus, this type of regulation is designed to set rules for the following components of the health system:

- individual providers, through licensing and certification;
- institutional providers, through accreditation;
- financing mechanisms, through rules for insurance funds and similar instruments;
- organizations in charge of the articulation function, through accreditation and supervision, so as to assure their accountability to consumers;
- educational institutions, through accreditation; and
- drugs, equipment and medical devices, through technology assessment; capital investments, through plans.

These regulatory activities must be carried out in a decentralized manner and with the active participation of all actors. In fact, the operation of many regulatory procedures can be delegated to organizations of civil society, with the appropriate safeguards so that the regulatory process is not captured by special interests. The final aim must be to create structural conditions for improving the quality of health care.

5. Consumer protection. The important information asymmetry that characterizes the health care market makes it necessary to have an explicit strategy for consumer protection. A first instrument in this respect is to offer public information about the performance of insurers and providers. Making this kind of information available to consumers and to OHSAs (as agents in the purchase of health services) would foster effective competition. Of course, the mere dissemination of information is not enough for fully redressing the power imbalance among providers and consumers. It is also necessary to develop a deliberate effort—until now very much neglected—for human rights protection and conflict mediation.

In sum, the type of modulation that structured pluralism calls for does not place obstacles to the market for health services, but is instead a necessary condition for it to function in a transparent and efficient manner. Indeed, structuring pluralism through modulation offers a balanced middle point that combines the operation of market mechanisms with a framework of public responsibility. In this way, it becomes possible to mobilize a variety of policy and managerial instruments to deal, in an integrated manner, with the heterogeneous character of health services. Careful design of rules, incentives and information systems can then correct the different market imperfections while maintaining the integrity of the care process.

This vision supersedes the conventional conception of states and markets as alternative ways of organizing the pursuit of goals. A recent *World Development Report* moves away from such a dichotomous perspective by recognizing that '... markets and governments are complementary: the state is essential for putting in place the appropriate institutional foundations for markets' (World Bank, 1997). The image of private rowing with public steering (Osborne and Gaebler, 1993) seems to capture the changing role of the state.

Conclusion

Like Janus, the state in the 20th century has two faces: one of outstanding achievements, the other of shameful abuses. On the positive side of its century-long balance sheet, the state can write down its main asset as a catalyser of collective will in the pursuit of progress. Life expectancy, literacy, science and technology, democracy and recognition of human rights are some of the spheres with the greatest improvements in history. Side by side with these accomplishments, the negative column of the balance sheet shows a social debt that seems impossible to pay: 35 million people killed in war and 110 million victims of genocide during this century (Reyes-Heroles, 1998) are the dark legacy of states that corrupted the force of nation, ethnicity or religion towards the annihilation of diversity. To such expressions of mass destruction, one must add the daily tragedy of the 1.3 billion persons (World Bank, 1996) who live in extreme poverty—another form of denigration of human dignity.

It is against this backdrop that we must try to chart a future for health care. More than ever, the world is in need of a revision—that is, a new vision—about the role of the state in health. The key concept in this vision is the urgent need to supersede the false dilemma between state and market. The issue is not a simple quantitative choice between more or less state. The problem is qualitative: we need a *different* state, one that no longer seeks its strength in the authoritarian control of social forces but in their catalytic mobilization towards a synthesis of economic growth and equity (Aguilar-Camín, 1997). As the former Socialist president of Spain, Felipe González (1988), has said, the state in the modern world must be agile, not fragile or obese.

It is too early to know how the relatively recent invention that we call the nation-state will respond to the pressures from above, from below and from within (Reich, 1997). What is certain is that it will experience a fundamental transformation as the world crosses the threshold into the next century. Whatever course that transformation follows, it will have a major impact on the health needs of populations and on the system that cares for them. The future of health will be shaped by the future of the state.

Acknowledgements

An earlier version of this paper benefited from insightful comments by Juan-Luis Londoño, Philip Musgrove, Michael Reich and several participants at the Eighth Annual Public Health Forum at the London School of Hygiene & Tropical Medicine.

References

Aguilar-Camín H. Crecimiento y equidad (Growth and equity). *La Jornada*, 20 October 1997 p11

Barber BR. Jihad vs. McWorld: *How the Planet is both Falling Apart and Coming Together*. New York: Ballantine Books, 1996

Barr N. Economic theory and the welfare state: a survey and interpretation. *Journal of Economic Literature*, 1992; **30**: 741–803

Bennett S. Health-care markets: defining characteristics. In: Bennett S, McPake B, Mills A (eds) *Private Health Providers in Developing Countries: Serving the Public Interest?* London: Zed Books, 1997: 85–101

Bennett S, McPake B, Mills A. The public/private mix debate in health care. In: Bennett S, McPake B, Mills A (eds) *Private Health Providers in Developing Countries: Serving the Public Interest?* London: Zed Books, 1997: 1–18

Cassels A. Health sector reform: key issues in less developed countries. *Journal of International Development*, 1995; **7**: 329–348

Chernichovsky D. Health system reforms in industrialized democracies: an emerging paradigm. *Milbank Quarterly*, 1995; **73**: 339–372

Ebban A. The United Nations revisited. *Foreign Affairs*, 1995; **74**: 39–55

Enthoven AC. *Theory and Practice of Managed Competition in Health Care Finance.* Amsterdam: North Holland, 1988

Foucault M. *The Birth of the Clinic: an Archaeology of Medical Perception* [transl Smith AMS]. London: Tavistock Publications, 1973

Frenk J. Dimensions of health system reform. *Health Policy*, 1994; **27**: 19–34

Frenk J. Comprehensive policy analysis for health system reform. *Health Policy*, 1995; **32**: 257–277

Frenk J, Bobadilla JL, Sepúlveda J, López-Cervantes M. Health transition in middle-income countries: new challenges for health care. *Health Policy and Planning*, 1989; **4**: 29–39

Frenk J, Donabedian A. State intervention in medical care: types, trends and variables. *Health Policy and Planning*, 1987; **2**: 17–31

Frenk J, Durán-Arenas L. The medical profession and the state. In: Hafferty FW, McKinlay JB (eds) *The Changing Medical Profession: an International Perspective.* New York: Oxford University Press, 1993: pp 25–42

Frenk J, Sepúlveda J, Gómez-Dantés O, McGuinness MJ, Knaul F. The future of world health: the new world order and international health. *British Medical Journal*, 1997; **314**: 1404–1407

González F. Siete asedios al mundo actual (Seven besiegements on the present world). *Nexos*, March 1998; **21**: 38–45

González-Block MA. Access policies and utilization patterns in prenatal and child delivery care in Mexico. *Health Policy and Planning*, 1994; **9**: 204–212

Guéhenno JM. *The End of the Nation-state* [transl. Elliott V]. Minneapolis: University of Minnesota Press, 1995

Hobsbawm E. *The Age of Extremes: a History of the World, 1914-1991.* New York: Pantheon Books, 1994, p2

Hsiao WC. Lessons for developing countries from the experiences of affluent countries about a comprehensive health financing strategy. Paper presented at the International Seminar on Comprehensive Financing Strategy in Selected Asian Nations, Bali, Indonesia, December 1990 [unpublished]

Jamison DT, Frenk J, Knaul F. International collective action in health: objectives, functions and rationale. *Lancet*, 1998; **351**: 514–517

Johnson TJ. *Professions and Power.* London: Macmillan, 1972

Lindblom CE. *Politics and Markets: the World's Political-economic Systems.* New York: Basic Books, 1977

Londoño JL, Frenk J. Structured pluralism: towards an innovative model for health system reform in Latin America. *Health Policy*, 1997; **41**: 1–36

Mathews JT. Power shift. *Foreign Affairs*, 1997; **76**: 50–66

McPake B. The role of the private sector in health service provision. In: Bennett S, McPake B, Mills A (eds) *Private Health Providers in Developing Countries: Serving the Public Interest?* London: Zed Books, 1997, pp 21–39

Meyer JW. The world polity and the authority of the nation-state. In: Bergesen A (ed) *Studies of the Modern World-system.* New York: Academic Press, 1980, pp 109–137

Mills A. Contractual relationships between government and the commercial private sector in developing countries. In: Bennett S, McPake B, Mills A (eds) *Private Health Providers in Developing Countries: Serving the Public Interest?* London: Zed Books, 1997, pp 189–213

Musgrove P. Public and private roles in health: theory and financing patterns. World Bank Discussion Paper No. 339. Washington DC: The World Bank, 1996

North DC. *Institutions, Institutional Change and Economic Performance*. Cambridge: Cambridge University Press, 1990

Omae K. *The End of the Nation State: the Rise of Regional Economies*. New York: Free Press, 1995

Osborne D, Gaebler T. *Reinventing Government: How the Entrepreneurial Spirit is Transforming the Public Sector*. New York: Plume, 1993

Pauly MV. Overinsurance and public provision of insurance: the roles of moral hazard and adverse selection. *Quarterly Journal of Economics*, 1974; **88**: 44–62

Pauly MV. Is medical care different? In: Greenberg W (ed) *Competition in the Health Care Sector: Past, Present, and Future*. Germantown, Maryland: Aspen Systems Corporation, 1978, pp 11–35

Perrot J, Carrin G, Sergent F. *The contractual approach: new partnerships for health in developing countries*. Macroeconomics, Health and Development Series, No. 24. Geneva: Division of Intensified Cooperation with Countries in Greatest Need, World Health Organization, 1997 (WHO/ICO/MESD.24)

Reich MR. Reshaping the state: from above, from within, from below. Paper presented at the 75th Anniversary Symposium of the Harvard School of Public Health. Boston, 27-29 April 1997 [unpublished]

Reyes-Heroles F. Diferencia y tolerancia hacia el siglo XXI (Difference and tolerance towards the 21st century). Paper presented as the 'Julio Cortázar' Lecture at the University of Guadalajara. Guadalajara, Mexico, 16 January 1998 [unpublished]

Roemer MI. *National Health Systems of the World. Vol. 1: The Countries*. New York: Oxford University Press, 1991

Slaughter AM. The real new world order. *Foreign Affairs*, 1997; **76**: 183–197

Starr P. *The Logic of Health Care Reform: Why and How the President's Plan Will Work*. New York: Whittle Books, 1994

Tilly C (ed) *The Formation of National States in Western Europe*. Princeton, NJ: Princeton University Press, 1975

Walzer M. The idea of civil society: a path to social reconstruction. *Dissent*, 1991; **38**: 293–304

Weber M. Politics as a vocation. In: Gerth H and Mills CW (eds) *From Max Weber: Essays in Sociology*. New York: Oxford University Press, 1946: pp 77–128

World Bank. *World Development Report 1993. Investing in Health*. New York: Oxford University Press, 1993

World Bank. *Poverty Reduction and the World Bank: Progress and Challenges in the 1990s*. Washington DC: The World Bank, 1996

World Bank. *World Development Report 1997. The State in a Changing World*. New York: Oxford University Press, 1997

4
Reforming state capacity: the demands of health sector reform in developing countries

Sara Bennett

London School of Hygiene & Tropical Medicine, London, UK

Parallel to the debate about the role and place of health sector reform there has been an equally substantive debate about the appropriate role of the state in development. Whereas the 1980s saw a general move to reduce the role of the state, the debate in the 1990s has been reframed in terms of the development of the 'capable state' (Hilderbrand and Grindle, 1994) or 'reinvigorating state institutions' (World Bank, 1997). Whilst part of the standard policy recommendations prescribed by international organizations such as the World Bank remains a reconsideration (and potentially downsizing) of the role of the state, much more emphasis has recently been placed upon the central role a capable state may play in promoting development (Minogue *et al*, 1997).

As discussed in other chapters in this book, health sector reform has also commonly entailed a rethinking of the role of government. Recognition of the significance of private sector provision (Bennett, 1991; Berman and Rannan-Eliya, 1993), the new models of public sector management embodied by New Public Management theory (Kaul, 1997) and ideological influences of the 1980s have converged in policy recommendations emphasizing the indirect provision role of government (including the importance of regulation, policy setting, and enablement). At the same time a less central role for government in the direct provision of services has been suggested.

A number of alternative theoretical frameworks have been proposed to help re-formulate the role of the state. Economic theory suggests that there is a direct link between the (economic) characteristics of a good or service and the mode through which it is provided. For example Musgrove (1996) classifies health care activities into three domains: public goods, low-cost private interventions and high-cost private interventions. These domains are distinct from each other as they suffer from different forms of market failure, and hence, may suggest alternative types of government intervention to correct the failure. Batley (1997) refers to this approach as an 'organizational design' approach: it implies that there are universal answers to questions about the appropriate role of government.

In reality the appropriate role for government will be heavily influenced by existing institutional structures: differing institutions in different contexts imply that alternative government roles will be suitable (Picciotto, 1995). North (1990) referred to this issue as 'path dependence'. Government capacity to perform alternative types of functions is certainly one (although not the only aspect) of the institutional environment which needs to be considered.

New Institutional Economics provides alternative theoretical frameworks for considering appropriate roles for government, which give greater importance to institutional structures. Introduction of the notion of transaction costs helps explain why alternative organizational arrangements for service provision may be desirable in different country contexts (North, 1990; Ostrom *et al*, 1993). Alternative organizational arrangements (e.g. direct government provision, contracting out of services, private market provision) will incur different production costs, but also different transaction costs. Transaction costs include both the costs of setting up a contract or agreement, and monitoring and enforcing that agreement. Hence transaction costs will vary according to aspects of the local institutional environment, including the capacity of various actors to undertake different tasks.

Hirschman's analysis of exit, voice and loyalty (or control) (Paul, 1992) also offers insights into the design of reform programmes and the role of government. Each of these phenomena creates a channel for accountability. Institutional reform which gives greater rein to exit, voice and loyalty helps exert pressure for improved service quality. Aspects of the design of health sector reform programmes, which re-articulate government functions, are linked to each of Hirschman's trio:

- *Exit*
  (i) Reforms which more closely link reward of public sector providers to performance create greater incentives for providers to respond to exit
  (these include introduction of managed markets, provider payment reform etc);
  (ii) promotion of private sector provision gives greater opportunity for exit, and
  (iii) provision of information to health care users about quality and price of care at alternative facilities helps create better informed choices between providers.
- *Voice*
  Public sector reforms aimed at institutionalizing scope for public participation in policy and direct management of health care include decentralization,

establishment of hospital boards, interventions aimed at improving consumer
knowledge about the health system structure.

- **Control**
  This is the traditional approach to health sector management and as such has
  perhaps received less attention as part of health sector reform efforts.

New Public Management captures the principles described above in pragmatic
policy recommendations. The standard recipe generally includes elements which
encourage innovation and competitiveness, greater responsiveness to consumers,
stronger incentives for performance and more output-oriented systems (Kaul,
1997).

This chapter adopts a broad notion of capacity. Our central concern is the
institutional capacity conditions necessary for alternative reform options to be
viable (or desirable). Whilst some of the discussion relates to loftier issues
regarding the necessary macro-level institutional structures (such as legal systems)
necessary for successful reform, the chapter is equally concerned with the basic
administrative and management systems necessary to sustain reforms. An
underlying hypothesis is that health sector reform generally requires governments
to perform roles to which they are not accustomed, or with which they have only
limited experience.[1] Hence in many instances government capacity to perform
these new roles is limited.

The next section provides relevant definitions and describes the scope of the
chapter. This is followed by discussion of the implications of health sector reform
for the functions which governments need to perform, and consideration of the
evidence concerning government capacity to perform new roles. The last two
sections present a discussion of the evidence and lessons for capacity building for
reform, and for reform programmes.

Scope and definitions

The question of government capacity is an important question in developing,
developed and transitional economies. This chapter focuses primarily upon the
developing world where capacity issues may be particularly acute.

Whilst most analysts have asserted that there is *'no consistently-applied,
universal package of measures that constitutes health sector reform'* (Cassels,
1995) there does appear to be some agreement as to the most commonly pursued
reform options. Typically these are said to include:

---

[1] This is the underlying hypothesis of the DFID funded Research Programme on 'The Role
of Government in Adjusting Economies'.

a) **organizational reform within the public sector**, including decentralization, the establishment of greater autonomy for provider organizations, restructuring of ministries of health;

b) **resource allocation reform**, including the adoption of 'new' provider payment mechanisms, purchaser-provider splits and managed competition, and reform of the benefit package;

c) **promotion of greater diversity in the provision of care**, including a greater role for private for-profit and private non-profit providers;

d) **reforms aimed at the role of consumers**, encouraging people to take greater responsibility for their own health, encouraging consumers to make informed choices between providers/insurers;

e) **resource generation reform**, including the promotion of user fees, social health insurance.

Reforms (a)–(d) typically involve the state engaging in non-traditional spheres of activity; moreover, this set of reforms is most clearly linked to the ideas of New Institutional Economics (concerning voice, exit and loyalty) and the principles of New Public Management. The analysis here focuses upon these four broad reform options. Reform (e) commonly entails an extension of state activities in certain spheres, but forms less of a radical departure from traditional state roles. It is not examined here.

The term capacity has been defined in numerous ways. This chapter adopts the definition used by the research programme on the Role of Government in Adjusting Economies and described in more detail in Batley (1997). Figure 4.1 sets out the three levels of capacity considered and the dimensions at each level. This chapter covers not only the narrow traditional territory of capacity (related to skills and the internal organization of bureaucracies) but also aspects of capacity external to the executing organization and issues related to communications between the different actors involved in implementing the function (referred to as the task network (Hilderbrand and Grindle, 1994)). Capacity is conceived to be task-specific; hence the different dimensions of capacity identified in Figure 4.1 are more or less important depending upon the precise nature of reforms.

Government functions: old and new

In order to address the issue of government capacity constraints on the sustainability of health sector reforms we need to understand the traditional functions of government and the new demands placed upon government by reforms. This section addresses these issues in a generic manner. The following section examines actual country reforms.

---

1. Aspects of capacity internal to executing organizations

■   organizational and administrative structures
■   skills and professionalization of staff, personnel policies
■   availability of capital and financial control

2. Communication between members of the task network

3. Aspects of capacity external to executing organizations

■   financial and economic conditions
■   civil–public interaction
■   private sector development
■   political structures and preferences
■   legal and administrative frameworks

Figure 4.1 Aspects of capacity

Several analysts have attempted to classify the functions of government within the health care sector. Musgrove (1996) identifies five distinct instruments of public intervention, namely; information provision, regulation, mandating, financing and provision. Londoño and Frenk (1997) propose four main functions: the familiar ones of financing and delivery of care as well as two less familiar functions, namely 'modulation' and 'articulation'. 'Modulation' involves *setting, implementing and monitoring the rules of the game for the health system'* and 'articulation' lies between financing and delivery and is meant to co-ordinate the different aspects of the health system, in particular by organizing and managing consumption. Out of these four it is stated that only modulation is a core government function, private actors may play key roles in all three of the other functions identified.

Figure 4.2 sets out a list of government functions used in this paper. This classification is more detailed than those described above as it is intended to serve as a basis for considering necessary government capacities.Whilst all the functions identified above are traditionally seen as functions of government to some degree, the extent to which they have formed part of the core work of government within the health care sector varies. Prior to reform the core government functions within the health care sector would most likely be policy setting and planning, the administration of provision, and the direct provision of services. Many functions such as the analytical function, enforcement of rules, information provision and

- **Policy setting, rule making, planning and co-ordination:** ensuring that clear policies are agreed and supported;

- **Analytical functions:** monitoring and evaluation, analysis for purposes of strengthening policy and implementation, feedback on impact of reform measures;

- **Enforcement of rules and regulations:** regulation of provider organizations, licensing of practitioners, pharmaceutical regulation, protection of consumer rights;

- **Information provision:** provision of information to key actors within the health care system, for example to help stimulate efficient purchasing, provision of information on policies and reforms, information to promote public health;

- **Administration of provision:** contracting of services (public or private), accreditation, standard setting etc;

- **Fiscal functions:** organization of insurance function, setting and collecting fees, taxes etc;

- **Direct provision**

Figure 4.2 Functions of government

fiscal functions, would clearly have been seen as part of government responsibilities, but may not have taken up much of government capacity either because they were only performed to a limited extent (as with analytical functions and information provision) or because they were relatively simple (as with fiscal functions). Reforms have required governments both to perform functions in a far more complex environment and to extend certain functions significantly. For example the administration of provision in a wholly public, centrally organized system is likely to be simple but once systems are decentralized, and payment and/or budgetary allocation methods are reformed, this function becomes a lot more complex to administer. Prior to reforms, information provision focuses largely upon public health messages, but reforms have often extended this function significantly to cover not only communication about the reform package but also communication which enables people to be more active consumers.

Experience with health sector reform and state capacity

This section reviews reform experiences in less developed countries and how capacity issues have affected the success of reform. As with any type of institutional analysis, the experiences are highly context-specific. This review is not comprehensive but highlights key features. It considers the elements of capacity set out in Figure 4.1, including aspects of internal capacity, co-ordination between the task network and external factors affecting capacity. The section is structured by each of the reform thrusts identified earlier.

Each of the reform thrusts discussed involves significant policy shifts. Government capacity to negotiate and manage this policy change is critical. A significant literature about the policy process of reform has developed (Walt, 1994; Walt and Gilson, 1994; Reich, 1995). There is not space to do justice to this literature here, but a number of government capacity issues relating to successful policy reform are worth highlighting.

Policy making inevitably involves a wide range of stakeholders and actors; effective communication between these actors is critical to success and requires substantial administrative capacity and personal skills. In low-income countries where donors are significant stakeholders, successful donor co-ordination has made a significant contribution to effective policy change. The importance of this factor has been noted in Ghana (Smithson *et al*, 1997), Guinea (Hopwood, 1994), Niger (Diop and Baguirbi, 1998), Sierra Leone (Siegel *et al*, 1996) and Zambia (Mahler *et al*, 1997). In Sierra Leone it was stated:

> Most important has been the DOH's creation of a National Health Action Plan and a fairly firm insistence that all health sector activities and investments be planned within that framework. By initiating development of its own reform agenda, the DOH has largely pre-empted any externally-imposed agenda.

Individual leadership and charisma within government is often important (see Hopwood (1994) on Zambia and Guinea, Fizbein (1997) on Colombia) but it does not appear to be an essential element of capacity. For example in Ghana there has not been any political championship of reforms but the reform process has nonetheless moved ahead significantly, albeit incrementally (Smithson *et al*, 1997).

Analytical skills are also required to set out and consider alternative policy options. Where local analytical capacity is limited it appears that foreign technical assistance has contributed to this function (as in Niger (Diop and Baguirbi, 1998)). This may work in the short term but is likely to prove problematic in the longer run. In countries with greater analytical capacity, local skills (although not necessarily within government) have been depended upon more. In Thailand the government-funded, but autonomous, Health System Research Institute has played an important role in assisting the MOPH consider alternative policies (see Chunharas and Harrison, this volume). In Colombia a Health Policy and Research Institute was proposed to assist with the reform process (Bossert *et al*, 1998).

Organizational reform within the public sector

Organizational reform within the public sector (together with financing reform which is not considered here) has probably been the most prevalent of reforms. Decentralization has been a key part of many developing countries' reform agendas, although it has been pursued to different degrees and in different ways. The creation of autonomous institutions has often been pursued for similar reasons to decentralization: by moving responsibility for decision- making closer to the service delivery point it is hoped to improve service quality and efficiency; by creating more accountable local governance structures greater consumer voice will be facilitated, and increased community involvement (which is commonly an element of organizational reform) will bring in scarce management skills.

Decentralization and the establishment of autonomous hospitals do not necessarily change the role or functions which government must perform, but rather shift the loci of decision-making and change the conditions under which decisions are made.

A frequent argument amongst those opposing decentralization reforms is that inadequate capacity—primarily internal capacity in the form of skills and systems—exists at the local level to manage a decentralized system. However evidence to support this is not strong. Capacity at the local level can only develop if new responsibilities are handed over. A study of local government in Colombia concluded that with a combination of greater responsibility, more resources and political reform, local capacity evolved over time (Fiszbein, 1997).

Perhaps a more critical concern focuses around the capacity of central government to support decentralized units through developing adequate guidelines and managerial systems to ensure their proper functioning. In Zambia during the early reform period, central government capacity to support districts was a key concern (Bennett, 1993). In Ghana it was observed that capacity weaknesses lay not only with hospital boards but also with the MOH itself which 'could not spell out what it wanted or what the respective roles of the MOH and the Boards should be' (Smithson *et al*, 1997).

This issue of lack of guidelines for decentralized bodies is closely linked to that of co-ordination between members of the task network. Where it is unclear which functions should be performed at different levels of the system, co-ordination problems will inevitably occur.

External aspects of capacity appear important constraints with respect to organizational reforms: a number of different dimensions are important. First it is commonly observed that governments pay lip service to the notion of decentralization or granting local level units greater autonomy but in reality politicians (and possibly central bureaucrats) are reluctant to cede power. In Sri Lanka political inertia was blamed for failure to decentralize health care services:

> perhaps the main barriers to reform are political interests at the centre and province which oppose further decentralization (Russell and Attanayake, 1997).

In Ghana (Smithson *et al*, 1997) researchers speculated that officials within the central Ministry were unwilling to cede power to autonomous agencies.

Second, many of the desirable effects of decentralization and autonomy are supposed to flow from civil-public interactions. Decision-making at lower levels of the health care system should lead to greater sensitivity to public preferences, and by co-opting individuals as members of boards (be it hospital boards or district health boards) it is supposed that more private sector management skills will be accessed. Even where formal structures for facilitating such civil–public interactions are established it is difficult to ensure that they function as anticipated. Several capacity constraints are observed:

a)   those with greatest skills to offer the private sector are often also those with least time to devote to altruistic roles within the public sector;
b)   effective representation of community interests is commonly hindered by very non-representative involvement on boards or committees;
c)   sustaining civil sector involvement in public sector affairs is often difficult, particularly if people are expected to volunteer for no compensation.

Third, the effectiveness of decentralization within the health care sector may be limited by external bureaucratic constraints. This is especially the case if health sector decentralization is implemented without concurrent reforms in other sectors: the benefits of improved local level co-ordination between agencies is unlikely to transpire unless other ministries also decentralize. Furthermore it is common for one of the most critical resources for health care—human resources—to be controlled by a centralized civil service agency. If decentralized units do not have effective control over promotions, transfers and disciplinary procedures then their realm of power is severely limited. In instances such as Zambia, where the Ministry of Health has attempted to extricate personnel from a centralized civil service, this has proved to be highly problematic.

Finally, without centralized control of the health system hierarchy, rules and statutes binding decentralized actors become more important (Foltz, 1997). In Zambia the National Health Services Act which created a legal basis for the District Health Boards and codified decentralization within the health care system followed (rather than preceded) de facto budgetary decentralization. Thus, due to limited capacity to formulate and pass new laws, the decentralized authorities in Zambia acted for a period without any legal foundation.

Resource allocation reform

Whilst there has been much discussion of purchaser–provider splits in low-income country contexts (such as Zimbabwe) and it is clearly part of government policy in Zambia, to date progress in implementation has been limited. In Zambia there has been significant reform of the resource allocation formula used to distribute resources between districts. District Health Boards and Hospital Boards now receive resources under a contractual agreement with the Central Board of Health, but to date there has been no contracting within districts. The limited progress in this area in low-income countries possibly relates to the high demands that purchaser–provider splits may place upon government, combined with the lack of demonstrated benefits to such reform in low income contexts. In particular, purchaser–provider splits place significant demands on government's analytical functions (information about costs and the appropriate benefits package are required) and on administration of provision (including setting quality standards, negotiating and enforcing contracts with providers etc.).

With respect to provider payment reform in middle-income countries more significant reforms have occurred as several countries have switched (or are in the process of switching) from fee-for-service retrospective payment or global budgets to case-based (for example, using diagnosis-related groups (DRGs)) and capitation payment. Those middle-income countries which are adopting the 'new' forms of payment mechanism (such as Chile (capitation), Brazil (DRGs and capitation), Thailand (capitation), and Taiwan (DRGs)) have greater administrative capacity than most low-income countries. Nonetheless both capitation and case-based payment impose new tasks in administering provision. For example capitation requires registering all insured persons with a provider (or provider network); DRGs require the validation of foreign DRG systems in the local context and the establishment of information systems which enable billing by DRG both within the social security scheme and within provider organizations.

Sometimes lack of capacity to administer these new forms of payment has proved an obstacle to successful reform. In Thailand where a new social security scheme was established using capitation payment, two principal types of problem were observed. First, constraints on administrative capacity at the Social Security Office led the Scheme to opt for employers choosing registered provider on behalf of employees. Whilst this limited the number of transactions that the Scheme had to make, it also limited employee choice and resulted, during the early days of the Scheme, in low utilization rates. As a consequence the Social Security Office has gradually switched to employee choice of health care facility and now employees rather than employers choose providers. Second, limited administrative capacity at the Social Security Office meant that the Scheme was very slow to get the proposed patient information system up and running. For several years the Scheme had very poor information about diagnoses and treatments provided under the Scheme; hence it was difficult to verify or deny accusations of under-treatment to Scheme beneficiaries.

Getting new payment mechanisms up and running requires considerable administrative capacity; ensuring that these new payment mechanisms deliver the desired effects is even more complex. For example, new payment mechanisms offer financial incentives to providers to improve quality and efficiency. However, without concurrent budgetary reform, and possibly incentives for staff, public health care facilities may not respond to financial incentives embedded in payment mechanisms. Alternatively, where the objective functions of providers do encourage a response to the cost containment incentives of certain payment mechanisms, cost-cutting measures may adversely affect the quality of care provided, unless adequate quality assurance systems are in place. The environmental and institutional factors facilitating desirable responses to payment mechanisms are too poorly understood to be able to say which capacities are necessary.

A significant external obstacle to provider payment reform is sufficient political will and social consensus about reform to overcome opposing vested interests. In Taiwan, for example, an agreement to reform the national health insurance scheme so that it paid for six key conditions on a DRG rather than fee-for-service basis was reconsidered so as only to cover one DRG (Su, 1995). In Chile, the way in which budgets are allocated to public providers is shifting towards a capitation basis, but for several years the capitation system has been used only as a benchmark against which to compare actual payment (not to compute budgets) (Bitran and Yip, 1998).

Promoting competition and diversity in provision

The main reforms implemented with the aim of promoting competition and diversity in service provision include:

- contracting out (of both clinical and non-clinical services);
- liberalization of the private sector (and consequently regulation and quality assurance within the private sector);
- enablement of the private sector (through measures such as private finance initiatives, joint ventures etc.).

This reform thrust is perhaps the most complex in terms of the extra capacities required to implement effectively. Reform in this area places heavy demands upon government with respect to administration of provision (notably the negotiation, implementation and monitoring of contracts, but also through non-regulatory measures to improve private sector quality), enforcement of regulatory rules, and fiscal functions (such as the negotiation of joint ventures). Moreover, this particular area of reform engages governments in spheres of activity which may be almost entirely new.

Contracting out

In a review of several case studies of contracting out of services, capacity concerns along each of the dimensions in Figure 4.1 have been identified (Bennett and Mills, 1998). Health officials are often unaccustomed to negotiating with private sector entities and commonly have weak negotiation skills. As a consequence, contracts for health care services often have a number of design problems including inappropriate distribution of risk (with government bearing too much), limited sanctions available to enforce contracts, and weak quality specifications within contracts. In some instances (such as examples from Papua New Guinea and India) basic systems to ensure effective contracting out were not present: for example copies of contracts were not always kept, governments had often failed to pay contractors in a timely manner and hence few private providers were interested in bidding on government contracts. Information systems to help monitor contracts were also often weak.

Co-ordination between the various actors involved in the contractual process was also found to be problematic. This was particularly the case where a central tender board was responsible for negotiating and awarding contracts and was distant from the place or institution where services were to be delivered.

Whilst the level of economic development was not found to be a significant barrier to contracting out in most instances, a number of key external factors were identified. First, a transparent and accountable government is imperative. Without such transparency contracting out of services will contribute to inefficiencies by allowing resources to leak from the health care sector, and more importantly, by allowing inefficient providers to receive contracts. The second important external element governing capacity to contract is human resource management policies within the public sector. In many instances civil servants have 'jobs for life'. If it is not possible to reduce the public sector wage bill through retrenching staff when services are contracted out, then contracting out will only make sense under highly specific conditions. In virtually all of the instances of contracting out reviewed by Bennett and Mills (1998), the contracted service was a new service or constituted an expansion in service provision, thus avoiding the issue of public sector redundancies.

Liberalization

In several countries where liberalization of the private for-profit sector has occurred (as in Malawi, Mozambique, Tanzania, Zambia and many countries of the Newly Independent States and Eastern Europe), the statutes liberalizing private practice have formed the easiest part of the reform process. The 'second generation' issues of how then to regulate private providers have proved much stickier. Regulation is, of course, not a 'new' function for the state. Most developing countries have statutes enabling them to regulate private providers (primarily through licensing and application of structural quality standards) However in most instances these regulations have been very weakly enforced (Bennett *et al*, 1994).

It is easy to cite examples suggesting limited organizational (internal) capacity to regulate. In Ghana (Smithson *et al*, 1997), Sri Lanka (Russell and Attanayake, 1997) and India (Bennett and Muraleedharan, 1998), and presumably many other developing countries, no database exists with information on the size, location and activities of private providers. Thus any government-initiated regulatory effort lacks information on exactly which organizations need to be regulated. In many developing countries information about quality of care in the public sector is limited: such information about the private sector is virtually non-existent. Often developing country regulatory authorities are underfunded. Sri Lanka has a total of 25 drug inspectors to ensure adequate drug quality and practice standards. In Tamil Nadu state, India, there are a total of 87 drug inspectors in the state, but they are supposed to cover 2 800 drug manufacturers, 11500 licensed sales outlets and an unknown (but probably larger) number of unlicensed outlets. In Sri Lanka (until recently) and in most states in India, there is no identifiable unit within government responsible for regulating the private sector.

Whilst it is obviously the case that low-income countries face binding resource constraints, low resource allocation to regulation also reflects perceived priorities and political constraints. Capacity for effective regulation is constrained by a number of critical external factors and co-ordination issues. A move to more effective regulation, in both developed and developing countries, is likely to encounter resistance from a range of vested interests. In many developing countries regulatory policies were not considered until after a substantial private sector had developed, and this made it all the harder to tackle concerns about regulation (Bennett and Tangcharoensathien, 1994). Second, in many developing countries the boundaries between public and private health care sectors are permeable: physicians may work in public sector posts during the day and in private sector posts during the evening (Chawla, 1994). Whilst public sector posts provide security, private sector income is critical to maintaining desired standards of living. Public sector clinical staff may therefore be one of the most vocal (and worrying) opponents for governments contemplating tighter private sector regulation. Studies in both Sri Lanka and India cited fear of strikes by government doctors as one of the primary concerns of policy makers wishing to address this area (Russell and Attanayake, 1997; Bennett and Muraleedharan, 1998). Furthermore, it is not uncommon for senior level policy makers themselves to have financial interests in the private health care sector (as is the case in Thailand) and this, too, is likely to inhibit stronger regulation.

It is common for regulation to involve a very complex set of actors. A common scenario involves several different statutory professional regulatory bodies (often with competing interests) who are empowered to regulate professional education and certain aspects of clinical practice. This is supplemented by direct government regulation of clinical establishments. The third regulatory prong is via the legal system under tort law. These regulatory strategies are supposed to be mutually reinforcing, but often the complexities of the system make it difficult for consumers to understand and for government to co-ordinate. In the Indian context, civil society organizations (particularly consumer organizations and health action groups) have played a critical role in mediating between the different regulatory bodies and guiding consumers through the system.

Systems which are most prone to problems of corruption tend to be rigid bureaucratic systems with sources of government monopoly power (Klitgaard, 1988). Most regulatory systems exhibit these characteristics, and indeed corruption and lack of transparency do appear to be important constraints upon regulatory capacity. Regulatory capture is a persistent problem in the health care sector and takes a variety of forms, from outright bribery of government officials to more subtle capture by penetration. In instances where there is widespread mistrust of government, the private sector is unlikely to abide by regulatory statutes and is most likely to try to avoid them.

Logically, a strong legal system is required for effective enforcement of regulations. There are many anecdotes suggesting slow procedures in seeking legal recourse against medical malpractice. However by nature, legal recourse in medical cases is likely to be cumbersome and difficult. A credible legal system is necessary to back up other forms of regulation, but many more basic aspects of regulatory systems are so weak that they form bottlenecks.

Encouraging private sector development

Most developing countries have fewer examples of positive efforts to encourage private sector development. Projects aiming at developing joint public–private partnerships such as a jointly funded (government, private sector) hospital project in Delhi, India, and efforts to develop a model of franchising in Lusaka, Zambia, have been projects rather than broader reforms and as such have drawn upon considerable external expertise in their design and implementation phases (Makinen and Leighton, 1997).

Other instances of incentives provided by government to encourage private sector expansion appear on occasion to have had adverse effects, primarily due to governments' inability to oversee such initiatives. For example, the Board of Investment in Thailand which provides tax breaks to large hospitals co-ordinated very poorly with the Ministry of Public Health, and this probably contributed to the current over-supply of hospital beds in Bangkok (Bennett and Tangcharoensathien, 1994). In India, a government commission is currently enquiring into abuse of a scheme providing tax breaks to private hospitals which set aside a percentage of their hospital beds for indigent patients to be treated free of charge (Bennett and Muraleedharan, 1998). Government inability to monitor the scheme had led to concerns about abuse.

Reforming the role of consumers

Reforms in the role of consumers in developing countries range from formal centralized mechanisms to create greater accountability of health staff to clients (such as patient bills of rights, and the strengthening of complaints structures), to greater involvement by community members in policy making and priority setting, to strengthening local level structures for community voice in service delivery. The latter may include community representation on hospital and district health boards (as discussed above), community participation through village health committees, and in many low-income countries 'community financing' involving some form of cost sharing and local management of funds. While these different strategies involve the establishment of alternative organizational structures, they rely on one common government function: the provision of information direct to communities.

A UNICEF-co-ordinated review of experience with community financing type initiatives in Sub-Saharan Africa found that several countries had failed to communicate effectively what the 'new' role of communities within the health care system was supposed to be (Hanson, 1997). In Zambia, for example, neither health staff nor communities understood the principles of community involvement in cost sharing to which the MOH aspired: there was a lack of community involvement and revenues were not used to improve aspects of quality valued by communities (Daura et al, 1998). The UNICEF review noted that, in Benin and Guinea, the lack of community development skills in Ministries of Health had been cited as a problem but this was probably also a problem elsewhere and had most likely contributed to failure to communicate policies and practices to communities effectively (Hanson, 1997). In addition to lack of skills in community development, it is very rare for Ministries of Health to have an effective public relations unit. Whilst consumer information campaigns on very specific aspects of health sector reform (e.g. Collins et al, 1995) have been mounted in developing countries, there appear to be virtually no examples of campaigns which have communicated the broad thrust of reform and the implications of reform for consumers.

The provision of information to community members is also critical under reforms which aim to stimulate competition through consumer choice. In systems where consumers register directly with a provider (as under the Social Security Scheme in Thailand) consumers require information about the price and quality of services available from alternative providers. Where consumers register with alternative insurance organizations (as with EPSs in Colombia, Obras Sociales in Argentina, IAMCs in Uruguay (Medici et al, 1997)) information is required about the benefit package, and the relative prices and performance of different insurers.

Developing country governments have taken on this function of information provision only to a limited extent. Part of the reason for this may be a lack of analytical capacity and reliable data sources to provide useful information to aid consumer choice (Medici et al, 1997). In Thailand, as already noted, the Social Security Scheme was very slow to get its information systems fully up and running, and routine data collected by the Ministry of Public Health provides very little assistance in guiding patient choice. Being able to provide information to consumers on quality of care offered by different providers is potentially very complex: few developing countries have in place routine review of professional or patient perceived quality of care of different providers.

While many European countries have adopted some mechanisms to help ensure greater accountability to consumers with regard to the quality of care provided (including the establishment of patient charters, legislation on patient rights, and the strengthening of formal complaints mechanisms (Saltman and Figueras, 1997)) and several developing countries have shown interest in such mechanisms, few appear to have actually implemented them. The enunciation of such principles appears relatively easy, but their enforcement, even in industrialized countries, is harder to ensure.

Like decentralization, one of the principal external constraints upon effective change in this reform area is political will. Consumer empowerment is likely to mean a shift away from civil service or medical profession dominance which powerful vested interests may oppose. In Sierra Leone an innovative attempt to involve community members in priority setting helped build support for reforms and enable the health system to respond better to consumer priorities. However, analysts of the reform process suggested that the priority setting exercises had dealt mainly with chiefs, who probably were not good representatives of the poor (Siegel *et al*, 1996). While it may be politically acceptable (or even desirable) to involve community members of high social standing in decision-making, giving voice to the poor and vulnerable is likely to meet greater opposition.

Lack of political will to empower consumers may be partially offset by strong civic institutions. In particular, an independent press and media, and strong consumer advocacy organizations may help nudge government to commit to well-meaning (but hollow) policy statements. In India for example, consumer rights organizations have played a critical role in informing consumers of their medical rights under law, supporting complaints against medical care providers and even providing training to help consumers identify quality providers and negotiate with them over their health care needs (Bennett and Muraleedharan, 1998). In many countries with a free press, the media have played a key role in informing the general population of reform processes in health care, and how these may affect the care received.

Discussion

There is substantial diversity across countries in institutional context, and capacity is not a one-dimensional attribute. In some instances Ministries of Health may have highly skilled individuals but a weakly identified organizational mission so skills are not put to good use; in other cases the opposite may be true. Moreover, it is insufficient to examine only internal capacity, many reforms have been handicapped by external capacity constraints. Sometimes capacities external to government (e.g. a strong civic society) may help offset internal weaknesses. For example, in India, active NGOs have assisted government pharmaceutical regulatory agencies by uncovering scandals within the pharmaceutical business (Bidwai, 1995). In other instances, however, external capacities cannot make up for limited capacity in the executing agency. This diversity of institutional capacity militates strongly against universalist prescriptions regarding appropriate roles for government.

This chapter started from the premise that reforms required change in the way in which government operated, and often expanded the sphere of government activity into new areas, or alternatively implied that government must carry out existing functions in new (and generally more complex) contexts. Given traditional concerns about weak government capacity, it was hypothesized that governments in developing countries might find it difficult to perform the new roles required. This was indeed found to be the case.

In practice, a range of different types of capacity bottlenecks have stifled reform. In some instances state capacity appeared so weak that basic functions such as maintenance of filing systems, timely payment of suppliers, etc. were not properly performed. In instances where this was the case, such 'in-capacities' prevented government from performing both its 'traditional' and 'new' roles adequately.

Some of the 'new' functions of government appear to be demanding ones which governments in developing countries (and some governments in industrialized countries) find difficult to perform well. In particular, regulatory functions and information provision appear to be tasks for which governments' capacity is often limited. However, the binding constraints upon government performance of such tasks often lie outside the control of the Ministry of Health. The review highlighted a number of common constraints:

- **Bureaucratic regulations** covering health sector operations, imposed by central government, often govern purchasing, budgeting, accounting etc. Reform within the health care sector may struggle to throw off these bureaucratic leashes. For example, it is commonly required that all contracts of a certain value are awarded by a central tender board: this removes effective control over the contract away from the recipient agency. In situations where the health sector is the only reforming sector, such constraints may be particularly troublesome. In instances where only limited reforms are made in the health sector, the persistence of centralized MOH regulations may hinder success.

- A particular and critically important example of centralized regulations constraining reform concerns personnel management. Many **centralized civil service structures** grant 'jobs for life', provide limited recourse in the event of non-performance and no incentives for good performance. For contracting-out, decentralization and establishment of autonomous hospitals, unreformed civil services can effectively block health sector reform entirely. Civil service reform is also important because personnel policies heavily influence organizational culture. Grindle (1997) concluded that effective organizations, almost universally, had bypassed standard civil service regulations in order to create a more goal-oriented organizational culture. Tendler and Freedheim

(1994) trace a number of channels through which a meritocratic recruitment process positively affected a primary health care project in Brazil. It seems that without direct control over the most critical input into health care, many health reforms will be sorely constrained.

- **Lack of commitment to reforms** amongst key actors (notably central ministry civil servants and politicians) appears a common phenomenon and is likely to impede the progress of a reform programme. It may be difficult to disentangle this effect from that of limited internal capacity: is failure to reform due to a lack of interest, or a lack of knowledge of how to go about reform?

- Whilst **corruption** may thrive in overly-bureaucratic cultures, partially reformed environments, where the relaxation of rules has not yet been counterbalanced by stronger mechanisms for downward accountability, are also likely to be susceptible to corruption. Corruption can be very costly not only in terms of direct leakage of funds but in terms of the efficiency of service delivery. Contracts awarded on the basis of bribery are unlikely to bring in efficient contractors. Corruption may also initiate vicious cycles: in instances where government is not trusted, it will be very difficult to get private individuals or organizations to comply with rules. For example, if it is widely believed that regulation is only to promote rent-seeking by government officials, then no one will register with authorities, in order to avoid regulation. This in turn raises the costs of regulation.

To make matters more complex, these external constraints are interrelated. For example the issue of corruption amongst public sector workers is unlikely to be resolved whilst many civil servant receive salaries on which it is impossible to survive.

Improved accountability to the public is at the core of many health sector reform efforts. The reform measures aim to strengthen the possibilities for both exit and voice. Although these features are clearly desirable, in the short run they commonly appear problematic. Systems of downward accountability take time to institutionalize and can never entirely replace upward accountability. Moreover reforms tend to make systems of accountability more complex. Under systems of contracting out, or decentralization, or autonomous hospitals, channels of accountability may run through multiple agents. Mapping a reform path which encourages the growth of downward accountability and greater bureaucratic flexibility, whilst maintaining some degree of upward accountability, is a complex challenge.

Lessons for capacity building for reform, and for reform programmes

There is no blue-print for capacity building for reform. Contexts and reform packages differ substantially; so must capacity building.

In some instances government failure to perform its 'traditional' roles has been rooted in incapacity to carry out even basic functions. Maintenance of records, basic financial and administrative systems etc., are just as critical to the 'new' roles of government as to the old. In contexts where these basic systems are not operating well, efforts to strengthen them are critical, regardless of the extent or nature of reform.

Whilst health sector reform does place new demands upon the internal capacity of executing organizations, some of the critical constraints appear to spring from external factors (such as corruption, rigid bureaucratic rules established by central ministries, weak civil society, etc.). Institutional capacity building efforts tend to focus upon internal aspects of capacity (through training, expatriate assistance, etc.) to the neglect of external aspects (Brinkerhoff, 1994). Yet external constraints are likely to be harder to overcome than internal ones. This is because they are outside of the control of Ministries of Health and because they may be very deeply entrenched in local society and culture. External constraints on capacity to reform need to be better understood, and reform programmes designed so as to take them into account.

The necessary functions of reformed Ministries of Health do require new skills; however, many of these skills are not '*communicable knowledge*' which can be transmitted from one person to another, but rather '*tacit knowledge*' acquired primarily by practice (North, 1990). Reform programmes need to be structured to allow opportunity for reflection and learning from experience. Similar arguments can be used at the system-level: institutional specificity of reform means that there are no clear-cut solutions before embarking on a reform path. Thus, having adaptive capacity, i.e. flexibility to reflect upon experience and adjust systems accordingly, is critical.

While efforts to build capacity are clearly important, the evidence reviewed here also has implications for how reform programmes are structured and phased. Different windows of political opportunity will inevitably mean that the pace and scope of reform differs between countries, but reformers should strategize carefully about the process of reform. How can reform programmes be phased so that they are best able to build upon the limited capacities which do exist? How might a major reform thrust be broken down into smaller, more manageable steps? Rather than bring a reform programme into direct confrontation with external constraints (such as government personnel policies) how can such constraints be worked around? These are topics which analysts are only just beginning to address. Our understanding of how the different elements of a reform package fit together is very limited. Fundamental questions about the interactions of institutions and the substance of reform urgently require addressing.

Acknowledgements

Sara Bennett is a member of the Health Economics and Financing Programme at the London School of Hygiene & Tropical Medicine which is supported by funds from the UK Department for International Development (DFID). Work on this paper, and several of the references cited in this paper, was also supported by the DFID-funded research programme on 'The Role of Government in Adjusting Economies'. The author would like to acknowledge the intellectual contribution made by colleagues working on the Role of Government research. In particular this paper draws upon discussions with and writings by Professor Richard Batley, Professor Anne Mills and Steven Russell. The facts presented and views expressed are those of the author and do not necessarily reflect the policies of DFID.

References

Batley RA. *A research framework for analysing capacity to undertake the 'new roles' of government.* Paper 23, The Role of Government in Adjusting Economies. Birmingham: Development Administration Group, 1997

Bennett S. *The Mystique of Markets: Public and Private Health Care in Developing Countries.* London: London School of Hygiene & Tropical Medicine, 1991

Bennett S. *An evaluation of the trial decentralized planning and budgeting project, Zambia.*[Unpublished] Consultancy Report to SIDA,1993

Bennett S, Dakpallah G, Garner P *et al.* Carrot and stick: state mechanisms to influence private provider behaviour. *Health Policy and Planning*, 1994; **9**:1–14

Bennett S, Mills A. Government capacity to contract: health sector experience and lessons. *Public Administration and Development*, forthcoming (1998)

Bennett S, Muraleedharan VR. *Reforming the Role of Government in Tamil Nadu Health Sector.* Birmingham: The University of Birmingham, 1998

Bennett S, Tangcharoensathien V. A shrinking state? politics, economics and private health care in Thailand. *Public Administration and Development*, 1994; **14**:1–17

Berman P, Rannan-Eliya R. Factors affecting the development of private health care provision in developing countries. Bethesda, Maryland: Abt Associates Inc., Health Financing and Sustainability Project, 1993

Bidwai P. One step forward, many steps back: dismemberment of India's National Drug Policy. *Development Dialogue*, 1995; **1**:193–222

Bitran R, Yip W. Provider Payment Reform: a review of experience in Latin America and Asia. Bethesda: Partnership for Health Reform, Applied Research Working Paper, 1998

Bossert T, Hsiao W, Barrera M, Alarcon L, Leo M, Casares C. Transformation of Ministries of health in the era of health reform: the case of Colombia. *Health Policy and Planning*, 1998; **13**: 59–77

Brinkerhoff DW. Institutional development in World Bank projects: analytical approaches and intervention designs. *Public Administration and Development*, 1994; **14**:135–151

Cassels A. Health sector reform: key issues in less developed countries. *Journal of International Development*, 1995; **7**: 329–348

Chawla M. Multiple job-holdings by government health personnel in developing countries. Bethesda: Abt Associates Inc., Health Financing and Sustainability Project, SAR Paper Number 17, 1994

Collins D, Quick JD, Musau S, Kraushaar D. *Health Financing Reform in Kenya: The Fall and Rise of Cost Sharing 1989-94*. Boston: Management Sciences for Health, 1995

Daura M, Mabandhla M, Mwanse K, Bennett S. An Evaluation of District Cost Sharing in Zambia. Bethesda: Abt Associates Inc., Partnerships for Health Reform Project, Technical Report, 1998

Diop F, Baguirbi I. 1998. Health Financing Reform in Niger. Bethesda, Maryland: Abt Associates Inc., Partnerships for Health Reform (draft), 1998

Fiszbein A. The emergence of local capacity: lessons from Colombia. *World Development*, 1997; **25**:1029–1043

Foltz A. *Policy Analysis. Anonymous Comprehensive Review of the Zambian Reforms: Technical Reports*. New York: UNICEF and World Bank, 1997, pp 2–28

Grindle MS. Divergent cultures? When public organizations perform well in developing countries. *World Development*, 1997; **25**: 481–495

Hanson K. *Strengthening the Health Sector in Africa: A review of the experience of Eight Countries*. UNICEF, 1997 [Unpublished]

Hilderbrand ME, Grindle MS. *Building Sustainable Capacity: Challenges for the Public Sector*. Boston: Harvard University, 1994

Hopwood I. Policy formulation and health sector reform: Lessons from Zambia and Guinea. Unpublished paper presented at the London School of Hygiene & Tropical Medicine, 1994

Kaul M. The New Public Administration: management innovations in government. *Public Administration and Development*, 1997; **17**:13–26

Klitgaard R. *Controlling Corruption*. Berkeley: University of California Press, 1988

Londoño J, Frenk J. Structured pluralism: towards an innovative model of health system reform in Latin America. *Health Policy*, 1997; **41**: 1–36

Mahler H, Chabot J, Ciardi P et al. *Comprehensive Review of the Zambian Health Reform: Main Report*. New York: UNICEF and World Bank, 1997

Makinen M, Leighton C. Summary of a market analysis for a franchised network of primary health care in Lusaka, Zambia. Bethesda: Abt Associates Inc., Partnerships for Health Reform Technical Report, 1997

Medici AC, Londoño JL, Coelho O et al. Managed care and managed competition in Latin America and Caribbean. In: Schieber G (ed) *Innovations in Health Care Financing. Proceedings of a World Bank Conference, March 10–11, 1997.* Washington DC: World Bank, 1997, pp 215–232 (World Bank Discussion Paper no. 365)

Minogue M, Polidano C, Hulme D. Reorganizing the state: towards more inclusive governance. *Insights*, 1997; **23**: 1–2

Musgrove P. *Public and Private Roles in Health: Theory and Financing Patterns*. Washington DC: The World Bank, 1996 (World Bank Discussion Paper no. 339)

North DC. *Institutions, Institutional Change and Economic Performance*. Cambridge: Cambridge University Press, 1990

Ostrom E, Schroeder L, Wynne S. *Institutional Incentives and Sustainable Development: Infrastructure Policies in Perspective*. Boulder, Colorado: Westview Press, 1993

Paul S. Accountability in public services: Exit, Voice and Control. *World Development*, 1992; **20**:1047–1060

Picciotto R. *Putting Institutional Economics to Work: From Participation to Governance*. Washington DC: World Bank, 1995 (World Bank Discussion Paper no. 304)

Reich MR. The politics of health sector reform in developing countries: three cases of pharmaceutical policy. *Health Policy*, 1995; **32**: 47–77

Russell S, Attanayake N. *Sri Lanka—Reforming the Health Sector: Does Government Have the Capacity?* Birmingham: The University of Birmingham, 1997

Saltman RB, Figueras J. *European Health Care Reform: Analysis of Current Strategies.* Copenhagen: World Health Organization, Regional Office for Europe, 1997 (WHO Regional Publications European Series no.72)

Siegel B, Peters D, Kamara S. *Health Reform in Africa: Lessons from Sierra Leone.* Washington DC: World Bank, 1996 (World Bank Discussion Paper no. 347)

Smithson P, Asamoa-Baah A, Mills A. *The Role of Government in Adjusting Economies: The Case of the Health Sector in Ghana.* Birmingham: The University of Birmingham, 1997

Su CL. The effect of case-based payment for hospital services on the performance or providers in Taiwan. 1995 [Unpublished]

Tendler J, Freedheim S. Trust in a rent-seeking world: health and government transformed in Northeast Brazil. *World Development*, 1994; **22**:1771–1791

Walt G. *Health Policy: An Introduction to Process and Power.* London: Zed Press, 1994

Walt G, Gilson L. Reforming the health sector in developing countries: the central role of policy analysis. *Health Policy and Planning*, 1994; **9**: 353–370

World Bank. *The State in a Changing World: World Development Report 1997.* New York: Oxford University Press, 1997

5
Readdressing equity: the importance of ethical processes

Lucy Gilson

Centre for Health Policy, University of Witwatersrand, South Africa and London School of Hygiene & Tropical Medicine, UK

Equity is again receiving attention in international health policy debates. Within the space of two weeks in November 1997, there were at least four meetings in different parts of the world focusing on issues of equity, and bringing together public health professionals from different countries and different disciplinary backgrounds.

Given the growth of interest in equity, what concepts and experiences can inform future equity-oriented health policy? This chapter seeks to address this question firstly by reviewing some key issues relating to the equity impact of current health care reforms. It then puts forward the understanding that ethical processes are critical in promoting equity, before identifying some practical areas of action through which this perspective can influence policy development.

Within the text primary attention is given to experience in low- and middle-income countries. However, high-income country ideas and experience are also used to provide insight on the issues raised—and the conclusions drawn are relevant across all countries.

Current health care reforms and equity debates

Three interrelated sets of reforms have dominated the last ten to twenty years of health policy debates across the world: financing reforms (such as user fees, prepayment and insurance); provision reforms (strongly influenced by the ideas of the 'new public management' and including the development of various forms of contracting as well as other reforms such as new provider payment mechanisms); and prioritizing public sector resource allocations using cost-effectiveness analysis. Although the three sets of reforms have been promoted across countries, financing reforms initially received more attention in low- and middle-income countries and provision reforms have been implemented to a much greater extent in high-income countries.

Unfortunately little can be learnt about how to promote equity from reviewing existing experience of these reforms. Many of them were introduced with the objective of enhancing efficiency rather than equity. In some cases there is simply too little experience to evaluate but there has also been little attempt to evaluate any aspect of their impact (Gilson and Mills, 1995; Kutzin, 1995; Politt, 1995). The reform area for which there is most evidence in low- and middle-income countries is that of health care financing. The initial enthusiasm for introducing user fees as a means of resource mobilization has been tempered by growing recognition of their negative impact on utilization by the poorest and most vulnerable.[1] The consequences have included investigation of the potential for protecting the poor whilst raising revenue through the introduction of exemption mechanisms (Gilson et al, 1995; Willis and Leighton, 1995) and both formal and informal risk-sharing mechanisms (Gilson, 1997a; Creese and Bennett, 1997).

At the same time, the experience that a fees-plus-quality improvement package may in some cases actually enhance utilization by poorer groups (Litvack and Bodart, 1993; Shaw, 1996) has been used in support of calls to prioritize public sector resource allocations better to meet the needs of these groups. Such 'targeting' of public resources is currently identified as the major strategy for promoting equity within health systems. The prioritization process involves identifying the 'essential package of health services' which can most cost-effectively address the conditions generating the greatest burden of disease for the majority of the population (Bobadilla et al, 1994; Bobadilla and Cowley, 1995; Londoño and Frenk, 1997; World Bank, 1993). Ideally, governments should take financial responsibility for the whole package, whether provided through the public or private sector, and so ensure that it is available to everyone. However, national affordability problems may prevent governments from fulfilling this requirement and so, at the very least, they should ensure that those services that have 'public good' elements are provided free to all and that the poor should receive all services within a 'minimum package' at little or no cost to themselves. In the latter case, exemption mechanisms will be required which relieve the poorest from the burden of payment whilst ensuring that the non-poor pay for the essential services. 'Discretionary' services (those outside the essential package) should always be financed entirely from out-of-pocket payments or through mandated social

---

[1] Although these groups are often defined solely in relation to income, some analysts are beginning to recognize the multi-faceted vulnerabilities of those at risk of poverty and ill-health—as highlighted by community members' own definitions of these groups (Booth et al. 1995; Narayan 1997).

insurance. Overall, it is suggested that this approach will not only preferentially address the needs of the poorest, as they suffer most from the conditions on which the essential package of services is focused, but will also improve the cost-effectiveness of public sector provision.

But will the 'targeting' proposals that have come to dominate health care reforms really promote equity?

Although questions of feasibility are clearly important, the answer to this question is critically dependent on the values which shape the respondent's understanding of equity. From both Utilitarian and Rawlsian perspectives, the proposals are equity-promoting. The application of cost-effectiveness and burden of disease analysis to determine how best to generate aggregate health gain, for example, appears to reflect the utilitarian goal of pursuing the 'greatest good for the greatest number' (Anand and Hanson, 1995; Doyal, 1995; Mooney, 1996). At the same time the essential package approach seems compatible with the Rawlsian notion of equity as requiring that the worst-off in society are provided with a decent basic minimum of health care. Inequalities in (public health care) distribution which support the delivery of a minimum standard of care to the most needy are, in this perspective, equitable.

However, both Utilitarian and Rawlsian perspectives are criticized by Egalitarians. They judge (in)equity by assessing the extent to which health care is, in practice, distributed according to need and financed according to ability to pay (Wagstaff and van Doorslaer, 1993). At the heart of this perspective is a concern for the distribution of health care between people and population groups. Egalitarians, thus, criticize the utilitarian position on the grounds that it requires no particular consideration of the situation of the poorest and most vulnerable. Aggregate health status gains for the majority may be achieved even whilst the poorest gain little or nothing, and as a result the situation of the poorest relative to other groups may even be made worse. Thus, recent research on the equity-promoting potential of community financing schemes following 'Bamako Initiative' principles shows that whilst there may have been gains for the majority rural poor, it is much less clear that the minority poorest have benefited to the same extent, if at all (Gilson, 1998). The essential package approach would also be criticized by egalitarians on the grounds that achieving an absolute minimum level of care for the poorest is simply not enough. The more wealthy will still be able to maintain or even increase their relatively better access to, and utilization of, health care in general as they can and will purchase private care when necessary. Indeed, they are encouraged to do so within the essential package approach. Experience shows that even within a strategy of re-targeting public resources on the poor, the promotion of the private sector increases inequity in access to care and some aspects of quality of care between income groups (Bennett, 1997). The egalitarian would, thus, caution that the minimum standards approach can easily allow the relatively worse situation of the poorest to be maintained over time even whilst this group makes some absolute gains in terms of health care access.

For an egalitarian, the targeting approach thus holds the significant danger of leading to the creation of a tiered and segmented health system. The withdrawal of public benefits from the middle income within this process may then create a vicious cycle as they, in turn, withdraw their political support of the public health system, further reinforcing differences in access and quality between income groups. Over time, the public sector becomes primarily the source of care for the poor whilst even lower-middle-income groups move towards use of private services. 'What starts as a service for the poor may become a poor service or a rump service, as pressure to lower taxes and cut spending whittles the service down further ...[and a] vicious cycle of decline in public services is created' (Patton, 1997; see also: Dreze and Sen, 1989 and Nelson, 1989; 1992, for discussion of relevant experience from low- and middle-income countries).

The architects of the targeting approach suggest that by promoting transparency in decision-making, it directly counters socio-political constraints on 'good decision-making' (Bobadilla *et al*, 1994; Bobadilla and Cowley, 1995). However, this ignores the fact that transparency, like minimum standards, may simply not be enough. The relative position and power of the disadvantaged is often the most critical factor determining whether or not their needs are even considered as an important issue within reform development and implementation (Aiach and Carr-Hill, 1989; Carr-Hill, 1994). The failure to consider the potential socio-political consequences of the targeting approach is in line with the quite technocractic approach to policy formulation that its proponents adopt. They appear to assume that technical experts design essential packages of services which are then simply delivered to (and accepted by) the target group. In practice, however, nothing is that simple. Three further constraints need to be noted.

First, the decisions about what services should be considered as part of the package are likely to be made by those who hold power and can anyway afford to purchase above basic levels. Without real effort to understand the situation of the poorest it is, therefore, probable that their decisions may be detrimental to the poor (Anand and Hanson, 1995; Loewy, 1997). For example, some health care interventions such as emergency care may be very expensive and relatively less cost-effective but may nonetheless become necessary to access. Focusing public resources only on cost-effective interventions ignores the value of public finance in protecting all groups, but particularly the poorest, from having to make 'catastrophic payments' for such interventions.

Second, the causes of ill-health for the poorest and most vulnerable are mostly structural, often a result of broad environmental factors such as 'exposure to unhealthy, stressful living and working conditions' (Whitehead, 1990; see also Mburu, 1983; Zaidi, 1988). Yet the particular importance of a wide range of public health measures in tackling such conditions and the associated health inequities is largely overlooked in current health care reform debates. They are not included as part of the essential health services package and the need to develop and strengthen traditional public health services has been overlooked in the face of the dominant focus on basic curative and preventive medical care. The development of the package is also rooted in the assumption that public resource levels for health care cannot be increased. Yet there is no single correct level of spending on health-related interventions. How much should be spent on health care and on health promoting action outside the health system is a matter of debate (Anand and Hanson, 1995; Doyal, 1995; Patton, 1997).

Third, targeting is trapped in the goals of promoting 'equal access for equal need' within the public sector and redistributing public supply to promote 'equal utilization for equal need'. Considering only public sector supply, it overlooks the private sector's role in health care distribution and ignores demand-side obstacles to health care utilization such as the perceived need for health care and related informational and cultural barriers (Gilson, 1988; Mooney, 1997). Even when strategies are put in place to protect or benefit the poor there is clear evidence that their effectiveness in reaching the target group is undermined by factors such as the power of local elites, cultural norms regarding who should benefit within local communities and their own marginal position in society (Gilson, 1998; Gilson *et al*, 1995; Gilson *et al*, 1998). As a result, and however well-designed, the essential health service package may simply not be used by those on whom it is targeted.

Although equity is inevitably bound up with ideology, the social values which shape the currently dominant 'targeting' approach to health care reform have never been explicitly stated or put forward for discussion. The need to debate the fundamental value base of any health system appears to be seen as irrelevant in the face of what are identified as empirical facts and pragmatic needs. The resolution of past problems, including inequities, is apparently seen as simply requiring the technocratic solutions of 'better management' or improved cost-effectiveness. Yet the evolution of health systems around the world indicates that promoting equity is never simple, and never a matter simply of analysis and straightforward implementation.

An alternative vision of equity: focusing on ethical processes

This chapter specifically acknowledges the range of socio-political barriers to equity-oriented health reforms and builds on an egalitarian perspective to equity. It has four starting points:

1. health inequity results from differences in health outcomes between groups that are unnecessary, avoidable and unfair (Whitehead, 1990);
2. equity-promoting action in the health sector must put the needs and interests of the poorest and most vulnerable at their heart, as the relatively worse health outcomes of this group in comparison with other groups are most often a function of circumstances beyond their control;
3. ill-health and poverty are interlinked and so a concern for health demands the development of strategies to combat poverty rooted in analysis of the factors

that influence the ability of the poorest individuals and groups to gain access to the range of resources which enable them to lead healthy lives;
4. the intended beneficiaries must be involved in identifying, formulating and implementing all equity-oriented health policy interventions as they always play a role in the implementation of any policy intervention, actively adapting and using it rather than passively receiving it (Long and Long, 1992).

Overall, the text is rooted in the understanding that ethical processes are critical in promoting equity. Three different, and yet related, groups of arguments both support this position and provide insight into the nature of the ethical processes promoted in this chapter.

Procedural justice

Health policy debates about equity usually start from the understanding that it is rooted in distributional justice (Calman, 1997). Particular attention has been given recently to the importance of the distribution of health outcomes, rather than, for example, access alone. However, Mooney (1996) proposes that 'Equity in health care arises because of the desire on the part of the members of that society to create a just health care service as part of a wider just society' rather than only from a concern for equality of health (see also Mooney and Jan, 1997).

This perspective draws extensively on Communitarian theory rather than the individualism inherent in utilitarianism and neo-classical economics. It is rooted in the understanding that social value is derived from being a member of a community and from the quality of our relations with other members of the community (procedural justice), rather than only from the distribution of benefits (distributional justice). Mooney argues that social value is generated both as individuals directly participate in decision-making by and for the community, and indirectly, as each individual benefits from the freedom to achieve or to participate that others have secured for him/her. An additional requirement is that procedural rules exist to deal with situations when 'social conditioning makes a person lack the courage to choose (perhaps even to 'desire' what is denied but what would be valued if chosen)' (Mooney and Jan,1997 quoting from Sen,1992). This implies that in an equity-oriented policy strategy, the diverse barriers which may prevent, or limit, individuals' demand for health care cannot be ignored or even addressed by 'protection' mechanisms such as those of targeting or exemptions. Instead, procedures are required to enable such individuals to demand and to choose for themselves what they want (see also Chambers, 1993).

The importance of valuing others

The importance of social values and relations to equity, and the danger of individualistic market-based relations, has also been emphasized by other perspectives. Seedhouse (1997) suggests that whereas the individualist views the pursuit of self-interest as both a moral good and the best means by which to achieve a good society, the counter perspective (which he labels 'socialist') is that a good society is only possible if self-interest is controlled. Similarly, Wilkinson (1996) argues that:

> If one were to pick out something close to the heart of the difference between more and less egalitarian societies, it would surely be something to do with the social nature of public life. Instead of merely market or self-interested relations between families or households, it appears that in more egalitarian societies the public sphere of life remains a more social sphere than it does elsewhere. It remains dominated by people's involvement in the social, ethical and human life of the society, rather than being abandoned to market values and transactions.

Applying these perspectives to the action required to achieve equity, Brecher (1997) suggests that two principles must be fulfilled:

> ...(a) that there be a reasonable degree of equity in respect of outcome concerning the distribution of basic resources and (b) that people treat each other as ends, and not merely as means. The first ... may be understood as a political and economic dimension of socialism, while the second constitutes a moral and social element.

Adopting an attitude of respect for other people is itself a strategy for the promotion of equity, and achieving equitable distributional outcomes may not be possible if people do not value each other.

Public action

Finally, writers on development policy have for some time highlighted the notion of 'public action' as important in understanding the processes of social change that combat poverty and deprivation.

Rooted in Sen's theory of capabilities (Sen, 1992), public action to combat deprivation can include public financing and delivery of health care (and education) as a means of enhancing living conditions and so human capabilities. But Dreze and Sen (1989) also promote a pluralist approach in which various mechanisms, including market mechanisms, might play a role in achieving the objective of social security.[2] Most important to the approach is, however, the

---

[2] Which is itself defined as 'an objective pursued through public means rather than a narrowly defined set of strategies' (Dreze and Sen, 1989) in contrast to current health care

understanding that public action goes beyond state action. Defined as 'purposive collective action, whether for collective private ends or collective public ends' (Mackintosh, 1992) public action is 'in a very big way, a matter of participation by the public in the process of social change' (Dreze and Sen, 1989). In the health sector, such participation might range from direct involvement in public health campaigns, to lobbying for policy action that meets the needs of the poorest, to local level action in support of the poor through the extended family, the community and non-governmental organizations (see also Susser, 1993; Thomas, 1997).

In combating poverty and deprivation the state does not define public need for people or on their behalf. 'Rather, public need is defined through the active participation, or exclusion of various groups in society... little or nothing will be done about the poor and the deprived if they are excluded from the processes which structure public need' (Wuyts, 1992).

Policy action: developing equity-promoting processes

An empirical example from Brazil provides a foundation for further discussion of the policy action that can be derived from these theoretical considerations. Tendler and Freedheim (1994) report an analysis of the successes of a rural preventive health programme implemented in Ceara State, located in the poorest region of Brazil. Initiated in 1987, this community health worker programme began life as part of an emergency employment-creating programme and involved the hiring of a new cadre of 'health agents' who received an initial three months' training followed by substantial on-the-job training, and were supervised by nurses. Although the specific impact of the programme on health status is difficult to determine, available data suggest that it made important contributions to health and health system improvements. By 1992 the state had benefited from a 36% reduction in infant deaths and a tripling in vaccination coverage for measles and polio (increasing it to a level of 90%); and by 1993 the health agents were visiting about 65% of the state's population in their homes every month.

Analysis of this experience began with the question: what allowed unself-interested behaviour to thrive?

---

reform debates which promote specific, technical strategies often without clear ends. Although Dreze and Sen (1989) specifically considered the role of health care within the broader 'social security' strategy required to combat hunger and deprivation, health policy appears to have been little touched by the arguments of those promoting public action.

Ethical professional behaviour: the importance of trust and caring

> The provision of social services has a strong personal element: the quality of service depends heavily on the attitudes of the people undertaking it, and it is hard to monitor. Service provisioning, furthermore, often involves a position of power over users. Hence the importance of professional ethics (Mackintosh, 1995).

An important factor underlying the success of the Brazilian programme was the promotion of trust between the health agents and their clients and of a sense of professionalism among nurse supervisors. Three key factors seem to explain these facets of the programme:

- the state initially created an aura of mission around the programme and respect for its workers among the community through a wide-ranging information campaign, merit-hiring and strategies such as prizes for those identified by the community as good workers; later moves to offer some security of job tenure to health agents only reinforced their sense of status;
- health agents were allowed to take on a wider range of tasks than was listed in their formal job descriptions, such as providing some basic curative care, implementing public health tasks and simply helping mothers with household chores, and so came to be liked and respected by their clients;
- the nurse supervisors were paid higher salaries than in their previous jobs and, equally importantly, developed a sense of professionalism by being given a fair degree of control over how they ran 'their' programme, even whilst working within a broad set of guidelines.

As a result, 'the agents saw their clients not only as subjects whose behaviour they wanted to change, but as people from whom they actually wanted and needed respect' (Tendler and Freedheim,1994).

A contrasting experience which, nonetheless, emphasizes similar lessons is the introduction of the 'new public management' (NPM) in various social sectors and its impact on the way front-line health and social service professionals operate. Although more widespread in high-income countries, this managerial approach underlies the contracting and other institutional reforms increasingly promoted for implementation in low- and middle- income countries (see Cassels, 1995).

Reflecting on the still relatively limited experience of the NPM's influence on social care provision in the UK, Mackintosh (1997) raises concerns about its potential to undermine the situation of the poor and vulnerable. She suggests that the emphasis given to clients as consumers who must make choices about their own care disempowers more vulnerable clients who, in practice, have too little information or confidence to be able to choose.[3] At the same time, the new

---

[3] She gives the example of an elderly man who has recently suffered a stroke and so now needs nursing and practical help in his home. The social services department of the local

procedures have undermined the ability and motivation of front-line workers to respond to the needs of their most vulnerable clients. As key decisions, particularly those over resource use, can now only be made by managers, these front-line workers have also been disempowered and so discouraged from acting as advocates on behalf of their clients (see also Jackson and Price, 1994). By offering front-line providers less secure employment conditions whilst enhancing the power (status and rewards) of managers, the NPM widens the divisions between personnel within the public sector and so undermines its cohesiveness and sense of purpose in confronting and tackling need. Finally, the emphasis on indicators to monitor performance in areas in which outcomes are notoriously difficult to define and measure, results in the use of 'simple' indicators of volume and resource use. These give weight to business values, particularly the profit motive, and so provide incentives to exclude expensive (often more 'needy') clients (see also Walsh, 1995; Moore, 1996). Such incentives may offset traditional health care values, at the heart of which is 'a belief in the fundamental importance of helping other people achieve as much of their potential as possible.' (Seedhouse, 1994; see also Cribb, 1995; Politt, 1995)[4]

Although professionalism has been used in the past to ensure the domination of providers over users, and so has rightly been challenged in recent reforms, there is a danger of 'throwing the baby out with the bath water' through new health care management approaches. 'Nurses, doctors and related carers need to be neither suppliers of a product nor the paternalistic professionals of old. Rather, there has to be a properly professional relationship based on equality of respect in both directions' (Brecher, 1997; see also Patton, 1997).

These experiences stress the critical importance of an almost completely overlooked area in health care reforms—front-line health workers and human resource development policies that support them. Whilst such policies must include adequate skills-development through appropriate and relevant training programmes, it is equally important that attention is given to generating a sense of 'mission' among workers, recognizing and strengthening the non-financial incentives to which people respond, whilst ensuring appropriate disciplinary procedures, and allowing these workers to control and develop aspects of the way they provide services and care for those in need (see also Hilderbrand and Grindle, 1994; Moore, 1996).

---

authority has given him a list of private providers and told him to arrange his own care through one of them. But he feels insecure about making the arrangements and would anyway be happier with care provided directly by the local authority services.

[4] On a positive note, findings from recent research in the UK suggest, however, that those within the National Health System have not yet succumbed to market values (Williams and Flynn, 1997).

Strategic action and broader policy advocacy

The Brazilian programme was nurtured and supported by strategic action, both deliberate and accidental, to offset potential opposition. For example, anticipating that local mayors would see the programme as a threat to their own independence, the central level (the state) sought to offset the mayors' influence by encouraging popular demand for the programme through a wide-ranging information campaign outlining its benefits. They also secured nurses' support by enhancing their status (whilst keeping doctors' opposition at bay by working only in the rural areas where few doctors were based) and generated a virtuous cycle of success-demand-success by expanding the programme slowly and carefully, in response to demand from local communities. Analysis of broader reform experiences also suggests that the processes and strategies used to develop and implement policies have a critical influence over their effectiveness. It is not only important to develop and mobilize support but also to generate strategies that inform policies as they are being implemented, and so allow appropriate adaptation of policies (Walt, 1994; Gilson, 1997b).

A specific area of advocacy required to redress inequities in health status includes the promotion of wider economic and social policy action in support of health (Whitehead 1995; Wilkinson 1996; Calman, 1997; Loewenson and Mumbengegwi, 1997; Patton,1997). Whilst there are clearly limits on what health professionals can do in taking forward multi-sectoral action, they can play critical roles in lobbying for such action, promoting collaborative action with other groups and monitoring broader policies in terms of their health equity impact. Health policy-makers might also seek direct involvement in the formulation of wider policies (such as those concerning employment, working conditions, education, housing, food and diet) to ensure that their potential health effects and their distribution are considered in policy making (Dahlgren and Diderichsen, 1986).

More broadly, Chambers (1983; 1993) argues that development professionals in all sectors should adopt a broad advocacy role in tackling poverty. Calling for a 'counter-ideology of reversals' in the way that the diverse set of 'development professionals' operate in low- and middle-income countries (be they national or expatriate workers, working at international, national or local levels), he has argued that such professionals should 'put the last first' in all their actions in order to promote social change in the interests of the poorest and most marginalized.

> The problem is not "them" (the poor), but "us" (the not poor). The massive reversals needed to eliminate the worst deprivation need professionals to fight within the structures in which they find themselves [...] The basic issue is power. Those with power— "us"— do not easily give it up. The challenge then is to find ways in which more and more of those who are powerful and privileged can be enabled to start and strengthen processes which in turn enable those who are weak and deprived (1993; see also Wuyts, 1992).

Accountability, participation and responsiveness: creating an enabling state

Underpinning other equity-oriented policy action is the need for a new vision of the role of the state. Chambers' paradigm of reversals is, thus, linked to a vision of an 'enabling and liberating state', at the core of which is decentralized process and choice. 'In terms of this paradigm, the state has often done those things which it ought not to have done, and has left undone those things which it ought to have done' (Chambers, 1993). Depending on the circumstances, action might sometimes be required to abolish the state regulations which exploit the poor, but elsewhere action might be required to 'decentralise while providing safety nets, secure rights and access to reliable information, and permitting and promoting more independence and choice for the poor.'

In this conception it is important to note that the message is not simply, decentralize and democratize. Local decision-making is often itself dominated by elites and the need to give patronage and '... the best interests of minorities are not necessarily safe in the hands of majorities. This is of particular concern if the minority in question consists of those too vulnerable through illness to defend themselves' (Doyal, 1995). What is required is both a balance of central and local level decision-making, and the creation of more diverse mechanisms of accountability.

Thus, a final important explanation of success in the Brazilian case was that the central level (the state) did not 'do less' in relation to the health agent programme, but remained interventionist whilst undertaking different tasks. It:

- retained central control over the hiring and firing of health agents and so reduced the opportunities for local mayors to use the appointment of health agents from within local communities as a means of exercising patronage (although nurse supervisors were employed by municipalities, they were often recruited from outside the area and were required to have both relevant training and experience so the potential for mayoral patronage in their appointment was limited);
- did not force the programme on reluctant municipalities at some predetermined pace and pattern, but allowed the pace and pattern of expansion to be determined by demand and interest (i.e. which mayors chose to employ nurse supervisors);
- conducted vigorous public information campaigns which promoted strong local demand for the programme and created careful watchdogs over its development and the performance of health agents.

Together these actions 'made it politically more rewarding to provide good service and more politically costly to hire the party faithful—thus changing the dynamic of patronage politics as it related to public service at the local level' (Tendler and Freedheim, 1994), whilst creating significant pressures for accountability to the community.

Moore (1996), similarly emphasizes the importance of developing accountability based on 'a productive tension between ... (i) "local embeddedness" and (ii) "centralised mistrust."' The former is a product of establishing relations built on trust between front-line providers and their clients, and leads the providers to be sensitive to the needs of those they serve. At the same time, central oversight mechanisms should help ensure that local level staff do not become self-serving (see also Brecher, 1997). Rather than supporting the NPM view that that accountability is simply a result of 'exit' mechanisms which allow clients to change service providers when they are dissatisified, this broader strategy for developing accountability suggests that it is a function of close interaction between citizens and providers within the local setting. Such interaction can be particularly strengthened by developing the overlooked mechanism of 'voice', i.e. public participation in decision-making, through actions such as:

- strengthening, establishing and securing citizens' socio-economic and health rights whilst developing popular statements of patient rights—such as a patients' charter—and conducting wide-ranging public information and education campaigns about these rights and how to claim them (Chambers, 1993);
- establishing mechanisms of direct democracy such as specific consultative and decision-making bodies which include representation from all parts of 'the community', as complements to representative democracy (Paul, 1992; Chambers, 1993);
- supporting and involving civil society bodies, such as community-based and non-governmental organizations, as voice mechanisms to express the interests and needs of the poorest (Thomas, 1997);
- flexible implementation strategies, combined with effective procedures for monitoring and evaluating the impact on equity of health and other reforms and mechanisms for feeding the information forward into lobbying (GHEI,1997; McCoy and Gilson,1997; WHO,1997).

In general, such actions seek to promote equity through the promotion of 'a (partly) public interest state, responsive to the needs of the poor' (Mackintosh, 1992).

Promoting equity through cross-subsidization

Health care financing mechanisms and strategies are critically important to the promotion of equity goals. However, in contrast with recent reform packages, the perspective of this chapter stresses the need to consider how such mechanisms can support ethical processes within the health system rather than how they can mobilize resources or promote efficiency. Such a perspective suggests that, rather than promoting divisions between population groups in the level, quality or source of care, financing mechanisms should promote social solidarity and cohesive health systems which give special attention to the needs of the poorest through, in particular, cross-subsidization between population groups.

Cross-subsidization can, firstly, be promoted within and between the public and private sectors through various specific financing mechanisms. These include:

- the progressive financing mechanisms of tax-financing or social insurance coverage, rather than the regressive private financing mechanisms of fees or private insurance (Gilson, 1997a; van Doorslaer and Wagstaff, 1997);
- a single insurance scheme in which payments by the poor are reduced or waived, rather than separate insurance schemes for different population groups or insurance only for vulnerable groups (Gertler and Hammer, 1997; Jonsson and Musgrove, 1997; van Doorslaer and Wagstaff, 1997);
- where public sector care is attractive to higher income users either because it is perceived to be good-quality care or there are few alternatives for specific services, allowing 'private practice' within public institutions whilst ensuring full-cost recovery for those services as a way of retaining the non-poor as users of the public system and so ensuring cross-subsidy within the system (Mackintosh, 1995).

Although progressive tax-financing has not been on the agenda of health care reforms in recent years, there are signs that some analysts are again affirming its equity-promoting potential (Burgess, 1997). The other processes of cross-subsidy may be more acceptable in the current reform climate but must be complemented by steps to prevent the development of private insurance or, where it already exists, to regulate the sector. It is particularly important to prevent competition on the basis of risk-selection within this sector and so avoid a situation in which certain population groups are, in effect, uninsurable. Fee-for-service reimbursement mechanisms should also be deterred as they lead to cost escalation in the sector and so limit its potential to cross-subsidize other sectors of health care (Mackintosh 1995; Londoño and Frenk 1997; van den Heever 1997).

These financing mechanisms can, finally, be supported by public sector resource allocation processes which promote cross-subsidy between geographical areas and their resident populations. Although not a major focus of current health care reform debates, the proponents of the essential package approach suggest that it could be used within a resource allocation mechanism (Bobadilla et al,1994). However, its use in this way would only ensure that resource allocations supported the same level of care to be established in all areas of a country. It would not ensure that more needy populations received the greater share of resources likely to be necessary to enable them to offset historical deficits in health. Drawing the notions of procedural justice and vertical equity into discussions about needs-based resource allocation mechanisms, Mooney (1996; 1997) instead proposes that resource allocation mechanisms should include explicit weights to reflect societal preferences about which groups should be prioritized in this process. From the Australian experience of great inequalities in health status between population groups which are not the result of random distributions of ill-health, he proposes that resource allocation formulae should include an extra weight for the particularly disadvantaged Aboriginal communities '... if [formulae] do not weight more highly health gains to the worse off, then they may not lead to a narrowing of health differentials' (Mooney, 1997) but will rather simply maintain the existing differentials. He also suggests that community surveys could elicit societal preferences about which groups should benefit from such allocations and how much weight should be given to their greater need in resource allocation formulae.

Although Mooney's approach seems to hold much relevance for low- and middle-income countries where health inequalities are also large, little attention has yet been given to developing such mechanisms within these countries. Yet recent work in South Africa has shown the potential of resource allocation mechanisms even in relatively data-scarce countries and at both national and sub-national levels (Doherty and van den Heever,1997; Gilson et al,1997; Makan et al, 1997). Indeed, in South Africa at least, the existing inequities are so great that even the use of crude population data would promote equitable resource reallocations. The South African experience also emphasizes that financial resource reallocations should not occur too quickly, because of limited capacity to absorb reductions or increases in funding, and must be supported by planning processes which allow financial resource reallocations to be accompanied by the physical and human resource reallocations that are necessary to ensure the real changes in service provision that will promote equity. In other words, any new approach to priority setting or resource allocation must be supported by old-fashioned planning processes to be effective in promoting equity (or allocative efficiency).

Conclusion: developing the social capital required to promote equity

In contrast to the more technocratic approach of current health care reforms, this chapter promotes the vision of an equity-oriented health system rooted in ethical processes. At the heart of these processes is the pursuit of procedural justice rather than only distributional justice, a fundamental respect for the innate worth of other people and a recognition of each citizen's own responsibility to promote equity.

The 'public action' required to secure this vision is, therefore, not solely the function of some combination of financing and provision reforms but, more importantly, a broader process of social change in which all groups play an active role. Perhaps the most critical factor underlying this public action is the development of an enabling state which protects and promotes the interests of the poor through 'public interest' institutions lying both within and outside the public sector. In order to combat heath need and material deprivation, such institutions 'must be sites of mutual solidarity and inclusiveness not top down patronage and social exclusiveness' (Mackintosh,1997) and so must, in effect, promote the 'social capital' that is increasingly emphasized as an important component of health egalitarian societies (Wilkinson, 1996). Defined as the 'features of social life—

networks, norms, and trust—that enable participants to act together more effectively to pursue shared objectives' (Puttnam,1995), this social capital can be developed through three critical sets of policy interventions: human resource development policies that support ethical practices and behaviour by front-line providers; institutional reforms that encourage a sense of loyalty and accountability to the wider community and particularly to the poorest within it; and financing reforms that promote cross-subsidization between population groups.

Acknowledgements

Some of the ideas incorporated in this chapter were first presented at the meeting, 'Towards Equity?: Health Sector Reform and Access to Basic Health Services', held in Oslo in November 1997 and organized by the Centre for Partnership and Development, Oslo and the Tropical Disease Research Programme of the World Health Organization. Lucy Gilson is a part-time member of the Health Economics and Financing Programme of the London School of Hygiene & Tropical Medicine, which receives financial support from the UK's Department for International Development. She would like to thank Di McIntyre, Anne Mills, Helen Schneider and Gill Walt for their continued support in thinking through the ever-elusive issues of equity, as well as for reading and commenting on earlier versions of this paper. As usual, however, only she can be held responsible for the ideas presented here.

References

Aiach P, Carr-Hill R. Inequalities in health: the country debate. In Fox J (ed) *Health Inequalities in European Countries*. Aldershot: Gower, 1989, pp 19–49

Anand S, Hanson K. *Disability adjusted life years: a critical review*. Working Paper Series No.95.06, Harvard Centre for Population and Development Studies. Cambridge: Harvard School of Public Health, 1995

Bennett S. Private health care and public policy. In Colclough C (ed) *Marketizing Education and Health in Developing Countries: Miracle or Mirage?* Oxford: Clarendon Press, 1997, pp 93–123

Bobadilla J-L, Cowley P, Musgrove P, Saxenian H. Design, content and financing of an essential national package of health services. *Bulletin of the World Health Organization*, 1994; **72**: 653–662

Bobadilla J-L, Cowley P. Designing and implementing packages of essential health services. *Journal of International Development*, 1995; **7**: 543–554

Booth D, Milimo J, Bond G, Chimuka S *et al. Coping with Cost Recovery*. Report to SIDA, commissioned through the Development Studies Unit, Department of Social Anthropology, Stockholm University, 1995

Brecher B. What would a socialist health service look like? *Health Care Analysis*, 1997; **5**: 217–225

Burgess RSL. Fiscal reform and the extension of basic health and education coverage. In Colclough C (ed) *Marketizing Education and Health in Developing Countries: Miracle or Mirage?* Oxford: Clarendon Press, 1997, pp 307–346

Calman KC. Equity, poverty and health for all. *British Medical Journal*, 1997; **314**: 1187–1191

Carr-Hill RA. Efficiency and equity implications of the health care reforms. *Social Science and Medicine*, 1994; **39**: 1189–1201

Cassels A. Health sector reform: key issues in less developed countries. *Journal of International Development*, 1995; 7: 329–348

Chambers R. *Rural Development: Putting the Last First.* London: Longman, 1983

Chambers R. *Challenging the professions: frontiers for rural development.* London: Intermediate Technology Publications, 1993

Creese A, Bennett S. *Rural risk-sharing strategies in health.* Paper prepared for the International Conference on Innovations in Health Care Financing, World Bank, March 10-11th, 1997

Cribb A. A turn for the better? Philosophical issues in health care reform. In: Seedhouse D (ed) *Reforming Health Care: the Philosophy and Practice of International Health Reform.* Chichester: John Wiley, 1995, pp 171–182

Dahlgren G, Diderichsen F. Strategies for equity in health: Report from Sweden. *International Journal of Health Services*, 1986; **16**: 517–537

Doherty J, van den Heever A. *A resource allocation formula in support of equity and primary health care.* Johannesburg: Centre for Health Policy, University of Witwatersrand, 1997. CHP Paper 47

Doyal L. Needs, rights, and equity: moral quality in health care rationing. *Quality in Health Care*, 1995; **4**: 273–283

Dreze J, Sen A. *Hunger and Public Action.* Oxford: Clarendon Press, 1989

Gertler P, Hammer J. *Strategies for pricing publicly provided health services.* Paper prepared for the International Conference on Innovations in Health Care Financing, World Bank, March 10–11th, 1997

Gilson L. *Government health care charges: is equity being abandoned?* EPC Publication No. 15. London: London School of Hygiene & Tropical Medicine, 1988

Gilson L, Mills A. Health sector reform in sub-Saharan Africa: Lessons of the last ten years. *Health Policy*, 1995; **32**: 215–243

Gilson L, Russell S, Buse K. The political economy of user fees with targeting: developing equitable health financing policy. *Journal of International Development*, 1995; 7: 369–402

Gilson L, van den Heever A, Brijlal V. *DHS development in the North West Province: district financing and financial management.* Report to the Health Systems Trust. Johannesburg: Centre for Health Policy, 1997

Gilson L. The lessons of user fee experience in Africa. *Health Policy and Planning*, 1997a; **12**: 273–285

Gilson L. *Briefing document: Key lessons from the experience of implementing and evaluating health reform processes.* Paper prepared for first SAZA workshop, Johannesburg, November, 1997b

Gilson L. *Promoting equity within Bamako Initiative Schemes: A three country study. Final synthesis report.* London: London School of Hygiene & Tropical Medicine (Draft) 1998

Gilson L, Russell S, Oratai R et al. *Exempting the poor: a review and evaluation of the Low Income Card Scheme in Thailand.* London: London School of Hygiene & Tropical Medicine, PHP Publication Series No 28, 1998

Global Health Equity Initiative (GHEI). *Proceedings: China Meeting* October 4–10, 1997

Hilderbrand ME, Grindle MS. *Building Sustainable Capacity: Challenges for the Public Sector.* Cambridge: Harvard Institute of International Development, 1994

Jackson PM, Price CM (eds) *Privatization and Regulation: a Review of the Issues.* London: Longman, 1994

Jonsson B, Musgrove P. *Government financing of health care.* Paper prepared for the International Conference on Innovations in Health Care Financing, World Bank, March 10–11th, 1997

Kutzin J. Experience with organisational and financing reform of the health sector. Current Concerns SHS Paper no.8, WHO/SHS/CC94.3.Geneva: World Health Organization, 1995

Litvack JI, Bodart C. User fees plus quality equals improved access to health care: results of a field experiment in Cameroon. *Social Science and Medicine,* 1993; **37**: 369–383

Loewenson R, Mumbengegwi C. *Human development report: a conceptual framework.* Paper prepared for the Poverty Forum Preparatory Meeting for the Poverty Forum/UNDP Human Development Report, Harare, 1997 (unpublished)

Loewy EH. What would a socialist health system look like? A sketch. *Health Care Analysis,* 1997; **5**: 195–204

Londoño J-L, Frenk J. Structured pluralism: towards an innovative model for health system reform in Latin America. *Health Policy,* 1997; **41**: 1–36

Long N, Long A. *Battlefields of Knowledge: the Interlocking of Theory and Practice in Social Research and Development.* London: Routledge, 1992

McCoy D, Gilson L. Indicators for monitoring the inequity of health care provision. Paper presented at a seminar on The attainability and affordability of equity in health care provision, Manila, June 1997 (unpublished)

Mackintosh M. Question the state. In: Wuyts M, Mackintosh M, Hewitt T (eds) *Development Policy and Public Action.* Oxford: Open University Press, 1992

Mackintosh M. Competition and contracting in selective social provisioning. *European Journal of Development Research,* 1995; **7**: 26–52

Mackintosh M. Public management for social inclusion. Keynote paper for the conference on Public Management for the Next Century, Manchester, June 29-July 3, 1997

Makan B, Morar R, McIntyre D. *District health systems development in the Eastern Cape Province: district financing and financial management capacity.* Johannesburg: Health Economics Unit, University of the Witwatersrand, 1997. Working Paper series no. 31

Mburu FM. Health systems as defences against the consequences of poverty: equity in health as social justice. *Social Science and Medicine,* 1983; **17**: 1149–1157

Mooney G. And now for vertical equity? Some concerns arising from Aboriginal health in Australia. *Health Economics,* 1996; **5**: 99–103

Mooney G. *Equity in future South African health care: a tale of minimally decent Samaritans or good South Africans?* Public lecture given at the University of Cape Town, October 1997.

Mooney G, Jan S. Vertical equity: weighting outcomes? or establishing procedures? *Health Policy,* 1997: **39**: 79–87

Moore M. *Public sector reform: downsizing, restructuring, improving performance.* Forum on Health Sector Reform, Discussion Paper No.7, WHO/ARA/96.2. Geneva: World Health Organization, 1996

Narayan D. *Voices of the Poor: Poverty and Social Capital in Tanzania.* Washington: World Bank, 1997.

Nelson JM. The politics of pro-poor adjustment. In Nelson JM (ed) *Fragile Coalitions: the Politics of Economic Adjustment.* New Brunswick: Transaction Books, 1989

Nelson JM. Poverty, equity and the politics of adjustment. In: Haggard S and Kaufmann RR (eds) *The Politics of Economic Adjustment: International Constraints, Distributive Conflicts and the State*. Princeton: Princeton University Press, 1992

Patton C. Necessary conditions for a socialist health service. *Health Care Analysis*, 1997; **5**: 205–216

Paul S. Accountability in public services: exit, voice and control. *World Development*, 1992; **20**: 1047–1060

Politt C. Justification by works or by faith?: Evaluating the new public management. *Evaluation*, 1995; **1**: 133–154

Puttnam RD. Tuning in, tuning out: the strange disappearance of social capital in America. *Political Science and Politics*, 1995; **28**: 664–683

Seedhouse D. Health care values or business values. *Health Care Analysis*, 1994; **2**: 181–186

Seedhouse D. Is a socialist health service possible? *Health Care Analysis*, 1997; **5**: 183–185

Sen A. *Inequality Re-examined*. Oxford: Clarendon Press, 1992

Shaw RP. User fees in sub-Saharan Africa: aims, findings and policy implications. In: Shaw RP, Ainsworth M (eds) *Financing health Services through user fees and insurance: case studies from sub-Saharan Africa*. World Bank Discussion Paper No. 294, Africa Technical Department Series. Washington DC: World Bank, 1996

Susser M. Health as a human right: An epidemiologist's perspective on the public health. *American Journal of Public Health*, 1993; **83**: 418–426

Tendler J, Freedheim S. Trust in a rent-seeking world: health and government transformed in Northeast Brazil. *World Development*, 1994; **22**:1771–1791

Thomas A. The role of NGOs in development management: a public action approach. Paper for the conference on Public Management for the Next Century, Manchester, June 29– July 3, 1997 (unpublished)

van Doorslaer E, Wagstaff A. Equity in the finance and delivery of health care: an overview of the methods and findings of the ECuity Project. Paper prepared for the Human Development Department of the World Bank, 1997

van den Heever A. Regulating the funding of private health care: the South African experience. In: Bennett S, McPake B and Mills A (eds) *Private Health Providers in Developing countries: Serving the Public Interest?* London: Zed Books, 1997, pp 158– 173

Wagstaff A, van Doorslaer E. Equity in the finance and delivery of health care: concepts and definitions. In: van Doorslaer E, Wagstaff A, Rutten F (eds) *Equity in the Finance and Delivery of Health Care: an International Perspective*. Oxford: Oxford University Press, 1993, pp 7–19

Walsh K. *Public Services and Market Mechanisms: Competition, Contracting and the New Public Management*. Basingstoke: Macmillan, 1995

Walt G. *Health Policy: an Introduction to Process and Power*. London: Zed Books, 1994

Whitehead M. *The Concepts and Principles of Equity and Health*. Copenhagen: World Health Organization Regional Office for Europe, 1990

Whitehead M. Tackling inequalities: a review of policy initiatives. In: Benzeval M, Judge K, Whitehead M (eds*) Tackling Inequalities in Health: An Agenda for Action*. London: King's Fund, 1995, pp 22–52

Wilkinson R. *Unhealthy Societies: from Inequality to Well-being*. Routledge: London, 1996

Williams G, Flynn R. Health-care contracting and social science: issues in theory and practice. In: Flynn R, Williams G (eds) *Contracting for Health: Quasi-markets and the National Health Service*. Oxford: Oxford University Press, 1997, pp 153–159

Willis CY, Leighton C. Protecting the poor under cost recovery: the role of means testing. *Health Policy and Planning*, 1995; **10**: 241–256

World Bank. *Investing in Health: The World Development Report 1993.* Washington DC: World Bank, 1993

World Health Organization. *Draft report of meeting on policy-oriented monitoring of equity in health and health care.* Geneva 29 September–3 October. Geneva: World Health Organization, 1997

Wuyts M. Conclusion: development policy as process. In: Wuyts M, Mackintosh M, Hewitt T (eds) *Development policy and public action.* Oxford: Oxford University Press, 1992

Zaidi SA. Poverty and disease: need for structural change. *Social Science and Medicine*, 1988; **27**: 119–127

6
Global health policy reform: misleading mythology or learning opportunity?

Theodore R. Marmor

Yale University School of Management, USA

The subject of this chapter is easy to describe, but difficult to deal with substantively. The chapter addresses the claim that recent health policy-making in a wide variety of countries reflects a common global understanding of health care and its reform: in the world of the OECD, of the rapidly developing nations, and in the former Communist bloc. The backdrop to this consists of at least two apparently widespread developments. One is the spread of what is called 'health reform' to all these countries; the claim by many commentators that reform is everywhere. Second is the speed-up of communication about 'reform' across borders, the really extraordinary way in which ideas about problems, options, and remedies move in what I call the intellectual jetstream. This 'globalization' of notions about health care and policy change is a technical complement to the worldwide distribution of scientific findings, devices, and drugs among the medical care community. But there is a substantial difference to consider. The process of apprehending what a policy reform is, interpreting the relevance of it for any particular national setting, adapting a policy proposal to local conceptions, and taking into account the implementation barriers—all of these considerations make cross-border policy learning very much more difficult than understanding an article on a new cancer therapy, importing a new device, and so on.

There are a variety of myths that can prevent the learning of important lessons from other countries' experience in financing, improving, and delivering medical care. There are many cases where cross-border attempts at learning, though needed and available, were both wildly unreliable and unhelpful. In other contexts, I have tried to show how that was the case in American interpretations of Canadian experience with universal health insurance.[1] The topic here is the more general one of health reform in a variety of settings and the possibilities and limits of cross-border learning.

Health policy, national schemes and global forces

Health reform, one is led to believe, is now a global trend. 'Countries everywhere,' according to one European health newsletter, 'are reforming their health care systems.' 'There cannot be a country in the world,' these enthusiasts go on to claim, 'which is not at least raising questions about the cost of delivery of health care.' Finally, we are told, that 'what is remarkable about this global movement is that both the diagnosis of the problems and the prescription for them are virtually the same in all health care systems'(Hunter, 1995).

It is hard to imagine a more breathless and flawed description of health policy making in 1990s Europe (or elsewhere). Indeed, within this brief paragraph are two central misconceptions held by those I would call the global marketeers in health policy. First, the marketeers assume that the diagnoses and remedies associated with so-called 'health reform' mean the same things in different settings. (This view is, a priori, implausible and, as we shall see, it is empirically unsustainable.) Second, there is the presumption that, since the problems are similar and the remedies analogous, cross-national learning is largely a matter of 'establishing a database and information network on health system reform'. This trivializes both the need to understand the differing contexts of health policy making and the real threats to mislearning that make appeals to easy cross-national transfer of experience seem so naive.

There is little doubt, however, that there has been globalization of commentary in the world of medical care. Indeed, none of us can escape the 'bombardment of information about what is happening in other countries', as Rudolf Klein put it (1995). Yet, in the field of health policy, there is now an extraordinary imbalance between the magnitude of the information flows and the capacity to learn useful lessons from them. Indeed, I suspect that the speed of communication *about* developments abroad actually reduces the likelihood of cross-national learning.[2] Why might that be so and what does that speculation suggest about more promising forms of international intellectual exchange?

---

[1] The ideas in this paper were developed still more elaborately in Marmor, 1994.

[2] This sceptical argument is advanced, with Anglo-American examples from medical care and welfare, in Marmor and Plowden (1991). On the other hand, there is very rapid communication of scientific findings and claims, with journals and meetings regarded as the proper sites for evaluation. As of yet, there is no journal in the political economy of medical care that has enough authority, audience, or acuteness to play the evaluative role assumed by the *New England Journal of Medicine, Lancet, British Medical Journal,* or *Journal of the American Medical Association.*

The political setting: health reforms everywhere on the public agenda

There is little doubt about the salience of health policy[3] on the public agenda of most industrial democracies. Canada's form of universal health insurance is a model of achievement for many observers, the subject of considerable intellectual scrutiny and the destination of many policy travellers in search of illumination. Yet a majority of its provinces in recent years have felt sufficiently concerned about the condition of Canadian Medicare (and general fiscal pressures) to set up Royal Commissions to chart adjustments. The medical care worries of the United States have perhaps been more obvious recently, as I noted earlier. For most of 1994, only the legal troubles of OJ Simpson could dominate health reform for the attention of the media, with the ubiquitous CNN ensuring that the world knew something about both topics. And ever since, health care turbulence has been marked, an example of change without choice. The Dutch disputes about policy choices and policy coherence are on-going[4] and the degree of interest in policy is, at least in the United States, unprecedented in its level, if not comprehension. One could obviously go on with examples of policy controversies in Germany (burdened by the fiscal pressures of unification), in Great Britain (competing with the scandals in the Major government), in Sweden (with fiscal and unemployment pressures of enormous force), in South Africa (with pressures to universalize child and maternal health care), in Taiwan (with national health insurance), and so on. These subjects, of course, constitute the very concerns of many of the national specialists in health care and related subjects.

The politics of cross-national claims: timing, use and misuse

The puzzle, I suggest, is not whether there is such widespread interest in health policy, but why now. And why has international evidence (arguments, claims, caricatures) seemed more prominent in the 1990s round of 'reform' debate than, say, during the fiscal strains of the early 1970s? What can be usefully said not only about the substance of the experience of different nations, but about the political processes of introducing and acting upon policy change? I raise these issues bluntly so as to distinguish these comments from the casual presumption that there really is something that could be termed a common global discussion of the same problems and class of remedies. The point here should not be missed. The

---

[3] Readers may be puzzled by my reluctance to treat 'reform' as the object of commentary. This paragraph's parade of substitutes—health policy, concerns, worries, etc.—reflects discomfort with the marketing connotations of the 'reform' expression. That there are pressures for change is obvious and understanding them is important, but reforming can obviously be a benefit, a burden, or beside the point.

[4] The European Health Reform's first bulletin has a report on 'why the Dutch health care system is now in chaos and confusion' (Hunter, 1995) p 8.

presumption that the diagnoses and remedies for health policy are similar is widespread; the Hunter argument (1995) summarizes this view clearly: there are 'common pressures to contain costs, attempts to keep pace with demographic and technological changes, and the need to improve the performance and quality of care provided to service users'. This diagnosis, of course, is utterly commonplace and undifferentiated. Every health system in the post-war world has addressed them, but in different formulations, with differing weights and emphasis. As for remedies, the globalist view is that contemporary 'reforms share a number of common elements: a separation of purchaser and provider functions, the introduction of market principles based on the notion of managed competition, and an emphasis on clinical effectiveness and on health outcomes'.

Here again we see the triumph of faddish commentary over analytical clarity. There is no doubt that these phrases—market principles, payer/provider splits, and managed competition etc.—have come into widespread use. But their use has been largely, with important exceptions, by parties attacking the welfare state, ideologically celebrators of market allocation, and appealing to business and managerial convictions that are seldom subject to empirical investigation. The reference to interest in 'health outcomes' is perhaps the most obvious of the renaming of what any competent medical policy maker has been interested in. Equally, the appeal to the idea of 'managed competition' is an example of an oxmymoronic slogan being substituted for thought. Competition is regulated (well or poorly), not managed. And human resources are managed. So it was that the real combination, regulating competition and managing human resources more sensibly, got reduced to a slogan that misleads. For further discussion of this point, see Marmor and Mashaw (1993) and a revised version (Marmor and Mashaw, 1994).

Why now?

There is a simple answer to this question that one hopes is not simple minded. Medical care policy came to the forefront of public agendas during the late 1980s and early 1990s for one or more of the following reasons. First, the financing of personal medical care has everywhere become a major financial component of the budgets[5] of mature welfare states and, when fiscal strain arises—as with the prolonged recession of recent years—policy scrutiny, not simply incremental budgeting, is the predictable result. Second, mature welfare states, as Klein and O'Higgins argued (1988) in the late 1980s, under almost all circumstances come to

---

[5] Technically, this is not strictly true, as is evident in the sickness fund financing of care in Germany, the Netherlands, and elsewhere. But, since mandatory contributions are close cousins of 'taxes', budget officials must obviously treat these outlays as constraints on direct tax increases. Moreover, the precise level of acceptable cost increases is a regulatory issue of great controversy.

have less capacity for bold fiscal expansion in new areas. This means managing existing programmes (in new ways perhaps, but in changing economic circumstances) necessarily assumes a larger share of the public agenda. Third, there is what might be termed the wearing out (perhaps wearing down) of the post-war consensus about the welfare state. By that I mean the effects of more than two decades of fretfulness about the affordability, desirability, and governability of the welfare state. The bulk of this ideological struggle took place, of course, within national borders, free from the spread of 'foreign' ideas. To the extent that similar arguments arose cross-nationally, as Kieke Okma has noted, mostly this represented 'parallel development'. But there are striking contemporary examples of the explicit international transfer and highlighting of welfare state commentary. Some of this takes place through think-tank networks; some takes place through media campaigns on behalf of particular figures; and, of course, some takes place through academic exchanges and official meetings. Charles Murray—the controversial author of *Losing Ground* (1984) and co-author of *The Bell Curve* (1994)—illustrates all three of these phenomena. The medium of transfer seems to have changed in the post-war period. Where the Beveridge Report would have been known to social policy elites very broadly, however much they used it, the modern form seems to be the long newspaper or magazine article and the media interview.

Criticisms of the welfare state began in earnest during the 1973–74 oil shock, were sustained by stagflation, and bolstered by electoral victories (or advance) of parties opposed to welfare state expansion. Critics assumed a bolder posture and mass publics came increasingly to hear challenges to programmes that had for decades seemed sacrosanct (Marmor et al, 1992)[6]. From Mulroney to Thatcher, from New Zealand to the Netherlands, the message of necessary change was heard. Accordingly, when economic strain reappears, the inner rim of programmatic protection—not interest group commitment, but social faith—is weaker and the incentives to explore transformative but not fiscally burdensome options become relatively stronger. That, I would suggest, helps to explain the clear international pattern of welfare state review, including health policy, over the past decade, a review that intensified as recession moved across national borders in 1990.[7]

Even accepting this contention, there still remains the question of why there appears to have been such increased attention in these reviews to other national experiences. The turning to American health policy experience seems particularly puzzling to those, like myself, preoccupied with American health care problems, ready, as laggards on coverage and cost control, to learn relevant lessons from

---

[6] The wider scholarly literature on the subject is the focus of a review essay, 'Understanding the Welfare State: Crisis, Critics, and Countercritics,' *Critical Review*, 1993; 7: 461–477.
[7] Here again, there is a need to distinguish between common pressures and common definitions of problems or remedies. The fact that welfare states everywhere faced strains does not entail a common definition of either problem or solution in health care matters. Canada and the United States faced quite similar fiscal strains over this period, but the policy-making debate differed enormously and results were vastly different.

others, and unclear about what American policy experience can teach about economy and effectiveness in delivery medical care.

But globalization of inquiry has undeniably taken place. Times of policy change sharply increase the demand for new ideas—or at least for new means to old ends. Just as many American analysts turned to Canada's example, so Canadian, German, Dutch, and other intellectual entrepreneurs turned their attention internationally in recent years. One sees why in the interests reported and expectations cited by conference participants at international meetings. For example, since 1994 there have been annual meetings of health policy analysts and commentators from Holland, Germany, Canada and the United States. When asked what they hope to learn from such gatherings, they reported the following. Many said they hoped to get better policy answers to the problems they face at home: how to find a balance between 'solidarity and subsidiarity', how to maintain a 'high quality health system in times of economic stress', even an optimistic query about 'what are the optimum relations between patients, insurers, providers, and the government'.

Understood as simply wanting to stretch one's mind—to explore what is possible conceptually, or what others have managed to achieve—this interest in comparative knowledge is unexceptionable. Understood as the pursuit of the best model, without further exploration of the political, social, and economic context required for implementation, this is wishful thinking.

The participants at many such international conferences see the opportunity for an informational version of this intellectual stretching: quests for exchange of 'policy information' of various sorts without commitment to policy importation, 'exchanging views with kindred spirits', and explicit calls for stimulation (as with the hope for 'specific initiatives [from other countries] to generate thoughts about Canada's system'). All of this is the learning anthropologists have long extolled—understanding the range of possibilities, seeing one's own circumstances more clearly by contrast, and so on.

But what about drawing policy lessons from such exercises? What are the rules of defensible conduct here and are they followed? The truth is that, whatever the appearances, most policy debates in most countries are (and will remain) parochial affairs. They address national problems, they emphasize historical and contemporary national developments in their particular domain (pensions, medical finance, transportation), and embody conflicting visions of what policies the particular country should adopt. Only rarely are the experiences of other nations, and the lessons they embody, seriously considered. When cross-national examples are employed in such parochial struggles, their use is typically that of policy warfare, not policy understanding and careful lesson-drawing. And, one must add, there are fewer knowledgeable critics at home of ideas about 'solutions' abroad, a further inducement once the will is there. In the world of American medical debate, the misuse of British and Canadian experience surely illustrates this point. The National Health Service was from the late 1940s to the late 1970s the spectre of what 'government medicine' and 'rationing' could mean. In recent years, the mythmaking about Canada has dominated the distortion league tables in North America (Evans *et al*, 1991; Marmor, 1994). The parochialism of national debates is the dominant truth, though this is less obvious in Scandinavia than, for example, in North America, or in discussions among German as against Dutch policy makers.

The reasons for parochialism are almost too obvious to cite. Policy makers are busy with day-to-day pressures. Practical concerns incline them, if they take the time for comparative inquiry, to pay more attention to what appears to work, not academic reasons for what is and is not transferable and why. Policy debaters— whether politicians, policy analysts or interest group figures—are in struggles, not seminars. Like lawyers, they seek victory, not illumination. For that purpose, compelling stories, whether well-substantiated or not, are more useful than careful conclusions. Interest groups, as their label suggests, have material and symbolic stakes in policy outcomes, not reputations for intellectual precision to protect. The political fight over the Clinton health plan vividly illustrates these generalizations. The number of interest groups with a stake in the Clinton plan's fate—given the nearly one trillion dollar medical economy—was enormous; there were more than 8,000 *registered* lobbyists alone in Washington and thousands more trying to influence the outcome under some other label. The estimates of expenditures on the battle are in the hundreds of millions; one trade association, The Pharmaceutical Manufacturer's Association, spent $7 million on 'public relations' by 1993. The most noted effort was that of the Health Insurance Association of America, the group representing the smaller insurers, who produced their infamous Harry and Louise advertisements.

None of these considerations are new, or surprising. But the increased flow of cross-national claims in health policy generates new reasons to reconsider the meaning of cross-national policy learning.

The real scope for cross-national learning

There is a sharp distinction, too seldom made, between learning about and learning from cross-national experience (Marmor and Klein, 1994). There are two possible bases for drawing strong policy lessons from the experience of others. Crudely put, one is what can be learned from quite similar collectivities. If conditions are broadly comparable—economically, politically, culturally—one can be reasonably confident that a particular policy is possible. That is to say, the policy might well be implementable, and, roughly speaking, the results in country A are likely to be the consequences in similar country B. In short, policy transplantability and structural similarity are closely linked. The Nordic nations, to the outsider, appear to provide many instances of this process. But with this form of learning comes constraints. The most promising, appealing, compelling policy 'answers' may, for instance, lie elsewhere, in a very different sort of society. What to do? Nothing necessarily, I would argue, but understanding that to be the case. That, of course, is another way of saying that learning about other national experiences is not the same as learning from them.

There is, however, one other form of lesson-drawing that is rare, but powerful. Some describe the enquiry as generalization from the widest variety of cases—the very opposite of a 'similar system' design. If a policy generalization holds over many divergent cases, some powerful factor is at work, something policy-makers and administrators ignore at their (and their constituents') peril. The logic is straightforward: if Q follows from policy Z in countries A to T, why should nation Z believe its experience will be different? Just as the most similar design narrows the range of findings, so too does the most different design narrow the scope. But in the latter instance the narrowing is not of countries, but of the likelihood that there will be a large number of such transplantable generalizations. One example might be that the costs of implementing new policies are always much larger than those estimated by their advocates. Another might be that wholesale transformation of the ways doctors are paid—a familiar yearning of health policy analysts—is almost never a practical option. If accepted, this lesson has practical importance for payment policy debates.

The following issues seem to me important in addressing these topics. What are the general rules, if any, that hold across seemingly different systems? What bearing do they have for the recurrent concerns that prompt international symposia and conferences in the first place? Have we learned something general about the persistence, prominence, and power of interest groups that transcends individual national stories? If so, on what sorts of policy choices are they most important, least important? And, finally, is it true that the exchanges involved in serious reviews of international experience are mind-stretching? If so, in what ways? (We know that much international discussion in health care is mind-numbing.)

These are the issues raised by this essay. They are not regularly found in the marketing hype that characterizes the 'global beat' in the health care media and consulting world. At the same time, this essay does not take up what for many poorer countries in the world is the main form of comparative health policy: namely, the transmission of model health care systems by funding agencies like the World Bank, the IMF, and the WHO. But that would be another chapter, one well worth doing.

Acknowledgement

This paper is based largely on a chapter by the author in *Health Policy Reform, National Variations and Globalization* (eds. Altenstetter C and Björkman JW) 1997, and is included by kind permission of the publishers: MacMillan Press in the UK and St Martin's Press in the US.

References

Evans RG, Barer ML, Hertzman. The 20-year experiment: accounting for, explaining, and evaluating health care cost containment in Canada and the United States. *Annual Review of Public Health*, 1991; **12**: 481–518

Hunter D. A new focus for dialogue. *European Health Reform: The Bulletin of the European Network and Database*, No. 1, March 1995, p 1

Klein R. Learning from others: shall the last be the first? (*Conference Report/Four Country Conference on Health Care Reforms and Health Care Policies in the US, Canada, Germany and the Netherlands, 23–25 February 1995*) The Hague: Ministry of Health, Welfare and Sport, pp 95–102

Klein R, O'Higgins M. Defusing the crisis of the welfare state: a new interpretation. In: Marmor TR, Mashaw JL (eds) *Social Security: Beyond the Rhetoric of Crisis*. Princeton: Princeton University Press, 1988, esp. pp 219–224

Marmor TR. Patterns of fact and fiction in use of the Canadian experience. In: Marmor TR (ed) *Understanding Health Care Reform*. New Haven: Yale University Press, 1994, pp 179–194

Marmor TR, Klein R. Rationing: painful prescription, inadequate diagnosis. In: Marmor TR (ed) *Understanding Health Care Reform*. New Haven: Yale University Press, 1994, pp107–119

Marmor TR, Mashaw JL. Rhetoric and reality. *Health Management Quarterly*, 1993; **15**: 21–24

Marmor TR, Mashaw J. Hype and hyperbole in health care reform. In: Marmor TR (ed) *Understanding Health Care Reform*. New Haven: Yale University Press, 1994, pp 170–175

Marmor TR, Mashaw JL, Harvey PL. *America's Misunderstood Welfare State: Persistent Myths, Continuing Realities*. New York: Harper Collins, 1992, esp. ch.3

Marmor TR, Plowden P. Rhetoric and reality in the intellectual jet stream: the export to Britain from America of questionable ideas. *Journal of Health Politics, Policy and Law*, 1991; **16**: 807–812

7
Reforms to financing systems in poor countries

Barbara McPake

London School of Hygiene & Tropical Medicine, UK

Financing alternatives describe routes for finance to flow from households (or external sources) to health service providers. Figure 7.1 describes, in a simplified manner, the alternative routes available.[1] Options can be divided into voluntary flows, flows related to the compulsory system, and external flows.

Voluntary flows include direct out-of-pocket payments and voluntary insurance. Direct out-of-pocket payments made to health service providers are unique among all the flows shown in that they do not involve an intermediate institution between the household and the service providers. Such out-of-pocket payments are most commonly made on a fee-for-service basis but under health maintenance organization (HMO) type arrangements, service providers directly act as insurers and receive payments in the form of premia. The well-known Bwamanda hospital insurance scheme in Zaire is an example of such a scheme in a poor country (Kutzin and Barnum, 1992; La Forgia and Griffin, 1993), a mission hospital-based insurance programme has been reported in Kenya (McFarlane, 1996), there are a number of further examples in Africa and Asia (Creese and Bennett, 1997) and many in South America (Tollman *et al*, 1990; Banco Interamericano de Desarollo (BID), 1996). To avoid confusion with characteristics specific to the USA, this chapter will refer to such arrangements as 'direct insurance'. Other types of pre-payment, such as payment for a set number of visits in advance, can be found in the literature (for example, Stormer, 1994). However,

---

[1] The figure is neither wholly original nor wholly derivative from any one source. Griffiths and Mills (1983), Evans (1981), and Hurst (1992) use similar diagrams to describe financing flows. The list of financing flow options used to develop the diagram was taken from WHO (1996).

voluntary insurance more usually involves a private insurance agency acting as an intermediary between households and service providers. Such agencies are common, for example, in Latin American countries (BID, 1996).

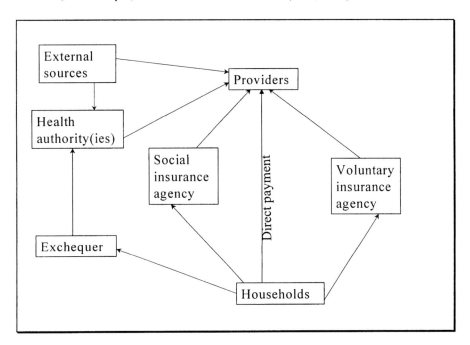

Figure 7.1

Compulsory flows require either a social insurance system or a tax-funded system. Social insurance systems imply separate identified payments for social insurance from those for tax, a separate system handling receipt and expenditure of premia (separate from the Ministry of Health), and 'earmarked' funds for social insurance benefits (increasingly, separate components of social insurance have separately earmarked funds but this is not universal). This implies at least one (and often many) social insurance agencies acting as intermediaries between households and service providers. In contrast, tax-funded systems route finances through the national exchequer, most funds are usually not earmarked and the health service budget is therefore subject to determination through periodic national (or sometimes sub-national) expenditure rounds, and there are at least two if not several layers (national, regional, district) of intermediaries between households and service providers. Some taxes are not directly paid by households (such as taxes on foreign investment for example) but may be indirectly so.

External financial flows reach service providers in a variety of ways. Multilateral and bilateral agencies most commonly make grants and loans to national government bodies. Non-governmental sources may directly support a single or group of service providers or operate their own projects.

While Figure 7.1 aims principally to express the options available to a country to direct flows of finance through intermediate institutions and to service providers, in some countries, especially some of the poorest, the diagram expresses the set of flows all of which are active. For example, BID (1996) describes the co-existence of all these types of flows as typical of the largest group of countries in Latin America and the Caribbean, and the routes can be seen to respond to the different categories of 'entitlement' (Frenk and Donabedian, 1987). In contrast, in many countries in Africa and Asia, both voluntary and social insurance are either absent or trivial in importance.

Much of the debate so far rehearsed on the subject of financing health services in developing countries can be seen to concern the implications of choosing each of these routes for equity, efficiency, appropriateness of services or other objective of health systems. The rest of the debate concerns the modalities and rules governing the flows: for example, whether the results are better (from any perspective) when insurance agencies (of any type), or public health authorities within a tax-based system, reimburse service providers by budgets (global or itemized), fee-for-service, capitation, or case-based payments (such as DRGs); what regime of co-payments and deductibles best controls moral hazard while avoiding important types of access loss; and so on.

Many health sector reform issues which are not typically considered as issues of financing are also captured as changes in flows of finances through the system and the rules governing them. All three flows which involve one or more intermediary financial institution can be organized as 're-imbursement', 'contract' or 'integrated' models (OECD, 1995). Whether or not public health authorities within a tax-based system, or insurance agencies of any type, directly own or contract with service providers determines the rules governing flows of finances between the two, but raises all the issues of 'managed competition' and 'purchaser-provider' splits. How funds within a tax-based system flow between exchequer, national, regional and district levels encompasses some of the debate on decentralization.

This chapter aims to broaden the debate about financing alternatives, to emphasize the interrelatedness of financing flows and of 'financing' reform with other components of reform programmes. Throughout, it will assume that the objectives of the health financing system are to support those of the health system as a whole which are to maximize the health status of the public. This implies both efficiency and equity concerns, since it emphasizes the role played by alternative financing mechanisms in allocating resources on the basis of need defined as: 'the minimum amount of resources required to exhaust a person's capacity to benefit' (Culyer, 1995). For shorthand, throughout the chapter this will be referred to as a 'public health objective'.

Reform options

This section aims to catalogue and briefly discuss the main options for organizing and regulating each of the four main financial flows identified in Figure 7.1 (external flows will be ignored because they are not fully under national policy control).

Taxation

Most of the poorer countries of Africa and Asia have planned that their health systems be dominated by a taxation-based financing flow to the extent of having legally abolished or severely restricted private provision in some (for example, Tanzania and Malawi[2]) and private insurance in others (for example, India). While in practice, tax-based funding has usually been less dominant than planned (see below), it remains important in all countries and strengthening this financial flow has high priority in the reform agendas of poor countries.

The largely public nature of the financing flow related to taxation implies greater likelihood of pursuit of a public health objective through this route. However, it is not an original observation that the incentives present do not exert strong pressure in favour of this role. Arguments commonly voiced in this respect are that the virtually unassailable employment rights and status of civil servants in many countries result in a lack of pressure for in-post performance; there are counter-efficiency incentives implicit in traditional budgeting systems; over-centralized systems are unresponsive to the needs of populations remote from the capital city; and there is a lack of market discipline enforcing efficiency throughout the public sector.

Examples of widespread inefficiency, corruption and pursuit of vested interests are not difficult to encounter. For example, Heiby (1996) provides a list of studies which consistently show the large gap between the care aimed to be provided and that actually provided in the public sector. This evidence suggests that deficiencies in incentive structures are not in general surmounted by the various planning, supervision and training measures traditionally advanced as the mechanisms to improve public sector performance. Where finance is public, poor performance tends to prevail even where provision is private (McPake and Hongoro, 1993). Public sector agents seem to fail as purchasers for the same reasons they fail as providers.

Recent years have witnessed a number of reform initiatives which aim to address such problems in achieving effective use of finances flowing through the taxation route. Civil service reform aims to reduce an overweight bureaucracy which undermines the efficiency of the system, and to introduce incentives to

---

[2] In both these countries the regulations have been relaxed (see Ngalande-Banda and Walt, 1995; Mujinja *et al*, 1993), an example of a policy discussed below.

improve the performance of public employees (Cassels, 1995). Beyond the health sector, it aims to improve the efficiency of the taxation system itself, one area where it has been seen to be highly effective in some countries (*The Economist*, 1996). Budgetary reform aims to introduce incentives to improved efficiency within budgeting systems by giving efficient managers more rather than less resources to manage and attempting to relate budgets to outputs rather than to previous spending levels (Issaka-Tinorgah and Waddington, 1993). Decentralization aims to move decision-making closer to the people affected and is intended to enable management, planning and policy functions to achieve greater efficiency and effectiveness (Mills *et al*, 1990; Collins, 1996). Movement from more traditional integrated models towards contract models has been argued to imply a different, 'market approach' to addressing the problems of the public sector (Mills, 1995), although it is possible to argue that reforms such as devolved budgeting have a similar 'quasi-market' orientation. 'Managed market reforms' aim to create competition among providers, and sometimes purchasers, by introducing contracting mechanisms and granting autonomous status to public actors while allowing purchasers or patients choice between providers (sometimes both public and private), and in some models, patients choice between purchasers (Enthoven, 1985; Mills, 1995).

Assessment of the effectiveness and efficiency of taxation-based financing flows therefore depends on assessment of the effectiveness and efficiency of the reform measures available to improve the management of public finances from their collection through to their application in purchasing health services for the population. While much of the evidence of the reviews cited above suggests that experience to date with such reforms has largely been disappointing, as yet experience is limited.

Social insurance

The defining characteristic of social insurance is that it is 'mandated': for at least some of the population, purchase of insurance is compulsory. This population usually constitutes a middle section of the market in poor countries. In most cases the agencies responsible for social insurance are public or quasi-public. Korea is unique in having achieved widespread coverage of social insurance based on private agencies (Chollet and Lewis, 1997). Social insurance agencies have a certain degree of autonomy given their independent financing and administrative structures, but are regulated by public codes of administration and influenced by substantial government participation and other types of political intervention (BID, 1996). The pressures to pursue a public health agenda are likely to be present but are less direct and likely to be weaker than in a tax-based system.

In comparison with ministries of health and health authorities, there is therefore likely to be greater incentive to respond to demand and perceived quality pressures.

However, much depends on the further rules governing financial flows and the institutions of social insurance themselves. In Latin American countries, those socially insured have traditionally had no choice regarding their insurer, and it is a prerequisite of social insurance that there is no opting out of the system (to the extent that recent reforms allow opting out entirely, they weaken their 'social' aspect). As in the case of public provision through taxation, there is an abundance of evidence of widespread dissatisfaction with social insurance provision in Latin America. Most countries in the region of Latin America are characterized by the coexistence of social insurance provision for formal sector workers, public health services for lower income groups, and private services for the richest and those excluded from the other services. In these countries, the problems of the public and social insurance sector health services are similar: poor and over-centralized resource management, poor quality, under-resourced services and low utilization (BID, 1996).

Inefficiency and cost-containment are major concerns influencing reforms to social insurance systems where falling income levels and rising costs have produced crisis in the systems of many countries (Mesa Lago, 1997) and lack of incentives for cost control alone is the dominant problem in others (Xing-Yuan and Sheng-Lan, 1995). At the same time, poor performance of social insurance institutions in the eyes of their affiliates has led in Latin American countries to the phenomenon of 'double insurance', in which richer population groups purchase private insurance in addition to paying social insurance contributions. These forces have prompted the marked current of reform in Latin American systems in favour of competition and affiliate choice of insurer, evidenced for example in Chile, where affiliates can now choose a private insurer in place of the relevant social one (Viveros-Long, 1986; Aedo and Larranaga, 1994; Jimenez de la Jara and Bossert, 1995), and in Colombia where all social insurance agencies and private agencies are now competing with each other for affiliates (Jaramillo, 1994; Fundación Corona et al, 1997). These types of reform also dominate the reform agendas of countries less advanced in the process such as Peru and Argentina, where private insurance companies are being allowed to compete with traditional social ones, for example (Government of Peru, 1997; Lloyd Sherlock, 1998). Such reforms introduce pressures for efficiency and consumer responsiveness that were absent before; at the same time, weakening other pressures previously exerted to promote public health objectives. Yepes and Sánchez (this volume) argue that epidemiological surveillance has suffered in the wake of the Colombian reforms.

Low coverage and lack of solidarity are usually identified as among the principal problems of social insurance systems in all poor countries (McGreevy, 1990; Kutzin and Barnum, 1992). Expanding coverage is therefore usually a primary explicit objective of social insurance systems and strongly influences the reform programmes and intentions of many social insurance systems such as that of Colombia which has set itself the goal of universal coverage by the year 2000 (Jaramillo, 1994; Mesa Lago, 1997). Some Latin American systems (for example, Uruguay, Chile, Ecuador and Costa Rica) extend the services offered by the main

social insurance institutions to indigents (Mesa Lago, 1997). Under both these
arrangements, the public health role of the social insurance institutes is much
stronger and the distinction between tax-based and social security-based funding
becomes very weak.[3]

Voluntary insurance

Voluntary insurance exists in the formal, urban sector, largely serving richer
groups of the population, and in the informal, rural sector as a means of extending
access to services to the poor. As with social insurance, it can be 'indirect' or
'direct' (direct arrangements are discussed in the following section), and can by
administered by public or private bodies, but voluntary insurance—especially the
formal, urban type—is more usually administered privately. Creese and Bennett
(1997) propose a distinction between 'Type 1' insurance which focuses on high
cost, low frequency events, and 'Type 2' insurance which focuses on low cost, high
frequency events.

Urban, formal voluntary insurance forms at most a small part of the market in
most poor countries. Within Africa, South Africa, Egypt, Côte d'Ivoire, Kenya,
Nigeria and Zimbabwe are the only countries where private insurance has a
significant presence (Chollet and Lewis, 1997). South Africa's Medical Aid
Schemes (voluntary and private) are the largest financial flow in the South African
system, contributing 43% of the total (van den Heever, 1997). There is very little
private, voluntary insurance in Asia. Even so, in India where despite severe
restrictions on private insurance, coverage is 3.3%, the resultant 33 million people
covered is the largest number of individuals covered in any poor country (Chollet
and Lewis, 1997). In Latin American and Caribbean countries, voluntary insurance
arrangements are extensive (Chollet and Lewis, 1997) and have also been growing
significantly, especially in the Dominican Republic (BID, 1996).

This type of voluntary insurance appears least conducive to cost control. In
South Africa, cost inflation averaged approximately 6.8% over the 1980s and was
approximately 17% and 12% in 1990 and 1991 respectively (van den Heever,
1997). These figures compare to the peak figures for insurance premium inflation
in the United States between 1988 and 1992 of 13.6% per annum (*The Economist*,
1998). The US provides the only prominent example of a voluntary insurance-
dominated system. Concern for cost control by private insurance agencies is
evidenced by low-benefit ceilings and many exclusions (in Turkey and Brazil for
example), or highly differentiated packages in which only the most expensive
cover 'catastrophic' care (in Argentina for example) (Chollet and Lewis, 1997).

---

[3] Normand (1997) makes the point that the two are analytically similar but distinct with
respect to attitudes and rhetoric. With respect to existence of specified rights, choice of
provider and greater patient participation in decision-making, social security systems more
closely resemble private insurance.

This implies 'Type 2' focus (Creese and Bennett, 1997) and implicit reliance on the public sector as the 'insurer of last resort' (Chollett and Lewis, 1997). In theory there should be some pressure for internal efficiency in this context. Much depends on the nature of the market and competition, and other conditions in which voluntary insurance agencies operate. In addition to adopting explicit priority setting mechanisms (usually the definition of intervention exclusion lists), private insurance companies ration using co-payments, deductibles and premium setting based on claims experience, while public agencies face overwhelming constraints in achieving explicit rationing rules (Bobadilla, 1996). It is arguable that the past failure to control costs of third-party insurance in the US owed as much to regulation of the industry and rules regarding tax exemption, which inhibited competition, as to the inherent characteristics of third-party voluntary insurance (*The Economist*, 1998). Like the US system, the South African system is dominated by employer contributions, fee-for-service reimbursement and tax deductions (van den Heever, 1997).

Urban, formal, voluntary insurance covers only richer groups of the population and is expected to generate problems of adverse selection (exit of lower risk affiliates in the face of imperfectly risk-adjusted premia) and of moral hazard (excessive use of services by the insured). Both these problems are prevalent in the South African system. According to van den Heever (1997), until 1989, medical aid schemes were legally required to offer premia levels based only on income and family size. Competition from insurance agencies not covered by the legislation attracted some of the lowest risk affiliates although restrictions on the type of insurance they were allowed to offer prevented major flight. Pressure from the increasingly profit-seeking agencies to change the legal basis on which premia could be set resulted in 1989 reforms allowing risk-based premia. This has resulted in competition between schemes based on 'cost shifting'. Identification of 'moral hazard' requires a definition of 'excessive use' of health services which is difficult to specify. Nevertheless, van den Heever (1997) estimates a health expenditure *per capita* among the highest income group, all of which flows through the medical aid schemes, to be 35 times as high as those of the lowest income group and reports concerns of moral hazard among those of the Commission set up to review private health care. There are strong incentives to individualize risk assessment through 'under writing', 'tiered rating' and 'durational rating' which run directly counter to the pursuit of public health objectives (Chollet and Lewis, 1997).

In any private sector context, the role of regulation is crucial in determining the nature of incentives affecting institutions, and the extent of pressure to pursue public objectives (Bennett *et al*, 1994; Kumaranayake, 1996). The effectiveness of the regulatory system, and the potential effectiveness of a reformed regulatory system, therefore have strong influence on the implications of increasing the role of voluntary insurance agencies. Van den Heever (1997) suggests that appropriate regulation could be used to pursue cost containment and expanded coverage of medical aid schemes by protecting community-rated arrangements, obstructing individual risk-rated arrangements and institutionalizing cross-subsidy between high- and low-income groups. However, Chollet and Lewis (1997) argue that regulation of private insurance in poor countries has focused principally on ensuring solvency and accountability rather than pursuing public health objectives, and has been generally weak as a result of inadequate regulatory frameworks and weak institutional capacity. Where Chollet and Lewis' rather than van den Heever's conclusions are likely to apply, discouragement of this type of voluntary insurance might be more conducive to achieving public health objectives. The World Bank's current health, nutrition and population strategy concludes that: 'Because of cost and the pronounced market failure that occurs in private health insurance, this is not a viable option for risk pooling at the national level in low- and middle-income countries' (World Bank, 1997).

At local level, there are a number of obvious difficulties in establishing insurance: it is difficult to identify beneficiaries; it is difficult to assess their incomes; it is difficult to collect contributions, and it is difficult to mandate coverage and thereby avoid adverse selection (Creese and Bennett, 1997). Despite this, commentators have reached more optimistic conclusions regarding rural and informal insurance arrangements (for example Chabot et al, 1991; Arhin,1995). Creese and Bennett (1997) have produced the most comprehensive review of rural risk-sharing strategies available. Their evidence suggests that the optimism of other authors is more usually based on enthusiasm for the theoretical advantages of the model of local risk sharing over user charges, than concrete evidence of the ability of such arrangements to perform against efficiency and equity criteria. Arhin (1995) argues that there is evidence of substantial willingness to pay for insurance packages within the rural informal sector although Normand (1997) notes that claimed willingness to pay may or may not prove real willingness to pay when tested.

Direct payments to providers

Service providers (whether public, private or quasi-public)[4] directly receive payments from patients where user fees are levied, managed and retained for use at the facility's discretion, and where direct insurance arrangements operate. This financing flow appears to be one of the most important in the health financing systems of poor countries. For example, a World Bank study found that 75% of total health spending originated from private out-of-pocket sources in India, 82% of primary health care (PHC) spending and 92% of curative PHC spending. The proportions were higher in rural areas and among the lowest income groups (quoted in Berman, 1996). Another World Bank study estimates that private expenditure constitutes 41% of the total in China, 53% in sub-Saharan Africa and 49% in Latin America and the Caribbean (Govindaraj et al, 1995). The latter

---

[4] An example of quasi-public health care provision organizations can be found in the Curative Care Organizations of Egypt (Berman, 1996).

estimates include indirect voluntary insurance. Much of the innovation in health financing systems in the poorest economies has increased this type of financial flow. User charges have dominated the health financing reform agenda in the majority of African and Asian countries (Creese and Kutzin, 1995), and direct insurance arrangements in Latin American countries such as Ecuador, Peru, Paraguay and Venezuela (BID, 1996), and South Africa (van den Heever, 1997) have been growing. Many policies to strengthen the role of private providers in the health care system also increase the role of this type of financing flow (direct from patients to providers) in the health financing system.

Experience with the introduction of user fees for public health service providers has generally been disappointing, resulting in falls in utilization with public health implications (for example user fees might have been responsible for a resurgence of TB in China (World Bank, 1993)), inability to raise sufficient revenue to meet minimal quality standards (Ogunbekun et al, 1995), failure to raise significant revenue (Creese, 1990) or even to collect money (Hecht et al, 1993), and failure to protect the poor through exemptions (Willis, 1993; Kutzin, 1994; Gilson et al, 1995). Much of the problem may derive from the weaknesses of public sector institutions discussed above. Thus better experience with user charges might follow from effective civil service reform, budgetary reform, introduction of market mechanisms in the public sector or decentralization. Supporting the idea that failure with user charge policy derives from more general public sector failure, more successful examples have tended to derive from externally supported projects (Litvack and Bodart, 1993; Diop et al, 1995) and projects operated on a 'community financing' basis (McPake et al, 1993) with which there is important overlap with external support. The greater success of community-level schemes may also support the notion that over-centralization is one of the crucial public sector failures involved. Design features of user charge policy itself are also important in determining its success or failure and sensible lists of such features have been proposed (Creese and Kutzin, 1995; Gilson and Mills, 1995).

In theory, direct insurance produces incentives for efficiency by forcing service providers to absorb the risk inherent in an insurance system (see Scheffler, this volume). Where independent insurance agencies play this role, providers who have most influence on resource use decisions have fewer incentives to control costs. Many are convinced of the effectiveness of the integration of the insurance and provision function in the USA where HMOs have been shown to reduce hospital admissions (Welch et al, 1984; Manning et al, 1984). However evidence that this strategy significantly reduces overall hospital costs is contested.[5] Experience of

---

[5] The conventional wisdom is that HMOs have reduced not only hospital admissions but also average length of stay and elective procedures (for example Scutchfield et al, 1997) However, the interrelationships between variables are complex: there may be selection bias in HMO populations and local HMO growth rates may be determined by differences in market characteristics and thereby cause false attribution of the effect of growth on market outcomes. McLaughlin (1987) estimates a slight but insignificant effect of HMOs on overall hospital costs, and suggests that other cost control strategies (physician supply and rate

direct insurance in the context of poor countries is less well documented. Best documented is another project which has had substantial external support, the Bwamanda health zone project in Zaire, which confirms the ability of such structures to control cost escalation (Kutzin and Barnum, 1992). Ramirez and colleagues (1997) report experience of an NGO pre-natal care clinic in Mexico in trying to operate a direct insurance programme. The clinic failed to attract sufficient demand for the insurance package owing to the development of cheaper competition in the area, and poor productivity. To survive, the clinic will have to improve productivity and reduce the cost of the insurance package offered, demonstrating the 'market sanction' side of the pressures for efficiency. While in the US, major concerns relating to HMOs focus on quality (employers choose which HMO to enrol with, so may overemphasize cost relative to quality (*The Economist*, 1998)), concerns voiced with respect to the Zaire programme focus on inequity in utilization patterns between the insured and uninsured, and probably adverse selection (Kutzin and Barnum, 1992). The Bwamanda project achieved a cost recovery rate of 79% in 1988 (La Forgia and Griffin, 1993) which compares to rates achieved using user charges in similarly locally based and externally supported projects. However, successful experiments with direct insurance in poor countries has been rare, with Bwamanda the exception rather than rule, and Creese and Bennett (1997) argue that this model is not to be recommended for rural, informal sector risk sharing.

Planning a mix of financial flows

Reforms and less deliberate changes relating to one financial flow cannot be expected to be neutral in their effects on others. Maceira (1996; analysis described in BID, 1996) analyses the effects of public sector changes on the other sub-sectors of the health system, and the nature of the recourse to health services of different population groups in a Latin American country characterized by multiple sub-health systems. The analysis assumes an initial tripartite system with a public sector serving the lower half of the income distribution, a social insurance sector serving an upper-middle income group, and a private sector serving the rich. Public sector expenditure reduction causes a richer section of the lower-income group to seek

---

setting) are more likely to explain reduction in premium inflation rates in the USA. McLaughlin (1988) suggests that even the effect of lower admission rates in HMOs is offset by resulting higher admission rates in the non-HMO sector. Zellner and Wolfe (1989) challenge the model specification but Hill and Wolfe (1997) also failed to detect a significant impact on cost of increasing HMO-type competition in the State of Wisconsin. Feldman *et al* (1993) estimate that firms which offer HMO options increase average health insurance premia. Both HMO and fee-for-service premia were higher in these firms. Nevertheless, Baker (1997) estimates that increase in HMO market share from 20 to 30% reduces expenditure on fee-for-service health care by 3 to 7%.

care in the private sector. Falling formal sector employment (perhaps resulting from civil service reform or otherwise from general economic recession) causes a group of those previously utilizing social insurance to shift to recourse to the public sector. The combined strain on the public sector results in an unserved population group among the poorest. Finally, growing NGO provision adds a further layer of services offered to poorer groups and reduces the extent of the unserved population to some extent. While this particular mix of options is most relevant to Latin American countries, other countries' systems such as that of Thailand appear to have similar features. Maceira's analysis demonstrates the interdependence of health sub-systems, and the need to consider the effects of proposed reforms on the whole health system.

Changing the rules governing one financial flow can be designed with the objective of controlling or influencing activity covered by another, or can have unintended effects on another. For example, Argentinean reforms may succeed in channelling social insurance finances into public hospitals by improving record keeping and billing and charging social insurance funds for care received in public hospitals by their members. If so, public finance flows may be more efficiently targeted towards their intended beneficiaries (Lloyd-Sherlock, 1998).

Musgrove (1996) describes the situation in Brazil:

> There is an overall ceiling on expenditure, not just for the whole country but also at the level of the states and, where cities administer services, at the municipal level as well. Once all the budget allocation for a state is spent, continued payment for services becomes the responsibility of the state government. In addition to this financial limitation, there is a physical cap: the Ministry limits itself to paying for hospitalisation for no more than nine percent of the population in each state. This policy was adopted as an incentive for ambulatory treatment as a substitute for hospital admission. If a state reaches the limit, it can continue to receive federal funds for ambulatory services until reaching the financial cap.

The intended impact of physical caps on hospital services spans public and private services since the Ministry of Health has contracts with both. It implies also unintended impacts on 'unmet need', purchase of private insurance and use of directly paid private services as implications of shifting public expenditures reverberate through the system. The complexity of the rules governing public flows makes these effects particularly difficult to predict and plan for.

Jönsson and Musgrove (1997) argue that if a single flow of finance is dominant, it is easier to control and plan financing systems, and risks of sub-optimization through inadequate co-ordination of flows are minimized. Given that most feasible changes to financing systems will be incremental, few countries will count the adoption of a single flow dominant system among their range of options. Nevertheless, some countries may consider moving in this direction as a goal. Brazil, Costa Rica and Nicaragua have achieved integration of their social security and public health systems, for example (BID, 1996) and other Latin American countries such as Mexico and Colombia aim for this.

However in countries which have inherited more unified health systems, current financing reforms often aim to create a more diverse mix. Many African countries are attempting to introduce or strengthen insurance mechanisms (for example, Kenya; see Mwabu, 1995), while India is relaxing restrictions on private insurance (*The Economist*, 1997). The implicit rationale is that more sources of finance imply greater total availability of resources for the system. This recognizes the limited tax base in some countries which may be fully or even overexploited, but may be misguided if the principal problem for the public health system is absolute shortage of health specific resources, especially health care professionals. Where this applies (it is not ubiquitous—doctors, at least, are in excess supply in some South Asian and Latin American countries), there is a danger that adding voluntary insurance options to the existing mix increases the already competitive environment for such scarce resources with the result that even less is available to the public sector. In these cases there is greatest need to justify diversification of the financing mix by demonstrating that activities financed by new flows will be public health oriented.

Conclusions

Financing reform has typically been considered to consist of changing sources of finance and changing the rules by which financial flows are governed. This chapter has argued that reform of the activities financed by each flow is in practice inextricable from reform of the flow itself. Thus, reforms to taxation systems and social insurance systems, and to the rules governing resource allocation in the public and social insurance sectors, will not be effective if broader 'public sector reform' is ignored. This implies tackling the causes of public sector failure through measures such as civil service reform, budgetary reform, decentralization and managed market reforms. This conclusion applies to the introduction of user charges, initial enthusiasm for which seems to have been premised on the assumption that public sector failure could be attributed to a single cause: lack of finance (Akin *et al*, 1987). The unimpressive results associated with pursuit of this policy, especially where external actors are not present to minimize the impact of public sector failure, can be attributed to the lack of such a 'multi-pronged' approach.

It is also now more commonly recognized that real policy choices are seldom about choosing user charges, insurance or a taxation system as the basis for a financing system, but about making incremental changes to a given mix of financial flows. Thus countries whose systems are dominated by taxation or social insurance, for example, are likely to gain most from considering reforms that will make those systems work better and only to a lesser extent, gain from changing the mix of financial flows, for example introducing more direct flows from patient to provider. Policy makers are now more likely to realize that the challenge is to plan a coherent financing mix which aims to maximize public health, with the efficiency and equity considerations that implies.

Whether reforming existing financing flows, or introducing new ones, the need to assess and direct (using regulation or complementary reforms) the nature of competition between and within financing flows is an overriding theme of reform across the world. Thus for financing flows with a public or compulsory nature, the introduction and management of competition is a main concern, whereas for financing flows with a private or voluntary nature, where competition has been the norm, the improvement and design of regulation have been dominant concerns.

These new and proposed arrangements imply a convergence of public sector incentive structures with private ones. Public service providers now have to 'sell' their services and at least some part of their budget depends on them doing so. This shifts the incentives they face towards trying to meet the demands of those who can pay. Whether this represents a significant movement away from trying to meet the needs of all, and especially the poorest, depends on the extent to which pressure to meet this objective had effectively been exercised under previous arrangements. In some cases, effective privatization of public sector activity pre-dates the formal implementation of reforms (Asiimwe *et al*, 1997)

Whether or not any of these arrangements will increase incentives to efficiency depends on the market situation and demand pressures of the service provider institutions. Lack of competition in rural areas of poor countries weakens the extent to which incentives to efficiency are exerted. The rules governing the payment of direct subsidies to public provider institutions, which in almost all cases continue under user charge arrangements and sometimes under insurance arrangements, also exert strong influence on the incentives to efficiency present. There is an underlying conflict between guaranteeing support to the institution and its surrounding community, especially when there is no competition, and exerting pressure for efficiency improvement through finance. Inevitably the continued provision of services to a given community takes priority over the effort to achieve efficiency improvements, and direct financing arrangements seem to have exerted extremely weak pressure for efficiency improvement. The evidence that competitive pressures, where present, effectively increase efficiency is in any case mixed and unclear (Bennett, 1996; 1997; McPake, 1997).

Regulation can be used to direct private sector activity (and other regulated activity) towards pursuit of a public health objective; and therefore towards meeting needs rather than demands. To the extent that it succeeds, pressures towards convergence of public and private sectors (and compulsory and voluntary financial flows) can be seen to operate in both directions. Equally, some policies to expand the role of private service providers, attempt to increase the incentives for private providers to pursue public objectives (Berman and Rose, 1996; Swan and Zwi, 1997). Experience with regulation has not been encouraging (Kumaranayake, 1996), but the issue has received very little attention in poor countries until recently. Regulation failure is itself a special case of public sector failure suggesting a simple conclusion: public sector objectives, including public health objectives, cannot feasibly be pursued in the absence of a competent public sector.

These two currents equally—the introduction of competitive pressures in public, compulsory health sub-sectors, and the strengthening of regulation in private, voluntary sub-sectors—might be classified as constituting the full range of 'managed market' reforms. In many, if not most countries, actual reform has been scarce, but these themes have almost universally marked debates and agendas. Their success will depend on the extent to which difficulties in achieving the objectives of managed competition and improved regulation can be overcome, in turn perhaps dependent on the success of other public sector reforms. Given the early stage of those few countries that have started to adopt reforms, it is premature either confidently to predict failure, or to proclaim an 'evidence base' for such reform efforts.

Acknowledgement

Barbara McPake is a member of the Health Economics and Financing Programme which is supported by the UK Department for International Development (DFID).

References

Aedo C, Larranaga O. *Sistema de entrega de los servicios sociales: una agenda para la reforma*. Chile: Banco Internacional de Desarollo, 1994

Akin JS et al. *Agenda for Reform*. Washington DC: World Bank, 1987

Arhin DC. Rural health insurance: a viable alternative to user fees. London: London School of Hygiene & Tropical Medicine. PHP publication no. 19, 1995

Asiimwe D, McPake B, Mwesigye F et al. The private sector activities of public sector health workers in Uganda. In Bennett S, McPake B, Mills A (eds) *Private Health Providers in Developing Countries: Serving the Public Interest*. New Jersey: Zed Books, 1997, pp 141–157

Baker LC. The effects of HMOs on fee-for-service health care expenditures: evidence from Medicare. *Journal of Health Economics*, 1997; **16**: 453–481

Banco Interamericano de Desarrollo (BID). *Progreso Economico y Social en America Latina, Informe 1996, Tema Especial: Como organizar con exito los servicios sociales*, 1996

Bennett S, Dakpallah G, Garner P et al. Carrot and stick: state mechanisms to influence private provider behaviour, *Health Policy and Planning*, 1994; **9**, 1–13

Bennett S. The public/private mix in health care systems. In: Janovsky K (ed) *Health Policy and Systems Development: an Agenda for Research*. WHO/SHS/NHP/96.1. Geneva: World Health Organization, 1996, pp 101–123

Bennett S. The nature of competition among private hospitals in Bangkok. In: Bennett S, McPake B, Mills A (eds) *Private Health Providers in Developing Countries: Serving the Public Interest*. New Jersey: Zed Books, 1997, pp 102–123

Berman P. The role of the private sector in health financing and provision. In: Janovsky K (ed) *Health Policy and Systems Development: an Agenda for Research* WHO/SHS/NHP/96.1. Geneva: World Health Organization, 1996, pp 125–145

Berman P, Rose L. The role of private providers in maternal and child health and family planning services in developing countries. *Health Policy and Planning*, 1996; **11**: 142–155

Bobadilla JL. Priority setting and cost effectiveness. In: Janovsky K (ed) *Health Policy and Systems Development: an Agenda for Research*. WHO/SHS/NHP/96.1. Geneva: World Health Organization, 1996, pp 43–60

Cassels A. *Health sector reform: key issues in less developed countries*. Forum on health sector reform, discussion paper No. 1. WHO/SHS/NHP/95.4. Geneva: World Health Organization, 1995

Chabot J, Boal M, da Silva A. National community health insurance at village level: the case from Guinea Bissau. *Health Policy and Planning*, 1991; **6**: 46–54

Chollet D, Lewis M. Private insurance: principles and practice. In: Schieber GJ (ed) *Innovations in Health Care Financing: Proceedings of a World Bank Conference*. March 10–11, 1997. World Bank Discussion Paper no. 365.Washington DC: World Bank, 1997

Collins C. Decentralization. In: Janovsky K (ed*) Health Policy and Systems Development: an Agenda for Research*. WHO/SHS/NHP/96.1. Geneva: World Health Organization, 1996, pp 161–178

Creese A. *User charges for health care: a review of recent experience*. Current Concerns, SHS Paper No. 1. WHO/SHS/CC/90.1. World Health Organization: Geneva,1990

Creese A., Bennett S. Rural risk sharing strategies. In: Schieber GJ (ed*) Innovations in Health Care Financing: Proceedings of a World Bank Conference*. March 10–11, 1997. World Bank Discussion Paper no. 365. Washington DC: World Bank, 1997

Creese, A, Kutzin J. Lessons from cost recovery in health. Forum on Health Development Discussion Paper No 2. WHO/SHS/NHP/95.5 Geneva: World Health Organization, 1995

Culyer AJ. Need: the idea won't do but we still need it. *Social Science and Medicine*, 1995; **40**: 727–730

Diop F, Yazbeck A, Bitran R. The impact of alternative cost recovery schemes on access and equity in Niger. *Health Policy and Planning*, 1995; **10**: 223–240

The Economist. Born again to gather Uganda's tax. 27 January 1996

The Economist. India looks east. 8 March 1997

The Economist. Patients or Profits, and Health Care in America: Your money or your life? 7 March 1998

Enthoven A. *Reflections on the Management of the NHS*. London: Nuffield Provincial Hospitals Trust, 1985

Evans RG. Incomplete vertical integration: the distinctive structure of the health care industry. In: van der Gaag J, Perlman M (eds) *Health, Economics, and Health Economics*, Amsterdam: North-Holland, 1981

Feldman R, Dowd B, Gifford G. The effect of HMOs on premiums in employment based health plans. *Health Services Research*, 1993; **27**: 779–811

Frenk J, Donabedian A. State intervention in medical care: types, trends and variables *Health Policy and Planning*, 1987; **2**: 17–31

Fundación Corona, Associación Colombiana de la Salud, Fundación FES de Colombia and Deutsche Gesellschaft für Technische Zusammenarbeit. El estado actual de la ley 100/93 en salud. Santa Fe de Bogotá, March 3, 1997

Gilson L, Russell S, Buse K. The political economy of user fees with targeting: developing equitable health financing policy. *Journal of International Development*, 1995; **7**: 369–402

Gilson L, Mills A. Health sector reforms in sub-Saharan Africa: lessons of the last 10 years. In: Berman P (ed) *Health Sector Reform in Developing Countries: Making Health Development Sustainable*. Harvard Series on Population and International Health. Boston: Harvard University Press, 1995

Government of Peru. Ley de modernización de la seguridad social en salud y su reglamento D.S. No. 009-97-SA, 1997

Govindaraj R, Murray CJL, Chellaraj G. *Health Expenditures in Latin America*. World Bank Technical Paper No. 274. Washington DC: World Bank, 1995

Griffiths A, Mills M. *Money for Health: a Manual for Developing Countries*. Geneva: Sandoz Institute for Health and Socio-economic Studies, 1983

Hecht R, Overholt C, Holmberg H. Improving the implementation of cost recovery for health: lessons from Zimbabwe. *Health Policy*, 1993; **25**: 213–242

Heiby J. Quality of health services. In: Janovsky K (ed) *Health Policy and Systems Development: an Agenda for Research*. WHO/SHS/NHP/96.1. Geneva: World Health Organization, 1996, pp179–190

Hill SC, Wolfe BL. Testing the HMO competitive strategy: an analysis of its impact on medical care resources. *Journal of Health Economics*, 1997; **16**: 261–286

Hurst J. The reform of health care: a comparative analysis of seven OECD countries, Health Policy Studies No. 2, Paris: OECD, 1992

Issaka-Tinorgah A, Waddington C. Encouraging efficiency through programme and functional budgeting: lessons from experience in Ghana and the Gambia. In: Mills A, Lee K (eds) *Health Economics Research in Developing Countries*. Oxford: Oxford Medical Publications, 1993, pp335–350

Jaramillo I. El futuro de la salud en Colombia: la puesta en marcha de la Ley 100. Bogota: Fescol, Fundación Corona, FES, and Fundacion Restrepo Barco, 1994

Jimenez de la Jara J, Bossert T. Chile's health sector reform: lessons from four reform periods. In: Berman P (ed) *Health Sector Reform in Developing Countries: Making Health Development Sustainable*. Harvard Series on Population and International Health. Boston: Harvard University Press, 1995

Jönsson S, Musgrove P. Government financing of health care. In: Schieber GJ (ed) *Innovations in Health Care Financing: Proceedings of a World Bank Conference*, March 10–11, 1997. Washington DC: World Bank, 1997

Kumaranayake L. Regulation within the health sector: a common framework. Draft mimeo. Health Economics and Financing Programme, London School of Hygiene & Tropical Medicine, 1996, unpublished

Kutzin J, Barnum H. Institutional features of health insurance programs and their effects on developing country health systems. *International Journal of Health Planning and Management*, 1992; **7**: 51–72

Kutzin, J. *Experience with Reform in the Financing of the Health Sector*. WHO/SHS/CC/94.3 Geneva: World Health Organization, 1994

La Forgia GM, Griffin CC. Zaire community health insurance schemes. In: La Forgia GM, Griffin CC (eds) *Health Insurance in Practice: Fifteen Case Studies from Developing Countries.* HFS Small Applied Research paper No. 4, Health Financing and Sustainability Project. Bethesda, MD: Abt Associates Inc., 1993, chapter 2.1

Litvack JI, Bodart C. User fees plus quality equals improved access to health care: results of a field experiment in Cameroon. *Social Science and Medicine*, 1993; **37**: 369-383

Lloyd-Sherlock P. Healthcare financing, reform and equity in Argentina: past and present. In: Lloyd-Sherlock P (ed) *Sickening for Change: Health, Policy and Poverty in Latin America*. London: Institute of Latin American Studies, 1998

Maceira D. *Fragmentación y dinámica de los sistemas de salud en America Latina.* Documento de trabajo. Washington DC: Banco Interamericano de Desarollo, Oficina del Economista Jefe, 1996

Manning WG, Leibowitz A, Goldberg GA, Rogers WH, Newhouse JP. A controlled trial of the effect of a prepaid group practice on use of services. *New England Journal of Medicine*, 1984; **310**: 1505–1510

McFarlane GA. *Chigoria Hospital Insurance Scheme.* Kenya: Chigoria Hospital, 1996

McGreevy W. *Social security in Latin America: Issues and Options for the World Bank.* Washington DC: World Bank, LAC Regional Office, 1990

McLaughlin CG. HMO growth and hospital expenses and use: a simultaneous equation approach. *Health Services Research*, 1987; **22**: 182–205

McLaughlin CG. The effect of HMOs on overall hospital expenses: is anything left after correcting for simultaneity and selectivity. *Health Services Research*, 1988; **23**: 421–441

McPake B. The role of the private sector in health service provision. In: Bennett S, McPake B, Mills A (eds) *Private Health Providers in Developing Countries: Serving the Public Interest*. New Jersey: Zed Books, 1997, pp 21–39

McPake B, Hanson K, Mills A. Community financing of health care in Africa: an evaluation of the Bamako Initiative. *Social Science and Medicine*, 1993; **36**: 1383–1395

McPake B, Hongoro C. Contracting out of clinical services in Zimbabwe. *Social Science and Medicine*, 1993; **41**: 13–24

Mesa Lago C. Provision social y salud en America Latina. In: Ministerio de Salud de Peru (ed) *Seminario Internacional: Reforma del Sector Salud*. Lima, Peru: Ministerio de la Salud, 1997

Mills A. Improving the efficiency of public sector health services in developing coutries: bureaucratic versus market approaches. London: London School of Hygiene & Tropical Medicine, PHP Departmental Publication No. 17, 1995

Mills A, Vaughan JP, Smith DL, Tabibzadeh I (eds) *Health System Decentralisation: Concepts, Issues and Country Experiences*. Geneva: World Health Organization, 1990

Mujinja PGM, Urassa D, Mnyika KS. The Tanzanian public-private mix in national health care. In: Report of the workshop on the public-private mix for health care in developing countries, 11–15 January 1993, London School of Hygiene and Tropical Medicine, 1993, unpublished

Musgrove P. Some personal reflections on a decade and a half of research in health economics and its application, Paper presented to the Inter-American Network of Health Economics and Financing, Regional seminar on research on health economics and financing in Latin America and the Caribbean: current situation and challenges. University of Chile, Santiago, November 21–22, 1996, unpublished

Mwabu G. Health care reform in Kenya: a review of the process. In: Berman P (ed) *Health Sector Reform in Developing Countries: Making Health Development Sustainable*. Harvard Series on Population and International Health. Boston: Harvard University Press, 1995

Ngalande-Banda E, Walt G. The private health sector in Malawi: opening Pandora's box? *Journal of International Development*, 1995; **7**: 403–421

Normand C. Health insurance: a solution to the financing gap?. In: Colclough C (ed) *Marketizing Education and Health in Developing Countries: Miracle or Mirage?* Oxford: Clarendon Press, 1997, pp 205–221

OECD. New directions in health policy. Paris: OECD, 1995, OECD Policy Studies 7

Ogunbekun I, Adeyi O, Wouters A, Morrow R in collaboration with Dokunmu OOK, Lewis IA, Ehimwenma PH, Apesin MA. *Costs and financing of improvements in the quality of maternal health services through the Bamako Initiative in Nigeria.* National Primary Health Care Development Agency of Nigeria and Johns Hopkins University School of Hygiene and Public Health, Baltimore, 1995

Ramirez T, Zurita B, Cruz C, Recio M, Vargas C. The role of an NGO in the market for maternal and child health care services in Mexico City. In: Bennett S, McPake B, Mills A (eds) *Private Health Providers in Developing Countries: Serving the Public Interest.* New Jersey: Zed Books, 1997, pp 174–185

Scutchfield FD, Lee J, Patton D. Managed care in the United States. *Journal of Public Health Medicine*, 1997; **19**: 251-254

Stormer M. Final Report on Tororo Hospital Cost-sharing Scheme. Kampala: DED/GDS, 1994

Swan M, Zwi A. Private practitioners and public health: close the gap or increase the distance? London: Department of Public Health and Policy, London School of Hygiene & Tropical Medicine, 1997

Tollman S, Schopper D, Torres A. Health maintenance organizations in developing countries: what can we expect? *Health Policy and Planning*; 1990; **5**: 149–160

Van den Heever A. Regulating the funding of private health care: the South African experience. In: Bennett S, McPake B, Mills A (eds) *Private Health Providers in Developing Countries: Serving the Public Interest.* New Jersey: Zed Books, 1997

Viveros-Long A. Changes in health financing: the Chilean experience. *Social Science and Medicine*, 1986; **22**: 379–385

Welch WP, Frank RG, Diehr P. Health care costs in Health Maintenance Organizations: correcting for self-selection. In: Scheffler RM (ed) *Advances in Health Economics and Health Services Research.* Greenwich, Connecticut: JAI Press, volume 5, pp 95–128

Willis C. Means testing in cost recovery of health services in developing countries, Major applied research paper no. 7, Health Financing and Sustainability Project. Bethesda, Maryland: Abt Associates, 1993

World Bank. *Investing in Health: World Development Report, 1993.* Washington DC: World Bank, 1993

World Bank. *Health, Nutrition and Population.* Washington DC: The Human Development Network, World Bank Group, 1997

World Health Organization. *Health Care Systems in Transition.* Copenhagen: WHO Regional Office for Europe, 1996

Xing-Yuan G, Sheng-Lan T. Reform of the Chinese health care financing system. In: Berman, P (ed) Health Sector Reform in Developing Countries: Making Health Development Sustainable. Harvard Series on Population and International Health. Boston: Harvard University Press, 1995

Zellner BB, Wolfe BL. HMO growth and hospital expenses: a correction. *Health Service Research*, 1989; **24**: 409–413

8
Managed care, risk sharing and health system reforms in the United States

Richard Scheffler

School of Public Health, University of California, Berkeley, USA

This chapter first explores the impact of managed care in the United States. It follows with a discussion on the use of risk sharing in the US health system, and the concept is then illustrated by applying it to primary care, specialty care and hospitals in an integrated delivery system. The financial incentives of risk sharing and the design's methods to improve the co-ordination of care and encourage efficiency are discussed. Finally, the chapter considers the proposed expansion of private insurance including Medical Savings Accounts (MSAs) and public insurance (Medicare and Medicaid) to solve the problem of the uninsured in the US. The public policy issues that surround these two solutions are then debated.

The impact of managed care

Between 1980 and 1995, the United States experienced a rapid increase in the rise of managed care plans. In 1980, only 10 million Americans were enrolled in managed care. By the year 1995, this had increased to approximately 141.9 million (Figure 8.1) (Interstudy, 1996). This rapid change constituted an approximate 14-fold increase in enrolment in 15 years.

Reasons for the rise of managed care are mainly attributed to the rapid increases in health care costs, the oversupply of providers and hospitals, employers' concerns over the rise in health care expenditure, and the Clinton administration's failure to reform the health care system in the early 1990s. The government's failure induced the unleashing of the private sector, which proposed alternative solutions to health care reform in the United States.

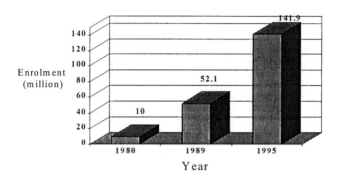

Figure 8.1 Growth of managed care in the US

The impact of managed care in the US health care system is most apparent in the drop in growth of health care expenditure in recent years. First, the growth of private health insurance premiums and the health care cost index dropped dramatically between 1992 and 1996 (Figure 8.2) (US Bureau of the Census, 1998), the growth in private health insurance premiums falling from 10.9% to 0.5%

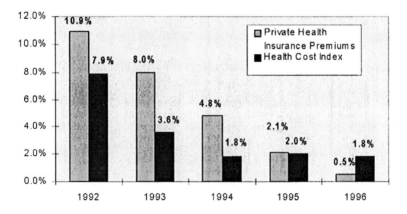

Figure 8.2 Increases in private insurance premiums and health care expenditures, 1992-1996

and the growth of the health care cost index from 7.9% to 1.8%. Interestingly, data showed that in 1996, the increase in private health insurance premiums actually lagged behind growth in health care expenditures. This discrepancy in growth was also found in the years 1997 and 1998 (data not shown).

Second, data accounting for real national health expenditure from 1961–1996 also showed an overall decrease in the growth of the nation's total health expenditure (Figure 8.3) (Levit *et al*, 1998). In 1961, health expenditure increased at an average of 6% per year; this figure was approximately 2% in 1996. In the two states experiencing the highest managed care penetration, the ratio of state *per capita* spending compared to the national average *per capita* spending decreased from 1.15 to 1.02 in California between the years 1980 and 1992, and from 1.09 to 1.0 in Minnesota.

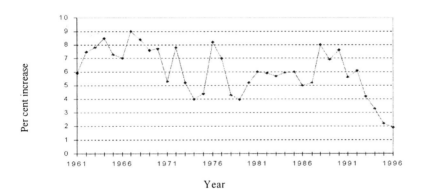

Figure 8.3 Annual increase in real national health expenditures, 1961–1996

These apparent decreases are attributed in part to managed care's impact on hospital utilization. From 1983 to 1993, a reduction of 12% in staffed beds was found in low health care maintenance organization (HMO) penetrated areas in contrast to a 24% reduction in high HMO penetrated areas of the United States. In-patient days were affected even more severely with low HMO penetrated areas experiencing a 29% reduction in in-patient days in contrast to high HMO penetrated areas that experienced a 44% reduction. In addition to reductions in in-patient days, the average patient's length of stay also decreased with the increase in managed care. In low HMO penetrated areas, a 19% reduction in average length of stay was observed, and a 20% reduction in high HMO penetrated areas. Finally, in-patient surgical procedures decreased by 35% in low HMO penetrated areas and 46% in high HMO penetrated areas (Robinson, 1996). The comparison between low and high HMO penetrated areas indicates the degree of impact of managed care; nevertheless, it should be noted that both types of area experienced decreases.

The expansion of managed care also affected the use of new technology in the delivery of health care in the United States. Technology, as measured by the adoption of cardiac catherization, open heart surgery, and CT scanner in one study showed a dramatic decrease in the elasticity between HMO enrolment and technology adoption in the years of 1980 to 1995 (Table 8.1) (Cutler and Scheiner, 1998). Thus, whereas in 1980, a 1% change in HMO enrolment was associated with a 6.2% increase in the adoption of all types of medical technology, in 1990 a 1% change in HMO enrolment was associated with a 2.7% decrease. Overall, a regression model suggests that HMO enrolment and the adoption of all new technologies are negatively correlated. The decrease in the adoption of technology can be perceived as an improvement in controlling the cost of health care; however, this impact of managed care may encourage stagnation of new medical innovations in the United States.

Table 8.1 Effect of managed care on technology adoption

Technology	HMO Enrolment*		
	1980	1990	1995
All new technologies	6.2	-2.7	-5.4
Cardiac catheterization	6.3	-7.5	-6.8
Open heart surgery	6.1	-2.2	-3.6
CT scanner	22.2	-12.9	-12.0

* Elasticity, measured as the percentage change in technology adoption over the percentage change in HMO enrolment

The considerable increase in managed care in the United States has raised concerns over potential abuse in the system, namely the sacrifice of quality and access for reductions in cost and utilization. In reaction to the increase in managed care, the federal and state governments have enacted a number of consumer protection laws, most notably the Anti-gag rule law. Passed in September of 1997, the bill prohibits HMOs primarily from enforcing 'gag rules' that prevent or discourage physicians and other health care providers from relaying certain information and opinions to patients regarding their medical conditions and treatment options, and the provisions, terms, requirements and services of the patient's health care plan. As a further response to the growth of managed care, the federal government has recently been considering a national patient bill of rights. The passing of this law will establish standards for patients' rights to proper and timely treatment in managed care plans.

The essence of risk sharing on the supply side

Managed care in the United States has been using mainly supply side reforms to control the rapid rise in health care expenditure and utilization. Techniques of managed care include the use of benefits, utilization, and risk management to achieve greater efficiency in the delivery of care. The new health delivery system differs from the pre-existing fee-for-service model in integrating the responsibility for delivering and containing cost of care, and combining the insurance domain with the provision of health care, thereby merging financial and health care delivery responsibilities under the same umbrella.

The newest evolution in managed care since its inception is the merger of clinical and financial risks as an integrated function in health care delivery systems. Basic notions of financial risks were first adopted from concepts used in the traditional health insurance industry, but unique characteristics of risk have emerged with the addition of clinical risk in the risk management pool.

The new risk pool consists of two sources of risk: operational risk and clinical risk (Conrad *et al*, 1996). Clinical risk in this case is not risk of disease as defined

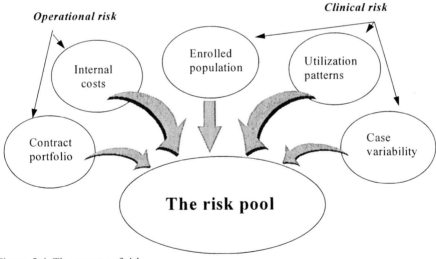

Figure 8.4 The sources of risk

in epidemiology, but rather risks in the delivery of health care services and coverage decisions surrounding care. Clearly, in an integrated health delivery system, risk of providing care can be intertwined with operational or management decisions. Operational risks arise as provider organizations become more complex, with an increased number of business entities and increased direct and indirect corporate liabilities. Clinical risk, on the other hand, demands control over the provision of clinical care, including credentialling physicians, risk management, rationing medical care, and utilization review.

Due to the interdependent nature of the two risks, reduction in operational risk may increase risk in clinical care. For instance, an operational or managerial decision to pay physicians by salary may remove incentives for physicians to under-treat patients, as no financial incentives exist to provide the most adequate care. On the other hand, paying physicians on a fee-for-service basis may create supplier-induced demand, or the induction of unnecessary utilization.

Operational risk can consist of two parts: 1) that arising from the contract portfolio of the managed care plans that comprise the organization's internal and external contracts for services such as pharmacy, beds, and other ancillary services; 2) that arising from the internal cost of operation, including the cost of managing low-risk, high-quality, cost-effective services within the organization. Gaining market share through acquisitions, expansion of contract agreements with payers, and through increased sales or service volume to achieve desirable economies of scale are yet other management strategies aimed at controlling risk. The primary goal of management of risk is to ensure financial stability by reducing inherent risks in the financing of the health care delivery system (Kongstvedt, 1997).

Total risk management, however, also considers the management of clinical risk associated with the delivery of care. Because management goals may not necessarily reflect those of clinical goals to deliver quality care and to achieve optimal patient outcome, managed care organizations must align operational and clinical goals to meet the challenges of a competitive market-place while delivering the highest quality care.

Managed care's financial solution to achieve economic goals as well as reduction in the risk of delivering poor services is the use of capitation arrangements in contracts between employers and health plans. Sub-capitation can be used to describe a financial arrangement between the health plans and the providers whereby a portion (thus 'sub') of the premium is allocated for each provider service. Since under most managed care insurance schemes, premiums paid to health plans are used to purchase an array of medical services (i.e. in-patient, out-patient, pharmaceutical, mental health, etc.) we refer to capitation arrangements with each of these provider entries as 'sub-capitation'. Thus, sub-capitation is a single fixed-sum paid to a group of providers for a defined set of services for an enrolled population. With a capitation amount, providers accept the actuarial risk for delivering all care to a defined population. This financial arrangement integrates the clinical and operational risk as providers accept a fixed financial sum, therefore accepting financial risk and clinical risk simultaneously.

Finally, other managed care techniques include:

- use of primary care gatekeepers to control referrals to expensive specialist and hospital services;
- creation of risk pools where a certain proportion of the total premium is set aside and later distribute to provide financial incentives for better performance;

- setting of expenditure targets to ensure proper use of budgets, and
- use of quality of care and outcome measures to evaluate the cost-effectiveness of treatment provided by contracted or salaried providers.

Illustrations of risk sharing

How it works

Implementation of risk sharing activities follows these basic steps:

1. people choose coverage from available plans;
2. people purchase insurance and pay a monthly premium to the health plan;
3. the health plan contracts or pays salaried providers either on a subcapitation or fee-for-service basis, or on some combination of the two, and
4. the health plan bears all operational and clinical risks for providing care.

However, risk is shifted from health plans to providers accepting subcapitation payment to deliver care. Under this construct, combinations of financial compensation arrangements exist to achieve the managed care organization's goals to control operational and clinical risk.

The Kaiser Model

The Kaiser Foundation Health Plan is the oldest and best known managed care organization in the United States. Currently, Kaiser serves over 9.1 million members in 19 states and the District of Columbia. As an integrated health delivery system, Kaiser Foundation Health Plan provides or co-ordinates members' care, including preventive services, hospital and medical services, and pharmacy services. Traditionally, Kaiser's organizational structure has been the predominant managed care model.

The Kaiser Foundation Health Plan receives premiums for enrollees and distributes the fund to the Kaiser Permanente Medical Group, a professional organization that employs salaried physicians (Figure 8.5). Regional Permanente Medical Groups are responsible for a group of providers in a defined geographic region. For instance, the Northern California Permanente Medical Group is charged with operational and clinical management responsibilities for providers in the area. The medical group is paid by the Kaiser Foundation Plan a per-member per month premium for each enrollee. In turn, the medical group accepts financial and clinical risk to provide all professional services, with the exception of unpredictable

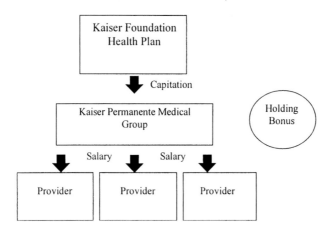

Figure 8.5 The Kaiser model

treatment needs that are high-cost, such as transplants, in which case the medical group will be paid on a dollar-per-dollar basis. A provider within the medical group provides care and receives a salary as compensation.

Under this construct, the Kaiser Foundation Health Plan shifts the clinical risk to the Kaiser Permanente Medical Group who then manages its financial and clinical costs through various managed care techniques. Unlike other risk sharing arrangements, however, the Kaiser Foundation Health Plan assumes full responsibility for any overruns in the initial budget granted to each medical group (calculated on a per member per month basis). The effects of overrun budgets, however, may have detrimental effects on the medical group in the long run. For instance, repeated overrun of budgets may cause the health plan to increase its insurance premiums. In a competitive managed care market, any small increase may reduce enrolment in the Kaiser health plan, thereby subsequently reducing the number of patients in the Kaiser Permanente Medical Group. Thus, although total risk lies primarily within the health plan, long term consequences of poor financial performances may affect the livelihood of the Medical Group. Recognizing such indirect effects, the physicians of the Kaiser Permanente Medical Group in 1996 volunteered a 10% pay cut to allow the health plan to lower premiums. The medical group, in fact, took into account the viability of the health plan in a price competitive market in their negotiated salaries (John Hellman, personal communication, 1998).

Currently, providers as individuals within the Kaiser system receive very few direct financial incentives to deliver high quality and efficient care. However, a small withholding bonus is available to providers with partnership status (defined as five or more years of service) if the medical group's total expenditure falls below that set by the health plan. The health plan maintains the right to retain the bonus if the expenditure target is not met.

In conclusion, the Kaiser integrative model has been the predominant managed care model in the United States. Currently, it uses some type of risk sharing to manage better its total operational and clinical risks—most risks do not fall on individual providers, but rather on the health plan. Whether the Kaiser risk sharing model has a similar impact on performance as other models merits further consideration.

The Virtual Kaiser

Kaiser, as an integrative entity, performs the following functions:

- financial management,
- medical management
- operations management, and
- marketing management.

In Kaiser, all functions are carried out internally. In newer managed care models, however, these core managed care organization functions may be contracted-out to the market place; some health plans out-source all services, while some may only out-source a few.

The virtual Kaiser model has increased in popularity in recent years and has gained a solid financial performance reputation. In 1996, the Kaiser-staff model HMO constituted only approximately 1.2% of all health plans, whereas integrated practice organizations (IPA) constituted 64.4% and network, group, and mixed together constituted another 34.4% (Interstudy, 1996). Clearly, these models are becoming more popular in the United States than the classic staff model HMO.

Virtual organizations represent a conglomerate of contracting or affiliated entities, each performing a certain managed care function for a negotiated price (Conrad *et al*, 1996). The approach avoids any ownership relationship between health plans and providers, thus allowing more flexibility to sever any sub-optimal relationships.

Risk sharing within non-staff model HMOs follow the Kaiser's risk sharing arrangements, although more risks are shifted to the provider. Under a generic model, the health plan retains approximately 20% of total premium dollars for administrative services such as information systems, quality assurance, billing, contracting, marketing, etc. The remaining 80% is distributed among the medical group's administration group (approximately 10%), primary care (10%), specialists (20%), and hospitals (40%) (Mayer, 1994). The actual amount received by these entities varies according to the risk-sharing scheme established to align incentives between different providers within the system. For instance, primary care physicians are paid on a per member per month basis and are allowed to make referrals to specialists and hospitals. Specialists, on the other hand, receive payment based on a prospective fee schedule outlining set fee-for-specialty services. An expenditure target is set for an individual or group of specialists based on the patient-mix, age, and other factors contributing to variability in cost of care within the population. A withhold, or a certain per cent of budget, is distributed equally among primary care physicians, specialists, and health plan when expenditure targets are met. Risk pool inclusion considers the extent to which the entity affects the total expenditure of the population. For out-patient services, primary care physicians maintain total control over the volume of specialist cases through the use of gatekeepers for referrals. Thus, specialists control the type of services provided while primary care physicians govern utilization patterns.

In risk sharing arrangements between primary care physicians and hospitals, hospitals are also held to an expenditure target that constitutes a percentage of the total fixed budget. The remainder is held in a risk pool shared equally by primary care physicians, hospitals, and specialists. Because both primary care physicians and specialists determine referral patterns to hospitals, their inclusion in the risk pool ensures responsibility over the use of hospital services. Once admitted, a patient's amount of utilization is determined by the hospital, which has incentives to provide the proper amount of services under an expenditure target. Risk pool distribution may be determined by measures of quality of care and ability to meet expenditure targets.

In conclusion, virtual Kaiser type organizations, as virtually integrated systems, perform all functions of financial, medical, operations, and marketing management. The virtual Kaiser models shift substantially more risk to providers through sub-capitation and provide incentives to deliver appropriate and efficient care by establishing risk pools. Kaiser, on the other hand, structures financial arrangements to shift some risk to the medical group; however, the ultimate financial responsibility still lies within the health plan. It is not the case that under the Kaiser model, no incentive exists for providers to deliver quality and cost-effective services; in the long run, overrun of established budgets may jeopardize the viability of the Kaiser Foundation Health Plan as well as the Kaiser Permanente Medical Group.

Public versus private solutions to the uninsured

A daunting problem facing the American health care system is the number of uninsured. In 1996, it was estimated that of the total US population, approximately 16% did not carry health care insurance. Of the remaining 84%, 72% were insured by private health plans, 13% by Medicare, 12% by Medicaid, and 3% through plans established by the military (US Bureau of the Census, 1998). Medicare (for adults over the age of 65) and Medicaid (for the poor, defined as a certain per cent below the poverty line) are two large insurance programmes through which the public sector has attempted to provide solutions to the uninsured. The ageing of the American population and the rise in health care expenditures has raised concerns over the financial viability of the Medicare programme, funded primarily by payroll taxes. As the ratio of older adults to the working population increases, the amounts of payroll tax money available decrease, thereby jeopardizing the future of Medicare. Nevertheless, President Clinton recently announced a potential reform proposal to include near-older adults (aged 55 to 64 years) to the Medicare programme in an attempt to resolve the growing problem of the uninsured. However, due to rising concerns over the financial viability of Medicare as it stands today, the future of expanding Medicare membership does not seem promising.

Reforms to the Medicaid programme also propose to expand its coverage to another population, all children under the age of 18. The CHIPS (Children's Health Insurance Provider Security) Act of 1997 encourages states through increased federal medical assistance to expand Medicaid coverage of children and pregnant women. The cost of this proposal is nearly $24 billion.

Finally, another federal effort to reduce the number of uninsured in the United States was the establishment of Medical Saving Accounts (MSAs), a project piloted recently and scheduled to end in the year 2000; over 750 000 Americans are participating in the project (US Internal Revenue Service, 1997).

An MSA is a tax-exempt trust or custodial account with a financial institution where money can be saved for future medical expenses. Under current regulations, an MSA must be used in conjunction with a high deductible health plan, defined as a plan with a minimum annual deductible of $1,500 for an individual and $3,000 for a family. The annual deductible must not exceed $2,250 for an individual and $4,500 for a family. The health plan must also have a high ceiling for annual out-of-pocket expenses (a maximum of $3,000 for an individual and $5,500 for a family). The goal of the MSA plan is to allow self-employed individuals or small employers to meet the cost of medical care without purchasing expensive, low deductible health plan memberships. In turn, MSA accounts grant individuals full control over using their accounts for meeting health care services costs which fall below a high deductible health plan.

The idea for MSAs originated in Singapore and its popularity is now growing in China. Nevertheless, in the United States under the current health care system, some caution must be taken before expanding MSAs to the rest of the population. Although MSAs may help reduce unnecessary utilization of health care services (moral hazard) by holding individuals accountable for costs, MSAs might exacerbate adverse selection as they may attract only healthy people to participate, leaving the unhealthy and the chronically ill in the health insurance plans.

Conclusions

We see that within the past two decades managed care, stimulated by rapid cost increases, provider and hospital oversupply and lack of sufficient government reform, has had a profound effect on the health care industry in the US. The health expenditure growth seen in both private premiums and at the national level have both shown notable decreases. The rate of increase in health care costs as reflected in technology adoption rates has also decreased. However, concerns have been raised over abuses in the system which sacrifice quality and access.

Managed care has sought to manage risk as an integrated function through the merger of clinical and financial risks using various techniques including sub-capitation. The virtual Kaiser HMO model, as a virtually integrated system, forces providers to accept both financial and clinical risk and has become more popular than the traditional staff model HMO.

Public solutions to decreasing the large percentage of uninsured involve expanding the Medicare and Medicaid programmes. Although proposals exist, the financial costs make their viability questionable. Pilot programmes such as those involving Medical Savings Accounts are underway, but their feasibility and drawbacks are as yet unknown.

Acknowledgement

Special thanks to Angela Ip, MPH for her extraordinary research efforts.

References

Conrad DA, Bonney RS, Sachs MA, Smith RJ. *Managed Care Contracting: Concepts and Applications for the Health Care Executive.* Chicago: Health Administration Press, 1996

Cutler and Scheiner. NBER 1998; Working Paper No. 6140

The Interstudy competitive edge: biannual report of the managed health care industry. Excelsior, MN: Interstudy, 1996

Kongstvedt PR (ed) *Essentials of Managed Healthcare.* Second edition. Gaithersburg, MD: Aspen Publishers, 1997

Levit KR, Lazenby HC, Braden BR and the National Health Accounts Team. National Health Spending Trends in 1996. *Health Affairs*, 1998; **17**: 35–51

Mayer, D. Coping with Capitation. *Northern California Medicine*, 1994; **5**: 24–25

Robinson JC. Decline in hospital utilization and cost inflation under managed care in California. *Journal of the American Medical Association*, 1996; **276**: 1060–1064

US Bureau of the Census, Current Population Survey – web page. Increases in Private Insurance Premiums and Health care expenditures, 1992–1996 [http://www.bls.census.gov/cps/cpsmain.htm. Link valid 9 Sept 98]

US Internal Revenue Service. Medical Saving Accounts (MSA), 1997: Publication 969 [http://ftp.fedworld.gov/pub/irs-pdf/p969.pdf]

9
Reforming integrated systems. The case of the UK: a balance sheet of the evidence on the impact of the internal market, 1991-1997

Nicholas Mays

King's Fund, London, UK

The internal market reforms of the National Health Service (NHS) introduced in 1991/92 separated the purchasing from the provision of health care in what had been an integrated system. Until that time, health authorities had been responsible both for service planning and for the direct management of hospitals and other organizations providing community health services for populations of about 250 000 people within their boundaries. The internal market changes were widely regarded as the most radical, 'big-bang' changes in the NHS since its inception in 1946. They were designed to alter the dynamics of the UK health system while preserving its method of mainly general tax financing, together with its hierarchical structure in which the Secretary of State for Health is accountable to Parliament for the way in which the NHS is run (Klein, 1995).

The changes generated an industry of comment and counter-comment from supporters and opponents. However, because of the highly politicized nature of the debate in the lead up to the changes and in the early stages after 1991, the government refused to mount a comprehensive programme of research to evaluate the consequences. Instead, it was left, initially, to independent organizations such as the King's Fund to support studies of the impact of the changes (Robinson and Le Grand, 1994). Subsequently, a complex body of scattered empirical evidence emerged.

This paper summarizes and attempts to interpret the findings from a comprehensive review, which began in 1995, of all the studies which contain empirical material relevant to assessing the effects of the three main planks of the internal market changes (Goodwin *et al*, 1998). The review focuses on:

- the performance of health authorities acting as purchasers of health services, together with the range of more local 'commissioning' organizations which developed in each health authority area;
- the consequences of a sub-set of general practices becoming fundholders by volunteering to purchase elective care for their patients; and
- the effects associated with the conversion of providers of hospital and community health services to NHS trust status separate from their local health authorities.

There have been other reviews of the research evidence on the impact of the internal market changes (Robinson, 1996) and numerous authoritative commentaries on the consequences for the health system of the internal market (Ham, 1996; Klein, 1995; Light, 1997; Maynard and Bloor, 1996), but the current review is more comprehensive and up-to-date, including empirical material produced up to the beginning of 1998.

Unlike previous reviews, the current review covers almost the entire lifespan of the internal market as conceived under the Conservative government of Margaret Thatcher, since the Labour government elected in May 1997 announced its plans for further change to the organization of the NHS in a White Paper in December 1997 (Great Britain Department of Health, 1997). The Labour rhetoric is that the internal market will be swept away in April 1999 and certainly key parts of it such as single practice general practitioner (GP) fundholding will disappear. However, the purchaser–provider split will remain, with an emphasis on co-operative relationships rather than competition and adversarial behaviour. Most health and community health services purchasing (now known as 'commissioning') will be carried out by Primary Care Groups (PCGs) which will be large groups of general practices covering around 100 000 patients in an area, somewhere between the size of local commissioning groups and current health authorities. Like fundholders, PCGs will hold budgets and will be able to retain any surpluses they generate. Clearly large parts of internal market thinking have been retained (Dixon and Mays, 1997), so this is a good moment to assess the extent to which Labour's vision for the future accords with the evidence of the last six years, and to look back at a period of unrivalled change in the internal organization of the NHS as it attempted to marry the operation of a competitive market with the goals of a publicly funded service.

Methods

Published and unpublished studies which included data on the impact of the three main planks of the internal market changes were searched for, using a combination of electronic databases, library catalogues at the King's Fund,[1] published bibliographies, reference lists of individual studies, a survey of Directors of Public Health in health authorities and by providing lists of identified studies to subject area experts at intervals to see if there were obvious omissions or work in progress which should have been included.

Any study which included relevant data was included and the strength of its evidence discussed at the relevant point in the review. Unsubstantiated writer opinion was excluded, but the review included indirect research (i.e. theoretically informed commentary and/or systematic hypothesis generating pieces) where these were helpful in explaining the empirical findings.

The effects of the internal market were considered in relation to their impact on the following broad criteria of health system excellence:

- efficiency;
- equity;
- quality;
- choice and responsiveness (for and to individual patients);
- accountability

which had been used in an earlier King's Fund assessment of the impact of the first two years of the changes (Robinson and Le Grand, 1994).

Results

The detailed results, based on synthesizing the findings of scores of studies, are available in book form (Goodwin et al, 1998). The findings from the review of fundholding, local commissioning and health authority purchasing have also been produced as a separate report available from the King's Fund (Le Grand et al, 1997). The sections which follow review the main findings.

The impact of NHS Trust status

As part of the introduction of the internal market, NHS hospitals and organizations providing community health services (but not family practitioners such as general

---

[1] The leading health services management and policy library in the UK.

medical practitioners and dentists which remained governed by a national contract) were separated from the health authorities, while remaining part of the NHS. They were turned into independent NHS trusts, each with its own governing body of executive and non-executive directors, accountable to the Secretary of State for Health. Trusts' income was dependent on their ability to attract the custom of the purchasers in the form of contracts. They were given certain freedoms including the ability to negotiate local pay agreements with their non-medical staff and to manage their capital expenditure. They were permitted to develop new services without the direct involvement of the health authority. Unlike fundholders, trusts were not permitted to retain budgetary surpluses. Perhaps the best way to think of an NHS trust is as a non-profit firm in which clinical directorates within the trust pursue the twin objectives of income and patient benefits (Bartlett and Le Grand, 1994). The White Paper, *Working for Patients*, was clear that freeing trusts from the control of health authorities, allowing them to manage themselves and permitting them to compete to attract patients would improve efficiency, quality and the responsiveness of services as well as creating 'a stronger sense of local ownership and pride'. There was no mention of equity in relation to trusts.

Within six years of the creation of the internal market, all providers of health care had become NHS trusts. Most conversions of former Directly Managed Units (DMUs) to trust status occurred in the first two years after April 1991.

NHS trusts have attracted relatively little research interest compared with the level of attention given to GP fundholders. The quality of the evidence is generally not high. The circumstances surrounding their introduction were not favourable to rigorous comparisons with hospitals and other providers which had not yet converted to trust status. The first wave of trusts was prevented from making major changes in the first year (1991/92). In the second year, the first and second wave trusts were dogged by the uncertainty of a General Election campaign in which opposition parties were committed to their abolition. By the third year (1993/94), the third wave of trusts had emerged and the remaining DMUs were too few and too unrepresentative to offer a meaningful comparison.

Table 9.1 provides a brief summary of the research evidence on the impact of NHS trusts in terms of the evaluative criteria set out at the beginning of the chapter. Despite the paucity of good research, it seems that few if any of the government's goals for trusts were met in any measurable way. In large part, this appears to have been because there was little meaningful supply-side competition despite the fact that the conditions for competition between acute hospitals existed in some parts of the country, at least at the beginning of the reforms (Appleby *et al*, 1994) and for some services. Rather than competing with one another for the business of the large health authority purchasers, a series of bilateral monopolies developed (Propper, 1995) as government increasingly stepped in to limit competition. Under these arrangements, block contracts were set for trusts under which they were given an annual budget for a service and expected to extract an ever increasing volume of patient care from it (Paton, 1995). In contrast, GP fundholders were marginal

Table 9.1 Impact of NHS trust status on provider performance

Evaluative criterion	Evidence
Efficiency	Some evidence of lower unit costs (higher productivity) in early trusts than Directly Managed Units (DMUs), but not clearly attributable to trust status. Some may have become trusts because they already had cost control mechanisms in place; others may already have had lower than average costs before becoming trusts General upward trend in NHS activity (though a very crude measure of efficiency) predated the reforms, but appeared to rise faster than increase in resources after 1991 (i.e. crude evidence of productivity gains) Contradictory evidence on whether trusts made greater use of supposedly 'efficient' techniques (eg. Day surgery) Evidence of increased management costs but not clear that all was due to the reforms - increases began before 1991, plus considerable relabelling of posts and shift of tasks from health authorities (HAs) to trusts No evidence on whether capital charging improved efficiency
Equity	Introduction of trusts not seen by government as about equity Some evidence that trusts gave preferential treatment to patients of general practitioner fundholders (GPFH) (shorter waits) and lowered prices where there was competition for marginal income. HAs also more likely to exhaust resources for elective care before GPFHs, so that HA patients had to wait longer No evidence (but little studied) of trusts 'cream skimming' (i.e. discriminating against high-cost patients)
Quality	Difficult to measure because of secular trends. No before and after studies. Clinical Standards Advisory Group study of emergency admissions found that DMUs admitted patients through A&E slightly more quickly than trusts No evidence that purchasers chose trusts on price at expense of quality. Some evidence that separation between acute and community health services trusts led to perverse incentives and cost shifting (e.g. premature discharge from acute trusts) which may have harmed continuity of care No evidence that rate of fall of waiting times was faster in trusts than DMUs though comparison only possible for a short time
Choice/responsiveness	Choice theoretically exercised not by patients but by HAs/GPFHs No evidence of trusts becoming more responsive or offering more choice though more trappings of 'customer care'. Reforms may not have reached the 'factory floor' of health care since patients remained a guaranteed commodity Trusts' lack of freedom to raise capital and set prices made creating new services difficult as a way of increasing choice Developments remained clinician-led or response to national policy initiatives

Accountability	No increase in local accountability though individual hospitals gained own boards of directors. Under the Conservatives, non-executive directors tended to share same political values including business orientation. Non-executives valued for their management skills not as community representatives
	Trust decision-making no more transparent to patients or public Providers made more centrally accountable to Secretary of State than before reforms. Increase in 1990s of central targets (e.g. Health of the Nation, waiting lists, Patient's Charter)

buyers of trust services with a budget for mainly elective (non-urgent) services which was protected from the pressures of rising emergency admissions which occurred during the 1990s. Thus they represented a source of additional income for trusts with tight annual budget constraints set by health authority purchasers. Particularly where the tight budget constraints meant that trusts might have spare capacity (e.g. in elective surgery), trusts were anxious to respond by either lowering prices or giving preferential waiting times to fundholders' patients (Propper *et al*, 1997; Ellwood, 1996) (see Table 9.1 for evidence of this).

Another feature of the implementation of the reforms was that trusts were granted far less freedom than their managers had expected. For example, originally the idea had been to allow trusts substantial freedoms to raise their own capital, but in the event their access to capital has been very restricted and they have not been free to borrow commercially in the normal way. National pay bargaining has largely been maintained, because trust managements have found local negotiations too time-consuming and risky financially. The pressure of central directives affecting the working of trusts intensified over the period as the NHS Executive pursued its goal of a 'managed market'. For example, trusts were required to earn a real return of 6% on capital employed, but in 1992/93 47% of first wave trusts failed to do so (Newchurch and Company, 1994). Finally, as discussed elsewhere in this chapter, NHS purchasers were less effective than predicted at putting trusts under pressure to assess the strengths and weaknesses of their services in comparison with others. This, combined with the lack of incentives for trusts to improve their efficiency such as the inability to retain any surpluses, may go some way to explaining the relatively weak effects of trust status on provider performance.

The impact of general practice fundholding

There is no doubt that of all the aspects of the internal market, general practice fundholding received the most attention both in popular debate and research since there was consensus that it represented a genuine novelty with the potential to alter previous power relationships, for instance between hospital specialists and primary care generalists. In addition, from the first wave of volunteer practices entering the scheme, fundholders were given significantly greater freedom than health authorities to innovate and to shift resources between providers if they saw fit. In part, this was possible because fundholders controlled only a small proportion (about 20% of the hospital and community health services, initially) of their patients' potential NHS resource consumption and each fundholding practice represented only a small part of each trust's income.

At variance with the top-down, population-based approach to purchasing represented by the health authorities, the NHS reforms introduced a rival model in which volunteer general practices would act as the clinically informed agents for their patients, purchasing a limited range of elective services and managing their own prescribing costs out of a single budget. Their budgets were deducted from the allocations of the health authorities. Fundholders were able to make savings from their budgets, which could be used at the convenience of the GPs either to purchase additional services from others or to improve facilities in the general practice. Initially, large general practices of 11 000 patients or more were eligible to volunteer. This was later reduced to 7 000 and subsequently even smaller practices could take part either by purchasing an even more limited range of services or by linking together into groups known as multi-funds in which they shared risk and management overheads. The range of services included in the scheme was also extended to include a wider range of community health services. By April 1997, just over 60% of the population of England was registered with fundholding practices.

The extent and quality of the research on the effects of GP fundholding is far better than that available on health authority purchasing together with the range of alternatives to fundholding which grew up below health authority level (see below). However, much of the research, perhaps inevitably, has focused on changes in the process of care and in activity generated by fundholding rather than on changes in the quality of patient care or patients' experiences. There have been very few studies which compared the performance of fundholders as purchasers with health authorities, or with non-fundholding schemes for involving GPs in the purchasing process. This is understandable since health authorities and fundholders were charged with a different set of responsibilities and regulated differently. Most crucially, health authorities had to purchase unplanned, emergency care for the whole population (including patients of fundholders) and elective or planned care for the patients of GPs who had chosen not to enter the fundholding scheme. Furthermore, fundholding practices were self-selected and tended already to have better facilities and to be in more affluent parts of the country than non-fundholding practices as a whole (Audit Commission, 1995; Petchey, 1995).

There have been a number of review articles examining the evidence on fundholding (Coulter, 1995; Dixon and Glennerster, 1995; Hoey, 1995; Petchey, 1995), but none was a comprehensive review of the evidence. The current review includes evidence up to the end of 1997 and includes material not covered previously.

The introduction of fundholding had an number of specific objectives according to government: to reduce inefficiencies in provider organizations; to create better quality secondary care; to place downward pressure on GP prescribing expenditure and on unnecessary referrals; to enhance facilities at practice level for patient care; and to promote greater choice and responsiveness to individual patients' needs. Table 9. 2 assesses the extent to which these were realized in so far as the research evidence permits.

As in the case of NHS trusts, it is worth attempting to explain some of the findings in terms of the wider management of the NHS in the period. For example, studies showed that GP fundholders were able to reduce the rate of increase of their prescribing expenditure more than non-fundholders, particularly in the first year, but that subsequently the relative reductions in spending declined until, after the third year, the increases in costs were similar for both types of practices. This may be explained in two ways. First, there may well have been a limit to the degree to which fundholders could find differential ways of curbing pressures on drug costs. Second, and indicative of the way in which the internal market was implemented, fundholders increasingly found that any savings which they were able to make were built into their next year's prescribing budgets by the health authority. This greatly reduced their incentive to continue to find ways of reducing their prescribing costs.

Another potentially puzzling conclusion is the consensus among more sophisticated commentators that 'cream skimming' or discrimination against high-cost patients (for example, by removing them from the patient lists of GP fundholders) was likely to have remained more a theoretical than an actual equity problem of the fundholding scheme. Although there is little or no evidence one way or the other, knowledge of the way in which the reforms were implemented suggests a number of factors which may have mitigated against systematic discrimination against high cost patients. First of all, there was a simple 'stop-loss' mechanism in the scheme, since the health authority became financially liable for any patient who cost the fund more than £6,000 per year. Second, most fundholders' budgets for most of the life of the scheme were based on historic expenditure patterns. Third, GPs were not personally financially liable for any overspending. The only sanction was the possibility that they would be removed from the scheme. Indeed, anecdotally, many fundholders had realized that, as doctors, in a tax funded service, they were in a strong position to defy the local health authority if they overspent, on the grounds that needed treatment should not be denied to their patients.

All in all, the extensive, if far from ideal, body of research on GP fundholding suggests that the scheme probably produced at least some of the intended consequences in relation to curbing the rate of increase of prescribing costs and producing more practice-level services. It seems, on balance, that trusts were more responsive to fundholders' demands than to those of other purchasers, though there was scope for any improvements in service to be generalized to other practices'

Table 9.2 The impact of general practitioner fundholding

Evaluative criterion	Evidence
Efficiency	No direct research on technical or allocative efficiency, but research on related areas
Prescribing costs	Considerable body of research showing reduced rate of growth of prescribing costs initially compared to non-FHs, probably due to greater use of generics and less repeat prescribing, but not sustained. However, absolute difference between GPFHs and non-FHs persisted. Some non-FHs able to reduce rate of growth similarly.
Referral rates	Number of studies, but vast majority showed little or no difference in trend of referrals compared with non-FH practices. No sign of effects of budgetary pressure or price sensitivity. No sign that GPFHs shifted costs to HA by increasing emergency admissions
Shift in location of care	Growth in practice level services (e.g. using savings) with smaller growth in non-FH practices. Mainly specialist outreach, but questions about cost-effectiveness of practice level specialist clinics
Financial management and savings	Greater savings than HAs. Underspent each year 1991-96, overall. Extent to which savings due to more efficient purchasing, economies, lower prices, more generous funding or healthier patients was not clear
	Majority of savings spent on practice premises, facilities and staff rather than secondary care, thereby giving GPFH practices advantage over non-FHs
Transaction costs	Consensus that transaction costs rose (though no detailed, direct data) due to more complex contracts than HAs and large number of small purchasers. Crude estimates suggest that additional costs were more than savings
Equity	
Level of funding	Evidence is mixed as to whether GPFHs were fairly funded versus HAs, though largely funded on basis of past spending. Likely that position varied across regions, though data were poor

Access to care ('two-tierism')	Focus of most criticism and large amount of anecdote and case study information. Best study shows significant difference in waiting times in favour of GPFHs though not possible to tell if non-FHs' patients were worse off as a result.
	Believed to be result of greater market power of GPFHs as marginal purchasers and earmarked budgets (see Table 9.1)
'Cream skimming'	Major concern initially, but no empirical studies. Hard to study directly, but less likely than theory suggested
Quality	Little attention and no comparisons with HAs, etc
Quality of secondary care received	One study which showed little change pre/post GPFH
Quality improvements in contracts with providers	Feature reported by GPFHs, HAs and locality commissioners, but GPFHs convinced that FH led to quality improvement in contracts (mainly better communication). No direct studies of service quality
Quality of practice-based services	Increase in practice-level services (see above, Efficiency), but no empirical evidence on quality or substitution
Choice and responsiveness,	GPFHs more willing to offer patients choice of hospital, etc., but patients indifferent to this. Few patients knew if GP was FH or not. No direct evidence about choice, but GPFHs reluctant to change hospitals
Accountability	Greater freedom than HAs. Accountability framework not introduced until 1994. This was criticized since still no assessment of value-for-money of GPFHs' purchasing

patients. However, the claim that fundholding had led to a 'two-tier' service, at least in terms of waiting times for in-patient treatment, appears to have been borne out. Finally, fundholding created a high administrative workload and higher transaction costs for trusts than other forms of purchasing, without necessarily being any more responsive to the preferences of individual patients.

The impact of health authority purchasing

In principle, the separation of purchasing from providing functions in the NHS was designed to free health authorities from the day-to-day preoccupations of running facilities, and enable them to reassess the health care needs of their populations unhampered by a commitment to any particular pattern of resource distribution. It was widely believed that it was especially important for health authorities to be able to challenge the primacy given to acute hospital services now that they were no longer responsible directly for them. In this way, they were to set new investment priorities designed to maximize the health of the population.

In polemical and research terms, health authority purchasing (and the sub-district variants on fundholding which it spawned such as locality and GP commissioning, see below) failed to capture the imagination. The early King's Fund research programme on the first two years of the reforms failed to include a study looking directly at the role of the health authority as purchaser. This relative lack of research, particularly compared with GP fundholding, can be explained in a number of ways:

- first, health authority purchasing seemed to bear a strong resemblance to the health authority planning of services which had preceded it, but with an internal market badge;
- second, health authority purchasing appeared more remote, strategic and long term compared with the immediacy of the idea of GPs 'shopping around' in the health service 'spot market' to reduce their waiting times;
- health authority purchasing was introduced everywhere from the beginning of the reforms rather than GP fundholding and trusts which came in 'waves', so there was little opportunity to compare it with anything else;
- in the first year of the internal market, health authorities were instructed by the centre (the NHS Executive) to aim for a 'steady state' as it was known in which their new contracts reproduced the existing pattern of referrals and activity. In contrast, GP fundholders were given freedom in 1991/92 to purchase the elective services within fundholding as they saw fit;
- health authorities and GP fundholders could not straightforwardly be compared since health authorities had a far broader remit, including purchasing emergency care for all fundholders' patients;
- additionally, the reforms themselves altered systems of routine data collection in the NHS so that straightforward monitoring of activity rates and spending by specialty, for example, became hazardous undertakings;
- finally, it could be argued that the ultimate test of health authority purchasing would be its effects on the health of the population within its boundaries. Yet such effects were likely to take years to demonstrate and would be confounded by many other influences on population health.

As a result, much of the research is either 'indirect' (i.e. theoretically informed commentary and prediction) or focuses on the process of purchasing such as whether purchasers had the necessary information systems to negotiate effective contracts. Table 9.3 attempts to summarize the evidence such as it is.

Table 9.3 Impact of health authority purchasing

Evaluative criterion	Evidence
Efficiency	Relates to the interaction between HAs and providers, so difficult to link to behaviour of HAs alone
Technical efficiency	29% increase in finished consultant episodes (FCEs) per bed, 1990/91 versus 1994/95. Reduction in acute stay from 11 to 8 days
	Cost-Weighted Activity Index (CWAI), which links activity to expenditure, rose faster than real resources and faster after reforms than before. Purchaser Efficiency Index (= yearly changes in activity in relation to changes in HA allocations) also rose since the reforms
	But problem with all measures because no link to outcomes, weight in-patient activity higher, based on episodes not patients, and reforms may have encouraged fuller recording of activity
Allocative efficiency	Little data on balance and content of what was purchased and changes of provider. None on whether changes between services or providers improved efficiency
Transaction costs	In 45 HAs, contracts tripled from 1,160 (1991/92) to 3,309 (1994/95) and became more sophisticated. Additional costs from Extracontractual Referrals (ECRs). Extra costs for HAs and trusts
	Extra costs from running HA and GPFH together
	But in relation to functions, HAs generated lower transaction costs than GPFHs (see Table 9.2)
Financial management	HAs more likely to be in deficit since the reforms than GPFHs, but not clear whether this is due to poor management or extra pressures they face (e.g. emergency services) or resource differences. HAs moved into deficit as growth of NHS revenue slowed
Equity	Concern that 'health gain' goal would ignore equity
	HA allocations moved increasingly to 'fair share' target based on capitation, but inequities in access to and use of specific services remained and HAs continued to purchase

	different combinations of services with local priorities. No evidence that reforms directly made inequities worse
	Panel survey data (BHPS) show no change in equity of GP and in-patient care standardized for need between 1990/91 and 1993/94
Quality	Emphasis on volume and price, though limited quality standards in contracts. 60% used outcomes in contracts, but only 20% related them to financial incentives
	Case studies showing quality/effectiveness gains through contracting
	Overall effects confounded by Patient's Charter and Waiting List Initiatives (centrally determined targets)
Choice and responsiveness	Increased emphasis on informing and consulting the public about plans stimulated by Local Voices initiative. Unclear whether views influenced HAs
	More responsive to government performance targets than individual patients/consumer representatives
Accountability	More 'upward' accountability for defined objectives (e.g. Patient's Charter targets) through a clearer framework
	No/little change in 'downward' accountability (see Choice and responsiveness, above)

The relatively muted discernible effects of turning health authorities into purchasing organizations requires some explanation. Health authorities remained part of a hierarchical management system in the NHS; indeed, the managerial changes associated with the reforms and their aftermath reinforced their position. Thus although there was variation (sometimes considerable) in the pattern of health services purchased by each health authority, this was largely the result of historical differences in local provision. The new drivers of change were the series of national initiatives such as the series of waiting list purges and the Patient's Charter (Great Britain Department of Health, 1991) with its waiting time targets (e.g. how long patients should wait to be seen once they had arrived in the out-patient clinic and, particularly, the avoidance of long waits for in-patient treatment). Evidence for this comes from a number of studies of the incentives facing health authorities as purchasers. For example, Hughes and colleagues (1997) studied the contracting of the nine health authorities in Wales in the mid-1990s and showed that their behaviour was influenced far less by market circumstances such as the choice of potential providers, opportunities to improve efficiency or a desire to reduce the transaction costs of complex contract negotiations, than by policy change at the centre. Health authorities were moving towards more collaborative relationships with their providers over time as a result of bureaucratic rather than internal market incentives.

In a similar vein, Propper (1995) examined the incentives facing health authority purchasers and pointed out that, irrespective of objective market conditions (e.g. the extent to which there was a choice of accessible providers), their regulatory environment was predominant. At an early stage of the reforms it had been shown that only 8% of acute hospitals in the West Midlands had a monopoly of their main surgical specialties within a 30-mile radius (Appleby et al, 1994), suggesting that health authorities potentially had considerable choice of providers, at least in the conurbations. Yet, where a particular aspect of performance was the subject of a performance target, the health authority could be shown to increase ouput in that dimension. For example, for much of the period of the reforms there was an emphasis on increasing activity at constant or reduced costs and some evidence that this is what health authorities gave priority to (see Table 9.3) rather than other ways of improving efficiency. In addition, the scale of resources deployed by health authorities may, on occasions, have inhibited them from making major changes of provider for specific services for fear of destabilizing other local services.

As well as responding to bureaucratic targets (such as waiting time) rather than internal market signals, the behaviour of the health authorities can also be explained by the wide scope of their purchasing responsibilities. Unlike fundholders, they were required to purchase across the entire range of hospital and community health services which put them at a relative disadvantage compared with fundholders. A study of health authority purchasing of specialized services revealed that, far from destabilizing such services either by ignoring them or by constantly challenging their providers to change what they provided or the way it was provided, health authorities lacked the expertise and/or resources to make many significant changes in these areas (Audit Commission, 1997). Few health authorities had put specialized services out to competitive tender or carried out thorough reviews of the cost and quality of their services which had led to decisions to change providers. Thus few of the predicted problems of health authority purchasing had materialized, but there had been few positive gains as well. This conclusion could apply to many aspects of health authority purchasing.

The Audit Commission (1997) concluded that one of the main problems remained the geographically unequal patterns of access to and use of highly specialized care which comparatively large purchasers like health authorities could begin to tackle. However, there was little sign that there had been much change in this respect since the reforms. It is interesting that this finding matches precisely recent evidence from a very different source, namely from the British Household Panel Survey (BHPS) analysed by Propper (1998). She compared the pattern of use of GP and in-patient services standardized for morbidity by household income group between 1990/91 (essentially before the reforms) and 1993/94 (after two years). Large changes could be interpreted as the result of major changes in the health care system, including the introduction of the purchaser–provider separation and contracting. The comparison indicated little difference between the two waves of the BHPS, and the overall distribution of the two forms of health care remained slightly in favour of the poor, allowing for need. Thus the broad picture was of little change in equity (or inequity, as shown by studies of specific services) in the delivery of care as a result of the reforms. Of course, these are relatively crude data which tell nothing about the quality or timeliness of the care received, nor do they include out-patient and other services. It may also be the case that three years was not long enough to produce discernible macro-level changes. Nonetheless, the findings from the BHPS provide further background corroboration for the conclusion that health authority purchasing was, for all the reasons discussed above, associated with relatively little change for good or ill.

The impact of non-fundholding: locality commissioning and general practitioner commissioning

Through most of the period 1991–97, GP fundholding received most of the attention as a mechanism for involving GPs in purchasing health services for their patients. However, a range of alternatives to fundholding emerged soon after 1991/92 as health authority managers and non-fundholding GPs sought ways of mimicking certain aspects of fundholding with which they approved (e.g. GP input to purchasing decisions) and of avoiding those aspects which they objected to (e.g. the divisiveness of fundholding, the cost of administering fundholding). Unlike fundholding, these were not central government initiatives and were not embodied in legislation.

The term health services' '*commissioning*' rather than '*purchasing*' was used to describe these schemes which operated below health authority level and within the framework of health authority purchasing (Mays and Dixon, 1996). The 'purchasing' undertaken by fundholders was defined by its critics as going out into the market-place in the short term with a sum of money and buying from the range of services already on offer. 'Commissioning', by contrast, was defined by its proponents as working strategically with providers over a period of time to develop the desired pattern of local services without necessarily directly controlling the budget which would be used to purchase the services at the end of the process. Thus the wide range of different models of commissioning operated without budgets which had been allocated to them as of right. The resources whose deployment they attempted to influence, or which they received in the form of an indicative budget or on a delegated basis from the health authority, remained the ultimate responsibility of the health authority.

There were two main types of commissioning distinguished principally by their origins (bottom-up versus top-down):

- *GP commissioning* in which groups of non-fundholding practices (at least initially, though over time fundholders began to join in) came together spontaneously in response to fundholding to propose service changes and developments to the health authority on behalf of their patients, and which the health authority incorporated into its contracts. Groups would normally be allocated an indicative or 'shadow' budget and might employ their own co-ordinator paid for by the authority. GP commissioning groups varied widely in size. They tended to emphasize internal democracy with regular elections of GP representatives to act in an executive capacity on behalf of their peers;
- *Locality commissioning* in which the health authority brought together all the practices in a geographical area (typically an area with a population of 50–60 000) to form a group charged with eliciting the views of all the GPs in the locality and channelling these constructively into the health authority's purchasing process either by influencing the plans of the health authority directly or by working with local providers to agree changes which could then be incorporated in health authority contracts. Again, locality commissioning groups could have indicative budgets to manage within the broader framework of the health authority's contracts, but would not contract independently. They would normally have a paid co-ordinator from the health authority.

In practice, the two types of scheme have much in common, being collective, non-budget holding alternatives to fundholding, working with and through the agency of the health authority on behalf of a sub-population of the authority. Both aimed to make health authority purchasing more locally sensitive to variations in needs and patients' views, using GPs as the main source of information and to overcome the perceived remoteness of the health authority bureaucracy. Both sorts of commissioning varied widely across the country in the details of how they were organized and their precise roles *vis-á-vis* the health authority. However, all relied heavily on their ability to influence local providers and the health authority without necessarily having the independent purchasing power to make their views count in the face of concerted opposition. In general, neither model has included an incentive that any 'savings' created by cost-conscious purchasing could be retained by the group to spend on additional services or facilities.

Both forms of commissioning organization are considered together in Table 9.4. Most of the limited body of evidence on locality and GP commissioning focuses on how the various schemes have evolved. There is only one study which attempted to compare commissioning with fundholding (Glennerster *et al*, 1996). For the rest, the studies attempt to assess the schemes against internal criteria such as the quality of their external relationships and their reported ability to change local services. A high proportion of the published material comes from participants in commissioning or proponents of the approaches.

Table 9.4 The impact of non-fundholding: locality and general practitioner commissioning

Evaluative criterion	Evidence
Efficiency	
Technical efficiency	Little data, but some examples of improvements negotiated in tests and elective surgery and reductions in prescribing costs
	Able to change services with HA support—local context is important
Allocative efficiency	No data, though able to shift providers
Management costs	Less costly to administer than GPFH
Transaction costs	Full costs not known, but probably less than GPFH
	Less costly schemes less effective in bringing about change
Equity	A high priority of participating GPs and built into design of organizations involving all practices in an area. Aim to benefit all patients equally. No 'two-tierism' (see Table 9.2)
	But no studies of access to services between practices within GP/locality group or in comparison with GPFH
Quality	Improvements reported, especially in primary and community health services and waiting, but no direct research on quality. Much depended on local HA
Choice and responsiveness	Schemes used by HAs to obtain patient/public views, but as in GPFH, GPs acted as proxies for patients. Not a high priority in schemes
Accountability	Formally part of the HA with HA legally accountable for budget
	Strong democratic accountability of GP representatives to their colleagues in many schemes (peer accountability)
	Local, 'downward' accountability not a priority

Although the evidence on locality and GP commissioning is not strong, there are valuable lessons to be learned since such schemes tended to operate somewhere between the extremes of single practice fundholding and large population-based health authority purchasing in terms both of scale and degree of direct budgetary control at local level. One of the key questions raised by locality and GP commissioning groups is whether it is possible to make the same sorts of quality and efficiency gains as were reported under fundholding, but at lower cost because of the absence of devolved budgets to manage and separate contracts to negotiate. The alternative scenario, which is also of interest in a cash-limited system, is one in which the commissioning group is able to achieve less, but at lower cost than the fundholder. Stand-alone studies of individual initiatives tended to conclude that it was possible (Willis, 1996), but the only study which attempted in any way to compare commissioning with fundholding came to a less favourable conclusion (Glennerster et al, 1996). It compared six schemes including a locality commissioning group, a GP commissioning group, a health authority-wide GP commissioning executive, a GP consultation group and a total purchasing scheme in which a group of fundholders had volunteered to take responsibility for a delegated budget from the health authority for a wider range of services than were included in the standard fundholding scheme (Mays et al, 1997). Although the study was small scale and did not directly measure the management costs of the six schemes, its findings are thought provoking. The schemes varied widely in their effectiveness as assessed by the GPs' reports of successful changes negotiated. Two factors appeared to be important in this: first, the extent to which the scheme had an infrastructure of a manager and information system ('minimalist' schemes had made little impact); and second, how far the health authority was prepared to take the group seriously and support its aims. The schemes which reported most success looked most like fundholding in that they gave the GPs some autonomy and control over a budget. Glennerster et al (1996) also compared the six schemes with the fundholders they had examined using the same methods in another study and concluded that, in general, the commissioning projects were less successful in resolving their local service problems than the fundholders. Finally, they noted that the strengths of the two broad approaches were somewhat different. Fundholding was associated with micro-efficiency improvements to services used by individual practice populations while commissioning groups were more effective in taking collective action to improve the quality and accessibility of local health services to an entire population. It appears that the answer to the question posed earlier is that relative success depends on the context and particularly on the posture of the local health authority, but that where there is a conflict of opinion or interest, the devolved purchaser/commissioner is likely to do better with control of a budget than without. It also seems likely that different types of GPs and practices were attracted into fundholding and non-fundholding schemes from the outset, motivated by different beliefs about what constituted a 'good' health system and even different beliefs about whether change could best be brought about using economic incentives or through building up relationships of influence. Equally, it seems plausible that in areas where the health authority was receptive to the views of GPs expressed through a commissioning group, there was little reason to take a budget and a local consensus grew that the expense of fundholding was unnecessary. In other circumstances (such as resistant providers and health authority) a very different consensus may have resulted. For instance, Glennerster *et al* (1998) claimed that where the health authority failed to take the role of the commissioning or consultation group seriously, practices tended to move into fundholding.

Interim findings from the national evaluation of total purchasing pilot projects (TPPs) shed further light on the ingredients of effective purchasing/commissioning in the internal market and particularly on the relative importance of economic incentives in bringing about change in a publicly funded health care system. TPPs were an extension of the fundholding scheme which allowed fundholding practices singly or in groups (average population 30–40 000) to take on responsibility for purchasing potentially all of the hospital and community health services for their patients. However, because the scheme was introduced on a pilot basis, the additional budgets received by the TPPs were delegated from the local health authority which remained ultimately responsible for the resources. As a result, the TPPs had much in common with those locality and GP commissioning schemes in which some degree of budgetary delegation occurred from the health authority.

Although comparative data on the performance of the TPPs versus other sub-district commissioning approaches and/or the health authority as purchaser are not yet available, there is considerable diversity between the pilots such that some 40% of the 53 'first wave' TPPs did not take a delegated budget in the first year and acted essentially as GP commissioning groups. Thus comparisons between the TPPs are instructive. TPPs with a delegated budget and at least some of their own independent contracts were more likely to report achieving their first year's purchasing objectives than the rest. However, 'success' was also associated with a higher level of health authority support and higher spending on the management infrastructure to bring about service change, particularly the investment in leadership and information systems needed to build links between previously separate general practices and good relationships with local trusts (Mays *et al*, 1998). For example, smaller, simpler TPPs were more likely to be able to manage their spending than larger, more complex TPPs in the first year because they had less organizational development work to do to encourage the GPs to take collective financial responsibility for their decisions. On the other hand, TPPs also found that they were too small alone to negotiate major service changes to local acute hospitals where these affected the services available to a far larger population. In these circumstances, they could make their views known, but the process of change was typically led by the health authority, often in collaboration with other authorities.

From the experience of locality commissioning, GP commissioning and total purchasing, it appears that effective service change requires some degree of budgetary control, but that this alone is insufficient in a Health Service which still sees itself as a 'system' (i.e. where the impact of one purchaser's decisions on the services used by other purchasers is a matter of collective concern, and where ensuring that a reasonable standard of service is available to all is as important as stimulating efficiency-improving innovations available, at least initially, to a sub-group of the population). The local context, the extent of health authority support, the quality of relationships with trusts and high-quality leadership are all necessary ingredients as well. Contracts in themselves may have potential importance in shaping health care, but it should not automatically be assumed that they are the sole or even the major influence. Other studies of purchaser-provider relations in the NHS internal market have reached similar conclusions, arguing that negotiating service change requires that there must be at least the *potential* for taking the business elsewhere ('*contestability*'), but that this must be supported on a day-to-day basis by the development of good communication and relations of trust between purchasers and providers (Flynn and Williams, 1997).

Discussion

On balance, does the highly condensed review contained in this paper indicate that the internal market was a success or a failure? How much change was there and how much can be attributed to the internal market? Whether the internal market can be seen as a success, a failure or somewhere between the two, now that it is coming to an end in its original form, what lessons can be learned?

Success or failure?

Perhaps the most striking conclusion from the review is how little, major, *measurable* change on the chosen evaluative criteria can be related unequivocally to the core structures and mechanisms of the internal market. Neither the prophets of doom nor the enthusiasts have been proved correct.

On *efficiency*, as Tables 9.1 and 9.3 showed, very crude measures of activity rose faster than the increase in NHS expenditure, even allowing for the increase in management spending and transaction costs in the period. The causes of this are not clear since similar trends were apparent before the internal market was introduced. The evidence using more sophisticated measures of efficiency is fragmentary.

On *equity*, the main equity concern, 'cream skimming' (discriminating against higher cost patients) did not seem to have materialized, but there is little doubt (though little good research) that 'two-tierism' (i.e. the preferential treatment of fundholding general practitioners' patients over patients whose services were purchased by the health authority) did exist in many places. Although the internal market did not appear to have exacerbated the existing inequities in access to specific types of health care, it did little or nothing directly to mitigate them.

On *quality*, there are very few studies which attempted to measure it directly. There is some evidence that fundholders used their budgets to provide more accessible services at practice level and negotiated shorter waiting times on average than health authorities. However, for all NHS patients, waits for in-patient treatment fell during the 1990s. This was particularly noticeable for long waits, but was not a direct product of the internal market so much as other initiatives. On the wider indicator of quality represented by public dissatisfaction with the NHS, dissatisfaction rose *before* the introduction of the internal market, fell during the early 1990s as more money was put into the system and resumed its upward trend after 1996.

On *choice and responsiveness* to the demands of individual patients, there is little evidence one way or the other. The internal market was designed to empower the main purchasers who would act as agents on behalf of patients rather than the patients themselves.

On *accountability*, there was a tightening of 'upward' accountability to the NHS Executive at national level in England, but little change in the modest level of 'downward' accountability to patients or the general public at local level.

These assessments based on an exhaustive review of the evidence concur in most respects with the less systematic views of the leading commentators. For example, *The Independent* newspaper argued in a leading article on 25 February 1997 that, 'The Thatcher–Clarke reforms—GP fundholding, the quasi-market—are neither pernicious nor notably efficacious.' Similarly, West (1997) summed up a recently published personal view of the reforms, 'There is no reason to believe that the NHS got manifestly worse under the Reforms.' While this may seem a paltry result given the effort and resources which were devoted to what was a huge organizational change, it is also reassuring given the potential for destabilizing the entire system inherent in the radicalism of the original reform proposals.

Although the internal market may not have produced the degree of measurable change predicted by opponents and supporters, it is clear that six years of the internal market have changed the culture and operating assumptions of the NHS in ways which are difficult to capture in largely quantitative studies. For example, for good or ill, the relations between GPs, health authorities and trust staff, especially medical specialists, have changed markedly due to GP fundholding. By passing secondary care resources to primary care professionals in the form of purchasing budgets, new forms of dialogue and relationships as well as new forms of health care have resulted (e.g. specialist out-patient clinics in community settings). It would now be almost inconceivable not to involve GPs and other primary care generalists in commissioning a wide range of services. Throughout the Service, there has been a considerable increase in cost-consciousness and a wide (but by no means total) acceptance that the device of separately identifying the purchaser role from that of the provider should remain in some form. There appears to be little desire among politicians, managers or clinicians to return to the NHS of the 1980s.

Why did these organizational and cultural changes not produce more demonstrable impacts in the areas investigated in the review? The answer must lie in how the reforms were implemented. From the perspective of those who believe in the feasibility of using quasi-market mechanisms to improve health systems devoted to social goals of equity, quality and efficiency, the incentives in the UK internal market were too weak and the constraints were too strong. Others such as Light (1997) have argued forcefully that the UK was quite correct in not letting market forces have much play. For example, competition between providers was strictly controlled by government even where it could have occurred in case its efficiency consequences, such as hospital closures, threatened other goals such as equality of access to services, or embarrassed the government politically. Though the internal architecture of the NHS had been substantially altered as if the NHS were any large business corporation, it remained the direct responsibility of central government and, therefore, the subject of party political controversy. When the potential effects of competition threatened to cause chaos in central London, for instance, the government stepped in with a review of services designed to limit the play of market forces (James, 1994). Ironically, central London was one of the few parts of the country where conditions for extensive competition between acute hospitals existed, though there is little doubt that there were competitive elements in the internal market in particular places and over specific services.

In fact, with the exception perhaps of GP fundholders, the NHS was driven through most of the period between 1991 and 1998 by a system of central directives and bureaucratic incentives covering topics such as waiting times, activity levels, priority services, and health promotion targets. For example, health authorities had little incentive to develop a budgetary surplus since the only guarantee was that it would be clawed back by the Treasury at the year's end.

The lessons to be learned

As Saltman (1997) has cautioned, health system reform is a 'socially embedded' process even when it appears to be driven by a strictly economic rationale. Similar seeming approaches will tend to be implemented in different ways and/or will produce different consequences in different countries as a result of their histories, starting points, political structures of accountability, etc. At the same time, it is increasingly being appreciated that effective contracting, especially in health care where the 'product' can be so difficult to define, depends on building relationships of trust, usually over a substantial period of time, between purchasers and providers.

The Conservative government appeared to recognize these sorts of insights from at least 1994 when it encouraged the Service to find the appropriate balance between competition and 'constructive co-operation' (Great Britain Department of Health, 1994). Labour's recent White Paper (Great Britain Department of Health,

1997) appears to go slightly further down the line of co-operation while maintaining key elements from the Conservative approach with a new collective version of the former fundholding scheme in the form of PCGs. No one now believes that a straightforwardly competitive internal market is feasible or desirable if it ever was. Ye at the same time, the experiment with such notions has apparently irrevocably changed the way in which publicly funded health care is thought of in the UK. The new Labour administration shows few if any signs of returning the NHS to the previous form of vertical integration. The purchaser-provider separation remains, albeit attenuated. The new PCGs will be allowed, not as a frontline strategy but *in extremis*, to switch between providers if they are dissatisfied with the services they are receiving. Their preferred operating policy should be to develop good relations with providers in order to bring about improvements by persuasion.

It is too early to know whether the gradual replacement of competition by collaboration and co-operation between purchasers and providers, which emerged under the Conservatives and which has been given more explicit recognition by Labour, will work. For co-operation to work consistently there have to be no conflicts of interest between purchasers and providers: this is unlikely, particularly at a time when much service innovation by purchasers concerns moving resources away from traditional places and forms of provision. After all, it was in recognition of the existence of such conflicts of interest that the internal market was designed. It is possible that keeping the potential for competition as a last resort (some form of last ditch contestability) becomes a mechanism for allowing co-operation to become the norm without losing sight of all incentives to greater efficiency. Given the difficulties in health care of maintaining a competitive environment and indeed its undesirability on many occasions, last resort competition may be a workable compromise. However, the precise effects on efficiency, quality, equity, etc will depend in large part on the detailed, day-to-day interpretation placed on future guidance and regulation from the centre by managers and clinicians throughout the NHS.

Acknowledgements

This paper is a personal summary of an extensive piece of collaborative work with colleagues from the King's Fund. A full account is given in Goodwin *et al* (1998).

References

Appleby J, Smith P, Ranade W, Little V, Robinson R. Monitoring managed competition. In: Robinson R, Le Grand J (eds) *Evaluating the NHS Reforms*. London: King's Fund Institute, 1994, pp 24–53

Audit Commission. *Briefing on GP Fundholding*. London: HMSO, 1995

Audit Commission. *Higher Purchase: Commissioning Specialised Services in the NHS*. London: The Stationery Office, 1997

Bartlett W, Le Grand J. The performance of trusts. In: Robinson R, Le Grand J (eds) *Evaluating the NHS Reforms*. London: King's Fund Institute, 1994

Coulter A. Evaluating general practice fundholding in the UK. *European Journal of Public Health*, 1995; **5**: 233–239

Dixon J, Glennerster H. What do we know about fundholding in general practice? *British Medical Journal*, 1995; **311**: 727–730

Dixon J, Mays N. New Labour; new NHS? *British Medical Journal*, 1997; **315**: 1639–1640

Ellwood S. Pricing of services in the UK NHS. *Financial Accountability and Management*, 1996; **12**: 281–301

Flynn R, Williams G (eds) *Contracting for Health: Quasi-markets and the National Health Service*. Oxford: Oxford University Press, 1997

Glennerster H, Cohen A, Bovell V. *Alternatives to Fundholding*. London: Suntory-Toyota International Centre for Economics and Related Disciplines, London School of Economics, 1996

Glennerster H, Cohen A, Bovell V. Alternatives to fundholding. *International Journal of Health Services*, 1998; **28**: 47–66

Goodwin N, Hamblin R, Mulligan J-A, Le Grand J, Mays N, Dixon J. *A Balance Sheet of the Evidence on the Impact of the NHS Internal Market, 1991–97*. London: King's Fund Publishing, 1998, in press

Great Britain Department of Health. *The Patient's Charter*. London: HMSO, 1991

Great Britain Department of Health. *A Guide to the Operation of the NHS Internal Market: local freedoms, national responsibilities*. London: HMSO, 1994

Great Britain Department of Health *The New NHS–Modern, Dependable*. London: The Stationery Office, 1997

Ham C. Managed markets in health care: the UK experiment. *Health Policy*, 1996; **35**: 279–292

Hoey A. GP fundholding: mixing money and medicine. *Consumer Policy Review*, 1995; **5**: 175–179

Hughes D, Griffiths L, McHale JV. Do quasi-markets evolve? Institutional analysis and the NHS. *Cambridge Journal of Economics*, 1997; **21**: 259–276

James A. *Managing to Care: Public Services and the Market*. London: Longman, 1994

Klein R. Big bang health care reform—does it work? The case of Britain's 1991 National Health Service reforms. *Milbank Quarterly*, 1995; **73**: 299–337

Le Grand J, Mays N, Mulligan J-A, Goodwin N, Dixon J, Glennerster H. *Models of Purchasing and Commissioning: review of the research evidence*. A report to the Department of Health. London: London School of Economics and King's Fund, 1997

Light DW. From managed competition to manged cooperation: theory and lessons from the British experience. *Milbank Quarterly*, 1997; **75**: 297–341

Maynard A, Bloor K. Introducing a market to the United Kingdom's National Health Service. *New England Journal of Medicine*, 1996; **334**: 604–608

Mays N, Dixon J. *Purchaser Plurality in UK Health Care: is a consensus emerging and is it the right one?* London: King's Fund Publishing, 1996

Mays N, Goodwin N, Bevan G, Wyke S on behalf of the Total Purchasing National Evaluation Team. *Total Purchasing: a profile of national pilot projects.* London: King's Fund Publishing, 1997

Mays N, Goodwin N, Killoran A, Malbon G. *Total Purchasing: a Step towards Primary Care Groups.* London: King's Fund Publishing, in press, 1998

Newchurch and Company. *Fourth Newchurch Guide to NHS Trusts.* London: Newchurch and Co, 1994

Paton C. Present dangers and future threats: some perverse incentives in the NHS reforms. *British Medical Journal*, 1995; **310**: 1245–1248

Petchey R. General practitioner fundholding: weighing the evidence. *Lancet*, 1995; **346**: 1139–1142

Propper C. Agency and incentives in the NHS internal market. *Social Science and Medicine*, 1995; **40**:1683–1690

Propper C, Wilson D, Soderlund N. *The Effects of Regulation and Competition in the NHS Internal Market: the case of GP fundholder prices.* Bristol: Department of Economics, University of Bristol, 1997

Propper C. *Who Pays for and Who Gets Health Care? Equity in the finance and delivery of health care in the United Kingdom.* Nuffield Occasional Papers, Health Economics Series: Paper No. 5. London: The Nuffield Trust, 1998

Robinson R. The impact of the NHS reforms 1991–1995: a review of research evidence. *Journal of Public Health Medicine*, 1996; **18**: 337–342

Robinson R, Le Grand J (eds) *Evaluating the NHS reforms.* London: King's Fund Institute, 1994

Saltman R. Convergence versus social embeddedness: debating the future direction of health care systems. *European Journal of Public Health*, 1997; **7**: 449–453

West PA. *Understanding the National Health Service Reforms.* Buckingham, Open University Press, 1997

Willis A. Commissioning—the best for all. In: Littlejohn P, Victor C (eds) *Making Sense of a Primary Care-led Health Service.* Oxford: Radcliffe Medical Press, 1996, 67–75

10
Reforming pluralist systems: the case of Colombia

Francisco José Yepes, Luz Helena Sánchez

Asociacion Colombiana de la Salud, Santa Fe de Bogota, Colombia

Colombia is a lower middle income country with 36.8 million inhabitants, of whom 73% are urban, and 91% literate. It has a GDP of US$1910 (1995), a life expectancy of 70 years, infant mortality of 26 per 1000, maternal mortality of 107 per 100 000 and total fertility rate of 2.8. Amongst the Latin American countries it ranks third in population, fifth in geographical size and ninth in per capita GNP (World Bank, 1997).

Though Colombia, a constitutional multi-party democracy, has had a relatively "stable" political system with uninterrupted elected governments for most of this century, it has been in a state of internal war for more than 50 years. This aggravates problems of governability and affects the government's ability to introduce reform. The civil population is caught in the crossfire of the main war actors: guerrillas, paramilitary groups, peasant self-defence forces and government armed forces. More than 1 300 000 war refugees are living in very inadequate conditions. For the last decade, the total number of homicides has been over 25 000 per year and 25% of the total burden of disease is attributable to homicides, a far greater proportion than for the world (1%) or Latin America as a whole (3%) (Republica de Colombia Ministerio de Salud, 1994).

Colombia's health system has its roots in pre-Columbian times as well as in the Spanish inheritance, and has been enriched over time with influences from Bismarck's Germany, the French and United States medical schools, and the PAHO/CENDES planning model, amongst others. Although from colonial times there have been government agencies responsible for the different health activities, the country had to wait until 1946 to have the first free-standing Ministry of Hygiene, later called the Ministry of Public Health, and more recently, the Ministry of Health. That same year, the Social Security Institute, which offered a

Bismarckian-style social security insurance to workers, was also instituted (Avila, 1988).

The Colombian health system has been reformed several times during this century, following the prevailing conceptions of the State and the influence of international organizations (Quevedo, 1990). In the second part of the 1970s, the National Health System was created, with a highly centralized structure and a powerful Ministry of Health at the top. This system, which was that existing prior to the most recent rounds of reforms, was a three-tier one. A private subsector served mainly but not exclusively the affluent. A social security system, which never reached beyond 20% coverage, was mainly concentrated in the largest urban areas and covered the workers of the formal sector, and a public sector with hospitals, health centres and health posts served the poor and uninsured. It was accepted by government that 20% of the population was not reached by any subsector.

There were three administrative (territorial) levels within the public sector, the Ministry of Health at the national level, the Department health services at the department level and the local health services at the municipal level. The Ministry of Health set the policies, defined the programmes, established the financing, actually delivered several services, nominated the Department health secretaries and supervised. The health services at the Department level had primarily co-ordinating functions, and the local (municipal) services actually provided care through community hospitals, health centres and posts. These were wholly run from the Department level with no participation from the municipal administration whatsoever, except in some large cities.

This health system was inequitable and inefficient. It was inequitable because real access to health services privileged those with least need. *Per capita* expenditures for the workers affiliated to the Social Security Institute were seven times those of the poor, taken care of by the Ministry of Health. Access to health services favoured the rich and those affiliated to social security: hospitalization rates for the higher income groups were almost double those of the lower income groups and those of the social security affiliates were more than double those of the non-affiliated (Yepes, 1990). Regional differences were also important to the point of having a five-fold difference in government *per capita* health expenditures between the Department getting the least and that getting the most (Molina, 1993). The system was inefficient because Colombia was already spending 7.4% of its GNP on health (Velandia, 1990), and the results were poor compared to other countries with similar or lower levels of spending, such as Costa Rica.

Nonetheless, the public system had been able to develop an acceptable public health infrastructure, the health information system had been considered a model for other developing countries, and there were examples of important social mobilization programmes with public health objectives led by the health sector, such as massive national immunization campaigns in the 1980s.

The reform

Starting from the late 1980s, there have been two main sets of reforms to the health system.

The first centred on the decentralization of the health services to the municipal level, as part of a general decentralization of the State. The prime concern of the decentralization process was to modernize administration, making it more efficient and strengthening democracy through widened citizen participation in the planning, management and control of municipal life (Manrique and Marín, 1987). After several unsuccessful decentralizing efforts which date from 1945, a series of Acts started a profound decentralization effort throughout the whole administration: Acts 14 of 1983, 11 and 12 of 1986 and a series of decrees, 77, 78, 79, 80 and 91 of 1987 (Manrique and Marín, 1987) which paved the way for a comprehensive decentralization process with political, administrative and fiscal reform components, incorporated as a constitutional mandate in the new Constitution of 1991.

Political reform involved actual transference of power to the department and municipal levels through the popular election of department governors and municipal mayors. Administrative reform involved the redefinition of roles and responsibilities of nation, departments and municipalities with the latter assuming many responsibilities that were before in the hands of the nation or the department. Construction of rural roads, schools, hospitals, health centres and posts, water supply and sewerage systems, previously undertaken directly by several national institutes, was transferred to the municipalities and the institutes closed. Fiscal reform involved actual transfer of economic resources to carry out the new responsibilities. Transfers to municipalities increased from 4.3% of GNP in 1990 to 7.7% in 1997.

Health decentralization was mainly established by Act 10 of 1990, complemented by Act 60 of 1993. Municipalities, which before decentralization had no responsibility in the health system, now became major actors. The municipal mayors are now the heads of the municipal health system; they must have a local health plan integrated into the municipal plan; and they are responsible for the health of their communities through the direct provision of health services, contracting with public or private providers, and developing public health activities.

The second set of reforms was that of the social security system which reflected changes in the role of the state in the face of economic opportunities and globalization trends. Act 100 of 1993, as a development of the new 1991 Constitution, established a National Health Insurance scheme with the goal of attaining universal coverage by the year 2001. This Act significantly transformed the health sector and introduced brand new actors and practices into the system (see Figure 10.1). It established the base of the reform, setting five guiding principles: efficiency, universality, solidarity, comprehensiveness and social participation.

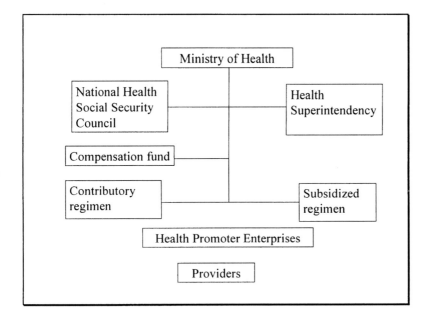

Figure 10.1 The Colombian health system

Efficiency

Efficiency is sought by managed competition and free choice of insurer. A two-layer system of managed competition has been created in which private and public, for profit and not-for-profit insurers compete in the market to offer a government-set standard health benefit package, and on the other hand, providers compete to sell their services to insurers. On their part, consumers are free to select an insurer, and to select providers of services from within those with a contract with their insurer. They have the right to change insurer once a year.

Universality

Universality is sought through compulsory social insurance with family coverage, funded by employer/employee contributions and by government subsidies. There are two ways of accessing the social insurance. The contributory regimen is for those with a formal labour contract irrespective of their income level, and for self-employed workers earning more than two minimum wages. They contribute 12% of their income (8% from the employer and 4% from the employee; the self-employed are responsible for the full amount). It is estimated that 70% of the population will fall into this regimen. Contributions are collected by the insurers (called Health Promoter Enterprises—HPE) who get paid by a risk adjusted premium (capitation) in such a way that a particular insurer, depending on the income/risk mix of affiliates, may generate a surplus or deficit in its actual premium collection. The law established a compensation fund where the insurers (HPE) either deposit their excess collections or are reimbursed for their deficits.

The subsidized regimen is for the poor. It is estimated that 30% of the population will be covered by this regimen. Municipal mayors are responsible for identifying the poor through the application of a targeting instrument (means test) which classifies the poor into three levels of poverty. Level 1, the poorest of the poor, will get a 95% subsidy, level 2 a 90% subsidy and level 3 a 70% subsidy.

All persons, in either regimen, will select an HPE which will be responsible for the provision of a standard health benefit package. HPEs may provide the required services through their own (but administratively distinct) network of providers or through contracted ones. Besides the HPEs, and exclusively for the subsidized regimen, the law allows the presence of other insurers which do not have such stringent requirements as the HPEs, are not-for-profit and in many instances are of community origin. These are called Subsidized Regimen Administrators.

The law allows the development of complementary health packages which can be purchased by anybody willing and able to pay extra for additional coverage or better amenities.

Solidarity

There are at least three solidarity mechanisms in the system. First, the contributory system has its own internal solidarity, since those earning more subsidize those earning less.[1] Second, one per cent of the contributory regimen payments is assigned by law to cross-subsidize the poor of the subsidized regimen. Third, the subsidized regimen is financed from general taxation.

Comprehensiveness

By setting a standard health benefits package, the government establishes comprehensive coverage of preventive and curative services, which all insurers must offer. Until the year 2000, subsidized membership provides a less comprehensive benefits package. Starting at 50% coverage of the contributory benefit package, it should increase through time as resources permit. In fact it is now around 60%. Both packages (subsidized and contributory) should include health promotion and preventive care. Furthermore, insurers are not allowed to

---

[1] The contribution of an individual to the contributory regimen, and his family capitation which will be paid to the insurer, would be equal to around 2.25 minimum wages for an estimated average family size of 3.64.

deny cover to anyone applying for insurance, and exclusion of pre-existing conditions is prohibited so as to avoid adverse selection practices.

Social participation

Acts 10 of 1990, 100 of 1993 and the 1991 Constitution explicitly laid down mechanisms and means for social participation and social control. Consumers may, at will, become constituted in consumer alliances at the level of insurers or providers, and citizen overseeing bodies must be created to control public investment. The law established a National Health Social Security Council as a central co-ordinating body for the system, with representation from the government, insurers, providers, professionals and community. This Council makes such decisions as setting the content of the standard benefit packages and the level of the capitation provided to insurers. It also established a Compensation Fund that manages all the resources of the Contributory Regimen. A consortium of accounting firms administers this fund. They act as fiduciary agent with four internal sub accounts: one to collect the surpluses from the HPEs and to redistribute to those with deficits, a second corresponding to the one per cent cross subsidy for the poor, a third for the promotion and prevention programmes of HPEs and the fourth for catastrophic events and traffic accidents.

The law also reformed the National Health Superintendency, enabling it to monitor the system and in particular its financial and quality aspects. Furthermore, it set the framework for the transition from supply financing to demand financing for public hospitals. In order to prepare for the competition with the private sector, they are to be transformed into State Social Enterprises with legal, administrative and financial autonomy and modernized management.

Under the decentralization process, municipalities have major responsibilities for the local operation of health insurance, particularly for ensuring that the poor receive a means test and are insured. They are responsible for convening the Subsidized Regimen Administrators interested in servicing the locality, paying them the corresponding capitation in accordance with the number of subsidized affiliates they insure, and supervising their operation.

The transition: growing pains

Both reforms have been difficult to implement and both are still in progress. Both have changed and will continue changing the relationships between the state, the population and the providers and, utilizing Frenk's categorization (Frenk, 1994) will have effects at systemic, programmatic, organizational and instrumental levels.

Decentralization has meant important power shifts among the territorial governments involved (nation, departments and municipalities). The national level has been freed of responsibility for the actual provision of services, allowing it to develop its role in policy formulation and technical assistance. The municipalities have assumed control over local health decisions and the departments have had their control reduced over municipal decisions. There has been both resistance and opposition from different actors, whose interests have been affected. Resistance at state level has not been uncommon, and there is a lack of adequate incentives for the departments and municipalities to decentralize[2] (Vargas, 1997). Development of institutional capacity at municipal level is still a major need, due to the complexity of the new responsibilities assumed, and the lack of expertise and experience at municipal level, particularly in the small localities.

As to the social security reform, the major limitation has been the lack of experience and of adequate information. It has been a process of learning by doing in a country which had no experience with capitation payments, or standard health benefit packages, and where cost information on health services was non-existent. The social security reform introduced new actors into the system who in many instances had to start from scratch. The health insurers (HPE) were totally new to the system, as were the Compensation Fund and the National Health Social Security Council. New and unfamiliar concepts were introduced. Capitation payment had not existed previously, since salary and fee-for-service had been the prevailing forms of payment. New also were the standard health benefit packages and the change from supply to demand subsidies. Appropriate software did not exist for the needs of the new institutions, which led to buying expensive solutions in Chile and Brazil which proved inadequate for Colombian requirements and had to be replaced with tailor-made packages.

Problems and difficulties

Most of the above problems are considered to be soluble through regulations without changing the law. There seems to be agreement on the adequacy of the macro design of the reforms (Jaramillo *et al*, 1998) and on the macro-economic viability of the system.

However, several observers have pointed to problem areas which need to be addressed to avoid future complications. Some of these are developmental. New institutions were created, and new concepts and processes adopted. Where there was no culture of national health insurance, there was a need to learn about the importance and the need to get insured. Where there was no tradition of capitation payment, it was necessary to learn how to contract based on capitation. The poor population needed to learn the advantages of being insured and the rights derived from it, and by the end of 1997 they were not yet utilizing services at a level that

---

[2] The departments are afraid of losing power to the municipalities and resist transferring control of the hospitals to them. Since the departments get the fiscal transfers automatically, there is no way of penalizing them. The municipalities also get the transfers automatically and do not have incentives to modernize their administration.

might have been expected. Public hospitals had to develop billing systems and learn how to bill for their services, and they are only starting to realize that the new system requires them to market their services. Development of adequate information has become a must.

There is an excess of norms and regulations (Vargas, 1997), which diminishes the transparency of the processes and increases the difficulty of citizen control. The financing mechanisms of the subsidized regimen are excessively complex and cumbersome (Jaramillo, et al, 1998). The way that part of the government funds are allocated geographically has been identified as highly inequitable; hence this is not encouraging a reduction in regional differences (Vargas and Sarmiento, 1997).

The process of transformation from supply to demand subsidies, which goes parallel with the transformation of public hospitals into State Social Enterprises, is moving slowly (Medina, 1997). In 1996, 87% of the public health resources were still assigned in the traditional way (Vargas and Sarmiento, 1997). This adds difficulty to the growth of subsidized coverage, which depends in good part on this transformation. On the other hand, public hospitals that for many years have been under the protection of the state and whose management has been below standard are in urgent need of developing modern management structures, a process that requires time.

Evasion, by non-affiliation of people who should be in the contributory regimen or by under-declaration of income, has been repeatedly identified (Sánchez and Yepes, 1997; Jaramillo et al, 1998) and might affect the economic viability of the reform model (Giedion and Wüllner, 1996). Estimates are that 35% or more of the population who should be in the contributory regimen are still not affiliated, and that there is at least a 30% under-declaration of income.

Public health programmes, one of the strengths of the previous system, have been affected first by decentralization and then by the social security reform. Municipalities have not completed the process of taking over their new responsibilities, and the information system and epidemiological surveillance are seriously affected (Jaramillo, 1997). An outbreak of equine meningitis in the northern part of the country went undetected until it was too late, and this has happened also with dengue fever outbreaks in the south-west.

Professional dissatisfaction is a general concern arising from several factors. There has been no strategy to prepare the professionals for the reform; financial negotiations with the insurers have not always been satisfactory; and professional autonomy has been affected by the relationship with the insurers[3] (Jaramillo et al, 1998). Health professionals in general, but physicians in particular, were unprepared for a reform which drastically changed their practices: as insurance coverage increases, fewer patients come individually on a fee-for-service basis and

---

[3] In order to control costs, the insurers submit certain diagnostic and therapeutic procedures to prior approval, and the prescription of drugs under compulsory insurance is limited to the official essential drug list.

more through the insurers on a prepaid basis. Middle-aged physicians with established practices have probably been more affected while recent graduates now find it easier to start a professional practice.

Public information and education have been grossly insufficient, and have affected people's ability to exercise their rights. During 1997, the Subsidized Regimen Administrators experienced a demand for services by their affiliates that was less than expected, reportedly because the insured lacked information about their rights. Since they are paid on a capitation basis and their profit margins were getting too high, they were required to use the 'excess profits' to create reserves.

Quality assurance is almost non-existent, and there is no information about what might be happening with quality of care in a system under significant pressure to control costs. There are also doubts about the macro-economic efficiency of the system. The reform brought new resources to the health sector. It is estimated that by 1996, total health expenditures were at 10.1% of GDP (4.2% private/5.9% public) (Vargas and Sarmiento, 1997), up from 9.1% in 1997 and from 7.0% (3.9% private/3.1% public) before the reform (Velandia et al, 1990; Harvard University School of Public Health, 1996). Yet 50% of the population is still uninsured. However, it is important to note that the 50% uninsured population is covered by the public system under the transitional arrangements.

There are population groups excluded from the system because the law has allowed special arrangements for them: the armed forces, schoolteachers and oil workers. It is considered on solidarity grounds that these exclusions should be eliminated.[4] Congressmen, who until very recently also had special status, have had it outlawed by a provision of the State Council.

The Social Security Institute, which existed before the reform as the largest public health insurer, was allowed to remain and to become another Health Promoter Enterprise. It is by far the largest, covering approximately 75% of the contributive regimen affiliates. By the way it is functioning without complying with all the regulations, the Social Security Institute is introducing serious distortions into the system.

Achievements

There have been a number of key achievements.

Social consensus

A first major achievement has been the construction of a consensus around the social security reform. In spite of all the difficulties, all major actors agree on the

---

[4] This applies to the oil workers, who are among the best paid in the country.

need for the reform for the country and consider it as a major social attainment, although many may have criticisms of specific aspects (Jaramillo *et al*, 1998).

Increased health insurance coverage

By the end of 1997, insurance coverage was at the level of 46.6%[5] for both regimens, a figure that more than doubled what the country had been able to achieve during almost 50 years of the previous system. The subsidized regimen is already covering 13% of the population (5 130 000), that is 43% of the estimated target (30%) while the contributory regimen covers approximately 33% of the population, up from 20% before the reform. The contributory coverage increase can be explained by the introduction of family coverage, which is now compulsory. This implies that, except for the effect of the inclusion of the family, there are not many new insured under this regimen. The subsidized coverage is particularly significant since it is reaching the poorer section of the population and is a reflection of the priority to equity given by the government.

Institutional development

There are 30 Health Promoter Enterprises[6] offering the contributory insurance, and approximately 231 Subsidized Regimen Administrators. All municipalities in the country have at least one insurer present, 70% at least two, and all state capitals at least five. The Ministry of Health and the department health secretaries have been relieved of responsibility for the direct provision of services, moving into activities connected with the direction of the system, and strengthening their policy formulation/monitoring capabilities.

Positive financial situation

During 1996, the private Health Promoter Enterprises which contribute to the Compensation and Solidarity Fund produced surpluses[7] of 88 million dollars, more than enough to compensate two deficit HPEs and leave reserves for future needs.

---

[5] Coverage figures are estimates from different sources and not completely reliable. More reliable data based on a national household survey should be available in 1998.

[6] Since the beginning of the reform, two HPEs have gone out of business.

[7] The difference between the contributions of the insured and the capitation rate.

Elimination of monopolies and captive clientèles

Under the old system there were captive clientèles for the Social Security Institute and the other social security institutions where employees did not have the choice to select an insurer unless they opted to pay twice. People are now free to select their insurer, and once a year they can exercise the right to move to a different one. However, the double contribution has not been eliminated, particularly for the higher socio-economic groups who are not satisfied with the choice of provider offered by compulsory insurance and choose to buy additional packages of prepaid medicine which may in part duplicate the basic insurance cover.[8]

The country still has a lot to learn in order to succeed with the new system. It is necessary to streamline norms and strengthen government institutions with improved information systems, to enforce and monitor compliance. Likewise, a very significant effort is required for a massive re-education of the human resources of the health system, and extended information and education of the public on the new system.

There are questions and worries still unanswered.

- What should be the future of the public network? Public hospitals are going through a profound change to adapt to the new system. As ordered by Act 100, they have been changing their legal status, becoming State Social Enterprises. In this way, they obtain administrative and financial autonomy which they did not have before. At the same time, the financing they used to get from government subsidies (supply financing) is progressively drying up, to be replaced by the income they are able to get by selling their services in the market. Undoubtedly, there are incentives in place for hospitals to modernize their administration, and become efficient institutions, and they are moving in this direction. However, since the law allows the insurers to own their own network of provider institutions, the question remains whether they will not move into developing their own networks, particularly in the more profitable services, eventually forcing the public network out of business or buying it.
- Will the government be able (willing) to enforce compliance with insurance, particularly for the high-income population, and control evasion? Otherwise the solidarity of the system and its economic viability will be seriously questioned.
- Will there be the necessary political decision to correct the inequity in the distribution of government resources to regions? Poorer regions do have a larger proportion of the poor among their population, and if they do not get a larger share of the transfers, they will not be able to provide subsidized insurance to their poor.

---

[8] This is a problem which could be solved by government regulations setting caps on the amount the insurers can charge for complementary services.

- There are questions about the role of the Social Security Institute, by far the largest Health Promoter Enterprise, which controls 70% of the subsidized regimen market. The Institute does not know exactly the number of its affiliates, and is not yet contributing to the Solidarity Fund. If and when it starts contributing, the question remains whether it is going to generate a surplus (contribution minus capitation rate) or a deficit.

It is still too early in the process to answer these questions, and we will have to wait some time for answers, but overall we will have to improve our ability to follow up the reform in such a way that we can provide appropriate and timely feedback to decision-makers. During 1998 there will become available the first household-based data on coverage and utilization after the reform, collected during the second half of 1997. This will provide important evidence on the success of the reform in improving access to and use of the health system.

References

Avila N. *Historia de las Instituciones de salud en Colombia.* Master's thesis. Health administration postgraduate program. Javeriana University. Bogota, 1988

Frenk J. Dimensions of health system reform. *Health Policy,*1994; **27**:19–34

Giedion U, Wüllner A. *La Unidad de pago por capitación y el equilibrio financiero del sistema de salud.* Fedesarrollo. Santa Fe de Bogotá: Editorial Guadalupe, 1996

Harvard University School of Public Health, Colombia Health Care Reform Project Team. *Report on Colombia Health Care Reform and Proposed master implementation plan. Draft final report.* February 26, 1996, p 66

Jaramillo I. *El futuro de la salud en Colombia. La puesta en marcha de la ley 100.* Fescol, Fundación FES, Fundación Restrepo Barco, Fundación Corona. Tercera edición. Santa Fe de Bogotá: Editorial Tercer Mundo, 1997, pp 341–343

Jaramillo I, Olano G, Yepes FJ. La ley 100. *Dos años de implementación.* ASSALUD, FESCOL, Fundación Corona, Fundación FES, GTZ. Informes técnicos # 2. Santa Fe de Bogotá: Editorial Guadalupe, 1998 (in press)

Manrique A, Marín F. Ley 12. *Descentralización administrativa y fiscal.* Serie: reforma Política N° 3. FESCOL, Procomún. Bogotá, Mayo, 1987

Medina A. La transición del sistema. In: Sánchez LH, Yepes FJ (directores). *Ley 100. Un año de implementación.* ASSALUD. Fundación FES. Informes técnicos # 1. Santa Fe de Bogotá: Editorial Guadalupe, 1997, p 80

Molina CG, Giedion U. *Cuantificación financiera de un sistema de Seguridad Social en Salud (informe final)* FEDESARROLLO. Santa Fe de Bogotá. 1993. Citado en Harvard University School of Public Health, Colombia Health Care Reform Project Team. Report on Colombia Health Care Reform and proposed master implementation plan. Draft final report. February 26, 1996.

Quevedo, E. (coordinador) *et al.* Análisis sociohistórico. In Yepes, FJ. (director) *La Salud en Colombia. Estudio Sectorial de Salud.* Ministerio de Salud. Departamento Nacional de Planeación. Ed. Presencia. Bogotá. 1990. Volume I

República de Colombia. Ministerio de Salud. *La carga de la enfermedad en Colombia.* Santa Fe de Bogotá: Editorial carrera séptima Ltda, 1994. p 25

Sánchez LH, Yepes FJ (directores). *Ley 100. Un año de implementación.* ASSALUD. Fundación FES. Informes técnicos # 1. Santa Fe de Bogotá, 1997

Vargas JE, Sarmiento A. *La descentralización de los servicios de salud en Colombia.* Comisión Económica para América Latina y el Caribe. Serie Reformas de Política Publica. 51. Santiago de Chile, 1997 p 41

Velandia F (cordinador) *et al.* Financiamiento. In Yepes, Francisco José (director) *La Salud en Colombia. Estudio Sectorial de Salud.* Ministerio de Salud. Departamento Nacional de Planeación. Bogotá: Ed. Presencia, 1990, Tomo II, p 87

World Bank. *Informe sobre el desarrollo mundial, 1997. El estado en un mundo en transformación.* Washington DC, 1997

Yepes FJ. *La Salud en Colombia. Estudio Sectorial de Salud.* Ministerio de Salud. Departamento Nacional de Planeación. Bogotá: Ed. Presencia, 1990. Tomo I, p 60

11
Private finance in public facilities—the experience of the UK

Allyson Pollock and Declan Gaffney

University College London, UK

Health systems are in transition. Countries like the UK are often seen as model makers in health and social care policy. Most recent market-based experiments in welfare are in no small measure ideologically driven, based on the beliefs that the individual should take responsibility and the private sector can do things better. This latter view emanates from business interests which see health and social care as market commodities to be exploited. In the first part of this chapter, using the example of long term care, we will show how, since 1979, government policy has been to substitute private for public finance in the building of facilities for health and social care and how this policy has been accompanied by the policy of devolving responsibility for funding and provision to individuals and their families and away from the state and society. In the second part of this chapter we will look at this policy in its most recent form, the private finance initiative, as it applies to NHS hospitals.

The 1948 NHS—its goals and values

The UK NHS is fifty years old. Sometimes described as a 'socialized' health care system, the NHS is both publicly funded through public taxation and has been for the most part in public ownership. The guiding principles of the UK NHS are to provide: universal coverage; comprehensive care from cradle to grave; services free at the point of delivery, and equity i.e. services delivered on the basis of need and not on ability to pay. The remarkable feature of the NHS has been its ability to deliver low-cost health care to the entire population of 60 million people for a relatively modest 7% of GDP. The system of central taxation, block budgets, public delivery and low administrative costs enabled the government to contain health care spending, and despite the introduction of user charges for a few services, charges account for less than 4% of the total NHS budget.

Capital investment in the NHS

Charles Webster, the official historian of the NHS, has recorded that the most notable feature of the 1948 NHS was the absence of any programme of capital investment:

> With remarkable smoothness and efficiency, NHS hospital authorities converted the ramshackle and obsolete institutions inherited from their predecessors into a first class, modern and integrated hospital network. All of this was achieved without the advantage of a major hospital building programme. The hospitals of the NHS were therefore usually grotesque conglomerates, comprising buildings and hutments, some dating from the eighteenth century and even earlier. Great ingenuity was exercised in adapting these antique facilities for housing the most advanced systems of diagnosis and treatment (Webster, 1988).

Throughout the 1970s and 1980s, public expenditure restraints and limited time horizons of government impeded progress in community care and primary care, and delayed programmes of hospital modernization in the UK. In its first decade, from 1948–58, capital investment in the NHS was estimated at only one-fifth the pre-war level of capital spending by local authorities (Webster, 1988). The Hospital Plan of 1962 was to have been a strategic programme of investment and modernization but, costed at an unrealistically low level, it was never fully implemented. The Community Care Plan of 1963 was sketchy in its resolve, unresourced in practice and never put into place.

Lack of capital investment became the fulcrum of a major shift in the policy of the Conservative government—the privatization of the delivery system itself substituting private finance for public funding in the building of replacement facilities for care. Prior to 1979, the debate on NHS privatization was mainly concerned with the possibilities for privatizing some of the *costs* of NHS care through user charges. The 1979 Conservative government under Margaret Thatcher marked a radical change in the direction of welfare policy with regard to the funding, provision and supply of services across the whole of the public sector so that by 1996, the climate had been so transformed that the Treasury was able to enunciate its principles as follows:

> government policy has been to:
> - reduce the size of the public sector through privatisation and contracting out
> - involve the private sector in providing existing and new services, through the private finance initiative and challenge funding (GB Treasury, 1996).

Although the private finance initiative has been around only since 1992, the concept of privatizing public services is not new as can be illustrated by what happened to long-term care and social care provision in the UK (Pollock, 1995a).

The privatization of long-term care

The responsibility for funding and providing long-term care continues to be divided between the NHS, social services departments under the control of local government and the individual. However, the relative balance of responsibility has changed from the state to the individual and from public to private provision (Harrington and Pollock, 1998).

Until 1981, the private sector played a relatively minor role in the provision of long-term care. This changed when the Conservative government used an amendment to the Social Security Act in 1980 to allow residents going into private institutional settings to claim board and lodging from the Social Security budget when those in local authority or NHS places could not. Cash-limited local authorities and health authorities encouraged residents to seek private sector alternatives, facilitating the closure and sale of public assets. Local authorities were restricted in the use of capital receipts from sales of land. The private sector showed a phenomenal growth accompanied by a decline in public provision across all the priority groups. From 1981 to 1995, the number of residential care places rose by 40% to 329 000, of which 57% were provided by the private sector. Places in nursing homes rose from 26 900 to 208 000 over the same period (1981–1995), of which 92% were provided by the private sector (GB Department of Health, 1996).

By 1993 the restructuring and privatization of the delivery of long-term care was nearly complete, thanks largely to the pump-priming of the private sector with the Social Security budget. But, as several influential commentators have noted, the goals of community care were not realized (although it is arguable whether community care was ever the goal of this particular government policy) (Henwood, 1991).

In 1993, the NHS and Community Care Act 1990 ended central funding for long-term care from the social security budget and transferred responsibility for long-term care funding to local authorities. The Social Security budget was to be used only for those with 'preserved rights', i.e. individuals funded by the Social Security system prior to 1997. Payment for residential care and nursing homes continued to be subject to means-testing, but as individuals 'spent-down' their assets they became the responsibility of local authorities. Local authorities receive block grants from central government to fund long-stay care, including a temporary ring-fenced grant (known as the special transitional grant). The receipt of the ring-fenced portion was made conditional on using private organizations to provide community-based services such as meals-on-wheels and home care. In 1996 the private sector provided 32% of total contract hours, compared with just 2% in 1992 (GB Department of Health, 1996).

Under the 1990 Act, the NHS has only a residual role in long-term care. Health authorities are required to draw up eligibility criteria known as 'continuing care criteria'. These are increasingly stringent and restrictive. The 1990 Act also required local authorities to introduce eligibility criteria at local level which are distinct and separate from the NHS continuing care criteria. These eligibility criteria are based on assessment of financial and social care needs. Individuals have to demonstrate both service need and financial entitlement. Local authorities began to fund the care of people who would formerly have been considered the responsibility of the NHS. Whereas formerly most local authorities did not means-test and charge for services, most now do so. Pressure on local authority budgets has meant that these eligibility criteria have also become more restrictive, targeting only those with greatest need. Compared to 1994, in 1995 local authorities were funding 15% more residents in residential care (139 000) and 72% more residents (43 200) in nursing home care. (In 1992 they had had no responsibility for funding nursing home places.) Although the intensity of services provided to individuals increased, reflecting the increasing dependency of the group, the numbers of households receiving community-based services such as home help and meals-on-wheels continued to fall, reflecting the increasing constraints of local authority budgets. There are no monitoring systems in place to establish how long-term care needs are changing and being met over time.

The NHS and Community Care Act 1990 finished what the 1974 NHS reorganization and 1974 Local Government Act had begun. Social care and long-term care is increasingly seen as a private good, the responsibility of individuals, their families and local communities. All this happened without public debate. The new Labour government is revisiting policies on funding long-term care through the Royal Commission on long-term care. It remains to be seen whether the Commission will look at the delivery of care as well as its funding.

The privatization of long-term care occurred in four phases (Pollock, 1995b). First, the 1974 structural reorganization separated the responsibilities for health and social care, allowing the transfer of services from the NHS where services were free at the point of delivery to a system with the potential to raise charges and means-test. Second, in 1980, the amendment to the Social Security Act was used at enormous public expense to pump-prime and stimulate the private delivery system, with restrictions on the public sector to prevent its participation in these schemes. The effect was to alter dramatically the relative balance of provision, away from public provision in a system free at the point of delivery to a means-tested private system. Third, the introduction of the 1990 NHS and Community Care Act, with its harsh and restrictive continuing care criteria, devolved the responsibility for funding, rationing and providing long-term care to local government and local people. Fourth, by switching off the national Social Security budget and restricting the expenditure of local authorities, the costs of care were transferred not just to local authorities and local people but increasingly to the individuals themselves through means-testing and charges. Finally, the government made central government funding allocations to local authorities conditional upon using the private and independent sector. Thus once again the public sector was restricted in its ability to participate and major subsidies were given to the private sector to stimulate its development.

The Private Finance Initiative

It was not until 1991 that the real assault was made on the acute hospital sector of the NHS. The implementation of the internal market and the purchaser-provider split effectively dismantled district planning structures, distancing district health authorities from local services and local people and introducing competition between trusts. The rapid ascendancy of managers unskilled in planning and needs assessment brought a halt to needs assessment and service development as health authorities and trusts wrestled with the new world of contracting and competition.

In 1992 the Treasury launched the Private Finance Initiative (PFI) as a programme of capital investment by the private sector across the whole of the welfare state including roads, prisons, hospitals and schools. Under the PFI for new hospitals for the NHS, private finance is used to replace existing NHS infrastructure. The private sector, including builders, bankers and facilities operators are invited to tender to design, build, operate and own the new hospital, and existing NHS assets are sold off or given to the private developers. Unlike the facilities which are being replaced, the new facility no longer belongs to the NHS but is leased back to the NHS for periods of up to 30 years. In effect, under the PFI, public assets are transferred to private ownership.

How PFI is paid for

The major PFI developments in the NHS are all 'design, build, finance and operate' (DBFO) schemes, under which the NHS makes annual payments from its revenue budget for the use of privately owned facilities over a 'primary concession period' of 25–40 years. The health service bodies which enter into these arrangements are NHS trusts, the public sector corporations which took over the provision of hospital services following the 1990 NHS and Community Care Act.

The cost of trusts' payments to the private sector are passed on to NHS purchasers (health authorities and GP fundholders) in the prices charged by trusts for clinical services. As part of the procurement process, it is necessary for a trust and purchaser to agree the future income level of the trust over the period of the PFI contract. In order for procurement to proceed, it is necessary that health authorities provide 'letters of purchaser support', guaranteeing sufficient income to allow the trust to meet its PFI obligations. (However, health authorities are *not* parties to the concession agreements between NHS trusts and consortia.) In most cases, health authorities have demanded that PFI hospital developments place no additional strain on their existing budgets and in some cases they have demanded reductions in annual costs.

The PFI procurement process

The PFI procurement process in the NHS is structured by the preparation and approval of two main documents. The first stage involves the preparation, and submission to the Department of Health, of an Outline Business Case (OBC). In this document the NHS trust makes the case for the proposed investment and gives an estimate of the capital cost based on standard NHS costings. The OBC thus provides a benchmark for the capital cost based on what the scheme would cost under traditional procurement. If the proposal is approved by the Department, the trust is required to seek a private finance partner. This is the beginning of PFI procurement proper. The Full Business Case (FBC), which has to be approved by both the Department of Health and the Treasury, presents the design offered by the private sector and compares its costs with those of traditional procurement, based on the estimates in the OBC.

The PFI unitary payment

The funding of annual PFI payments comes (in principle) from the annual budgets and the disposal of existing assets of the NHS trusts concerned. Annual PFI payments have two principal components: an 'availability payment' which covers the repayment of debt incurred by the private sector and returns on the investment, and a 'service charge' which covers the 'facilities management' side of the operation of the hospital. In general, all staff other than those directly providing NHS clinical services are transferred to the private sector.

The main budgetary element available to trusts to service PFI debt (availability payments) is the funding currently used to meet NHS capital charges (see below). After existing capital charges and the value realized by disposal of assets are taken account of, any further funding must come either from external sources (through increased health authority funding or from the Department of Health) or through reductions in the hospitals' other costs (in effect, staff costs).

Capital charging—resource accounting

The PFI payment system is intended to fit seamlessly into the existing capital charging regime in the NHS, under which returns on capital are made to the Treasury (Shaoul, 1998; Pollock and Gaffney, 1998). NHS trusts have a financial duty to make an operating surplus of 6% of relevant assets after inflation, as well as to make a straight-line depreciation charge over the lifetime of the assets. These charges are passed on to purchasers in the prices charged by Trusts, while purchasers' funding in turn includes a component equivalent to average capital charges, creating a closed loop.

The mechanisms of the capital charging regime are crucial to an understanding of PFI procurement in the NHS. It is often mistakenly assumed that capital charging is intended to allocate public sector capital costs to the operating units employing that capital. In fact the capital charge was never intended to reflect the cost of capital to the public sector: 'The practical choice of 6% ... for the cost of capital ... is an operational judgement, reflecting for example, concern to ensure that there is no inefficient bias against private sector supply' (GB HM Treasury, 1997). In other words, the capital charging regime was designed to reflect the cost of capital to the private sector rather than, for example, the rate of interest on government debt.

The stated aim was to enable comparisons of cost both between different NHS bodies and between public and private sector supply, at the level of individual operating units. The theory was summed up by the former Secretary of State for Health, Stephen Dorrell:

> ..every trust in the Health Service pays a capital charge which reflects the amount of capital which is employed within the trust and that, broadly speaking, reflects the cost of capital to the private sector as well. That allows the trust to make a comparison between buying the service from the private sector and doing the thing itself directly, including meeting the cost of capital which would be employed[1] (GB House of Commons Treasury Committee, 1996).

Apart from providing a comparative benchmark for private sector bids, the circulating funding for existing capital charges also provides the major source of funding for PFI investment. This leads to two problems. First, it creates a leak of funding from what was previously a closed system (Mayston, forthcoming). Second, any gap between what is available from current combined operating surpluses and depreciation charges and the future annual costs of PFI investment will need to be met from within the trust, from within the local budget for health care, or from regional or national budgets.

---

[1] Mr Dorrell was replying to the question 'How do you in your department go about monitoring the impact of switching between traditional funding and PFI within the budget of your department?'

The cost of the PFI

By comparing Outline Business Case capital cost estimates for the 'first wave' PFI hospital schemes with Department of Health estimates from July 1997, and where possible with costs given in publicly available Full Business Cases, we have shown that costs had escalated by 55% from Outline to Full Business Case (Table11.1). The effect of these cost escalations is to create an affordability gap between what the private sector charges and the public sector can afford (Gaffney and Pollock, 1997).

Table 11.1: Outline business case and current capital cost estimates for 'first wave' NHS PFI schemes

Trust	OBC capital cost	Current cost (£m)	Increase (%)
Bishop Auckland	26 000 000	52 000 000	100
Bromley	80 000 000	120 000 000	50
Calderdale	55 000 000	77 000 000	40
Carlisle	48 000 000	63 000 000	31
Dartford*	97 000 000	115 000 000*	18
Hereford	50 000 000	63 000 000	26
Norfolk*	110 000 000	214 000 000*	94
N.Durham*	60 000 000	86 000 000*	43
S. Manchester	40 000 000	89 000 000	123
S. Bucks	35 000 000	38 000 000	9
S.Tees	65 000 000	106 000 000	63
Swindon	45 000 000	148 000 000	229
Wellhouse	30 000 000	40 000 000	33
Worcester	45 000 000	91 000 000	102
Average			55

Outline business case cost estimates were confirmed by regional offices of the NHS Executive; current estimated capital costs are from Department of Health press release, 10 June 1997, with the exception of those marked *. Dartford & Gravesham NHS Trust and North Durham Acute Hospitals NHS Trust costs taken from FBCs; Norfolk and Norwich Hospitals NHS Trust costs taken from Department of Health press release 6/4/98

The affordability gap and the impact of cost escalations on the Trust's income can be quantified by comparing availability payments with current operating surpluses and depreciation charges: i.e. a comparison can be made between the cost of capital currently and future costs. This is shown in Table 11.2.

Comparing the current surplus and the depreciation charges with the availability payment gives an indication of the way the cost structure of hospitals is changed by PFI development. This comparison is more informative than with the actual capital charges (interest and dividend) paid since those Trusts which do not make the necessary surplus may have the dividend part of the charges waived. It can be seen that the cost of capital to the Trusts as a share of income rises quite dramatically. The only way it can be paid for, if revenue does not increase substantially, is by redundancies and job losses since 70% of Trust income is currently spent on staff salaries and wages. Advisers to the UK Department of Health estimate that the problems in bridging the affordability gap will result in significant job losses. The example given is of a £200 million capital investment on a new PFI hospital which they predict will result in job losses of 25% among doctors and nurses across the whole of the local health economy. This is at a time when the NHS is experiencing a recruitment crisis and faces serious shortages of doctors and nurses across many specialities (Newchurch and Company, 1997).

Table 11.2: Comparison of current operating surplus plus depreciation with projected PFI availability payment as a % of 1996/7 income

Trust	Income 96/7 (m.)	Operating surplus (o/s) 96/97 (m.)	Depreciation (Depn) 96/97 (m.)	OS + Depn as % of Income	PFI Avail. Charge (m.)	Avail. Charge as % of 96/97 income
Bromley	£74 430 000	£3 560 000	£2 890 000	8.7	£10 740 000	14.5
Calderdale	£77 730 000	£1 670 000	£1 570 000	4.15	£8 740 000	11.3
Dartford & Gravesham					£10 500 000	
N.Durham	£61 410 000	£2 640 000	£1 780 000	7.2	£7 010 000	11.4
Edinburgh	£157 780 000	£6 020 000	£6 060 000	7.6	£25 590 000	16.2

Sources: Income, operating surpluses and depreciation: *The Fitzhugh directory of NHS trusts 1997–8: financial information*
Availability payments: Bromley: 'Documents reveal costs of hospital' *Bromley News Shopper* 8 April 1998
Calderdale: Calderdale Healthcare NHS Trust, *Executive Summary of Full Business Case.*
Dartford, North Durham and Royal Infirmary of Edinburgh FBCs.
North Durham Acute Hospitals NHS Trust, *Addendum to the Full Business Case* (1998) p3 and *Full Business Case* (1997) p52; Dartford and Gravesham NHS Trust *Addendum to the Full Business Case* (1998) p51.

Included are non-financial services fees and non-works costs. 'Rolled-up interest' and financial services fees are excluded. VAT is excluded from all costs.

Subsidies

Using data on estimated capital costs of hospital PFI schemes and bed numbers in the first wave schemes at Outline and Full Business Case and other publicly available material, our research has showed that the affordability gap was being bridged at local and national level by: reductions in acute bed numbers; switching of funding from locally available (trust and health authority) budgets; and finally from subsidies from the Department of Health regional and national budgets.

i) Reductions in acute bed capacity

Table 11.3 compares total available bed numbers (excluding mental health beds) for the last two years for which information is available with projected beds under PFI development. 'Available' bed numbers include staffed in-patient beds only, and can therefore fluctuate from year to year, as beds and wards close and reopen in reaction to changes in demand and funding. By contrast, the planned bed numbers represent the maximum number of beds that will ever be available. Daycase spaces, which count as beds only in promotional literature produced by health authorities and trusts engaged in downsizing, have been excluded in accordance with Department of Health practice, as have private patient beds.

Table 11. 3: Changes in bed numbers at NHS Trusts under PFI development: selected sites—excluding mental health beds

Trust	1995/6	1996/7	Planned
Bishop Auckland Hospitals NHS Trust	306	348	262
Bromley Hospitals NHS Trust	610	625	507
Calderdale Healthcare NHS Trust	688	654	460
Dartford & Gravesham NHS Trust	524	506	400
North Durham Acute Hospitals NHS Trust	665	597	408
Norfolk & Norwich NHS Trust	1,120	1,207	809
Swindon & Marlborough NHS Trust	632	625	450
Worcester Royal Infirmary NHS Trust	524	526	390

Sources: Department of Health, *Bed Availability for England Financial Year 1995/6* ; *Bed availability for England 1996/7*; OBCs, FBCs and other documents provided by NHS Trusts and Community Health Councils

ii) Other service reductions

'Knock-on' effects on services other than those provided by the trusts in question were explored and are illustrated in the case study in Table 11.4. This shows, for West Kent Health Authority, how planned investments had to be revised when the Full Business Case was endorsed.

iii) Block capital allocations and equipment

The use of regional block capital allocations to subsidise PFI developments was the subject of interviews with civil servants at regional offices of the NHS Executive. 'Block' capital allocations for the first wave Trusts are given in Table 11.5. This table shows how block capital which is intended to be used for the repair and maintenance of the public asset base is now being diverted away from the NHS estate to pay for the new PFI build. The table shows the annual block capital allocations to individual trusts from the regional budgets for 1996/97.

Table 11.4: West Kent Health Authority: effect of affordability gap on health authority funding allocations

Service	Planned investment A	Planned investment B
Child resource centre	£ 249 000	£0.00
Relocation physical disability services	£200 000	£0.00
Relocation mental health services	£485 000	£0.00
Community nursing	£600 000	To be reviewed
Community hospital services	£1 000 000	To be reviewed

A = before endorsement of FBC by West Kent Health Authority (October 1996)
B = after endorsement of FBC by West Kent Health Authority (November 1996)
Sources: West Kent Health Authority, *Report of the director of commissioning, north to the meeting of the board on 31 October 1996* and *Report of the director of commissioning, north and director of finance to the meeting of the board 28 November 1996.*

Table 11.5: 1996-7 annual capital allocations for NHS trusts with PFI schemes

Trust	Region	Annual capital allocation (£ million)	Capital cost (£ million)
Bishop Auckland	Northern & Yorkshire	£9.6	£52
Bromley	South Thames	£1.075*	£120
Calderdale	Northern & Yorkshire	£1.5	£77
Carlisle	Northern & Yorkshire	£1.2	£63
Dartford & Gravesham	South Thames	£0.85	£137
Hereford	West Midlands	£1	£63
North Durham	Northern & Yorkshire	£1.7	£96
South Manchester	North West	£3.7	£89
South Tees	Northern & Yorkshire	£3.7	£106
Swindon	South West	not available	£148
Worcester	West Midlands	£1	£91

Source: Regional offices of the NHS Executive.

iv) The smoothing mechanism

By 1996 it had become apparent that none of the major health care PFI schemes was affordable within the annual budgets of the trusts concerned. A support scheme was arranged by the Department of Health and the Treasury. Eleven hospital trusts were approached by the NHS Executive and offered access to a scheme (known as the smoothing mechanism) under which PFI payments could be subsidised. The amounts allocated are shown in Table 11.6, and represent the annual sums available from the first year of the contract to reduce the PFI payments. This comes to £7.3m in the first year of the hospitals' opening. It is intended that the impact on purchasers should remain constant throughout the period. It is not intended to extend this subsidy to future PFI schemes.

Table 11.6: Subsidies to PFI schemes under the 'Smoothing Mechanism'

Trust	Annual funding (year 1) £000s
Bishop Auckland	317 000
Bromley	1 048 000
Calderdale	427 000
Carlisle	633 000
Dartford & Gravesham	1 059 000
Hereford	562 000
North Durham	757 000
Swindon	1 402 000
Wellhouse	358 000
Worcester	763 000

Source: Department of Health Private Finance Unit.

Discussion

The costs of PFI

Our study showed enormous escalations in capital cost (Table 11.1) which are *not* typical of NHS capital development. The monitoring of differences between outturn and original approved tender sums by NHS Estates shows average cost overruns of between 8.8% and 6.26% between 1990 and 1997.[2] Second, the increase in capital cost for the majority of these schemes is almost certainly understated due to the removal of equipment from PFI schemes (see below).

There is no obvious reason why the construction cost of PFI hospitals should be greater than that of traditionally funded schemes: after all, publicly funded

---

[2] Cost performance on capital construction projects over £1m. within the NHS (three year moving averages) provided by NHS Estates.

hospitals are also built by the private sector. Part of the rationale for the PFI was that the private sector was likely to propose original design solutions, which would be likely to prove *less* expensive than those produced using traditional design approaches.

One factor which has undoubtedly influenced capital costs in certain schemes has been the need for projects to be of a certain scale in order to obtain private investment (given the time and expense of bidding for PFI contracts). However, examination of the structure of costs for those projects where business cases have been made public shows the influence of a more general factor: the borrowing costs of the PFI consortium, which are included in the capital cost estimate.

The capital cost estimates quoted for PFI schemes typically include 'rolled-up' interest and financing costs incurred by consortia during construction. The rationale for this lies in the nature of PFI concession agreements. No fee is paid to the private sector consortium engaged in providing a new hospital until such time as the hospital is available to be occupied by the trust. The consortium, however, incurs interest charges throughout the construction period, which might be as long as five years. These are therefore capitalized and added to the construction costs, along with fees for financial services.

The affordability problem

As we have seen, the initial planning of the first wave PFI schemes—and the support of health authorities for those schemes—was based on the costs associated with traditional public sector procurement. At the same time, the revenue impact of the proposals was assessed at this stage in terms of the capital charges consequences: the need to make a 6% return and to charge depreciation, leading to revenue costs of roughly 7.5%. Any excess of annual PFI costs over the capital charges assumed in the OBC would place the viability of schemes in question. The cost estimates in Outline Business Cases (Table 11.1), on the basis of which health authorities originally gave their support, thus proved quite unrealistic. Not only have the costs of capital escalated from Outline to Full Business Case but the annual availability payments are considerably more than the capital charges paid currently, and around 3% greater than NHS capital charges would be for the same level of investment.

Bridging the gap—land transfers

Department of Health approval for major investments turns on their ability to deliver structural changes to the local health-care system, through reconfiguration of existing services and centralization of acute services on single sites. This gives rise to opportunities to dispose of buildings and sites deemed surplus to requirements which can be made over to PFI consortia in exchange for lower annual availability payments.

There is evidence that the need to free up land for development has had a significant impact on planning at a number of schemes, leading to decisions to relocate hospitals to cheaper 'green field' sites, as has happened with the developments for the Princess Margaret Hospital in Swindon and the new Royal Infirmary of Edinburgh, or failing that, reducing the area of the hospital to enable part of the existing site to be disposed of, as has happened at Carlisle, Durham and Bromley.

However, any hope that existing assets would eliminate the gap between existing capital charges funding and PFI availability payments would be mistaken. The impact of disposals of assets on scheme affordability is limited by Treasury accountancy rules in a way which was not anticipated (Dartford and Gravesham NHS Trust, 1998).[3] In order to avail themselves of the proceeds of land deals, trusts are obliged to amortize the economic benefit gained, leading to annual revenue costs. The logic is inescapable: allowing trusts to dispose of assets in order to fund PFI deals (without facing any revenue consequences) would mean that PFI had allowed capital to revert to being a 'free good', the very phenomenon that the capital charging policy was intended to eliminate and one of the planks of the rationale for PFI.

The Dartford and Gravesham NHS Trust was thus obliged to introduce an amortization charge of £920 000 into its financial projections, compounding its already severe affordability problems. This was later reduced to £383 000 by increasing the amortization period to 60 years (Dartford and Gravesham NHS Trust, 1998). In order to meet the cost, funding was diverted from the regional capital budget (see below).

Bridging the gap—generating savings at local level

i) reductions in hospital bed numbers:
The striking feature of the current hospital development programme is that dramatic increases in capital costs are combined with significant reductions in bed capacity (Tables 11.1 and 11.3). Debate on the relationship between the use of private finance and bed reductions has all too often been misrepresented in terms of a dichotomy between claims that PFI is uniquely responsible for bed reductions, and claims that they result rather from policy imperatives to change 'models of care'.

Some of the currently prioritized schemes show a decrease in projected in-patient bed numbers between the OBC and FBC, even though OBCs typically included large scale reductions (Calderdale Healthcare NHS Trust, 1997; King's

---

[3] Information provided by the South Thames Regional Office of the NHS Executive.

College London Centre for Mental Health Services Development, 1997).[4] These bed reductions go against current trends, where NHS acute beds have reopened in the last two consecutive years to accommodate rising caseload and emergency admissions. This reversal in the long-term trend for hospital bed numbers to reduce is reflected in the Secretary of State for Health's recently stated aim of reopening 2 000 hospital beds (GB Department of Health, 1997; *Financial Times*, 8 June 1998).

ii) reductions in other services
Reductions in bed numbers increase pressures on primary care and community health services. Moreover, the need to transfer land to the private sector to make schemes attractive to investors can have the effect of displacing existing community services, which are often provided in facilities on the sites of district general hospitals.

There are worrying indications that the costs of investment are leading to reductions in hospital capacity without any investment in substitute services. One business case, for a scheme involving considerable devolution of activity to community facilities, notes: '... the levels of devolved activity assume that the appropriate range of facilities available on the Worcester Royal Infirmary site will also be available in the community. This is unlikely to be the case......' (Worcester Royal Infirmary NHS Trust, 1996; Pollock *et al*, 1997).
As Table 11.3 shows, the new Dartford and Gravesham PFI schemes in West Kent will involve the loss of 124 beds (24% of current available beds). While there was no significant revision of projected beds in the course of procurement, there *was* an increase in projected caseload (Dartford and Gravesham NHS Trust, 1996). During the procurement process, West Kent Health Authority allocated funding for investment in community services which would be displaced as a result of the PFI deal (Table 11.4). In order to bridge the PFI affordability gap which emerged at the time of the Full Business Case in October 1996, the projected funding for investment in community services was largely withdrawn (Dartford and Gravesham NHS Trust, 1998).

Bridging the gap: regional capital allocations

'Block' capital allocations, disbursed by NHS regions directly to hospital trusts, are intended to cover maintenance and replacement of assets (Table 11.5). It was originally expected that block capital funding would be released to the rest of the NHS as trusts divested themselves of their assets through PFI deals. The costs of maintenance and replacement would then be factored in to the charges to be paid to the private consortium and would thus be paid out of the NHS revenue budget.

---

[4] We have not included day-case spaces and private patient beds.

However, NHS regions have considerable discretion in allocating block grants, and as affordability problems arose, means were sought to make use of block funding in order to reduce the cost to purchasers. To address the affordability of the Dartford and Gravesham scheme, South Thames NHS Executive agreed to convert the trust's block capital allocation into an annual subsidy to the PFI payment stream. The original allocation was worth £850 000. This was later reduced to £383 000 as a change in the amortization period for assets made over to the consortium reduced the affordability gap (Dartford and Gravesham NHS Trust, 1998).

A less direct way of providing subsidy is to remove equipment from a PFI scheme. This approach has been taken for all schemes in the Northern and Yorkshire region (Bishop Auckland, Carlisle, North Durham, South Tees) and for the Bromley scheme in South Thames. It is under discussion in the West Midlands (Hereford, Worcester) and South and West (Swindon) Regions.

Cuts in NHS capital budgets have led to reductions in the amount of block capital at the disposal of NHS regions. In the South Thames region this has led to reductions of 50% in allocations, which are expected to rise again in coming years. However in two regions (Northern & Yorkshire and West Midlands), capital allocations for PFI schemes have been maintained at the normal level, leading to further withdrawal of capital funding from other trusts.

Bridging the gap: the 'smoothing mechanism'

The economic rationale for the smoothing mechanism was that 'a number of the early PFI projects are expecting to face affordability problems ...despite offering good value for money.' This was attributed to the fact that the private sector would seek to recover the capital cost over the lifetime of the initial contract (25 to 40 years) 'whereas an equivalent public sector scheme would depreciate the asset over 60 years....... The support scheme is designed to equalise the payment streams for privately financed and publicly procured projects by spreading the capital costs across 60 years rather than the primary concession period.'[5]

The plausibility of this explanation is not enhanced by the way in which some NHS trusts have adopted quite different assumptions on asset lifetimes in business cases which have been approved by the NHS Management Executive. In its FBC, which was completed several months before the letter went out, the Dartford and Gravesham Trust had assumed a 40-year asset lifetime when comparing the costs of PFI with traditional procurement. The effect was to overstate the annual revenue

---

[5] Letter from David Revell, Branch Head, Private Finance and Capital, NHS Management Executive to Mr R McLachlan, Chief Executive, Bishop Auckland NHS Trust n.d. Letter of Colin Reeves (Director of Finance and Performance, NHS Executive) to NHS Trust chief executives etc. 14 January 1997. We gratefully acknowledge the assistance of the NHS Executive Private Finance Unit in providing copies of these letters.

impact of public sector procurement, eliminating the disadvantage on the side of the PFI option (Dartford and Gravesham Trust, 1996).[6] The trust nonetheless received an annual subvention of £1 059 000 under the 'smoothing mechanism' and went on to become the first NHS trust to sign a major PFI contract.

The subsidy thus has little to do with asset lifetimes and is more convincingly explained as an attempt to manage the difference between NHS capital charges—the 6% return on relevant assets—and PFI returns on capital.[7]

It is worth noting the subsidy of £42.6m to the Princess Margaret Hospital in Swindon, which will result from the annual smoothing payments (Table 11.6). This scheme has a total capital cost of £148m, and the OBC projected cost was £45m (Table 11.1). The NHS will be paying almost as much in this one subsidy as it would have paid to proceed with the original publicly-funded scheme.

While the 'smoothing mechanism' has been dropped for new PFI schemes, there is no reason to assume the need for subsidy will disappear. One solution may be for the Exchequer to directly fund part of a scheme, and this has happened at South Manchester University Hospitals NHS Trust, one of the 'first wave' schemes which did not receive a subsidy from the previous government (South Manchester University Hospitals NHS Trust, 1997).

Conclusion

What is the ultimate goal of the policy of substituting private finance for public and transferring ownership to the private sector? There can be no doubt that the effect of substituting private for public finance in the building of facilities for public use has had the effect of raising the costs of infrastructure development in the health service. The assumption that higher capital costs would be offset by savings resulting from the involvement of the private sector has proved simply incorrect. Rather, NHS trusts and health authorities have been obliged to make savings on other budgets in order to make the high costs of investment affordable. PFI has thus exacerbated existing pressures to reduce the costs of clinical services, but without passing the benefit of any savings back to the NHS or the Exchequer.

As 'affordability' problems could not be completely bridged using locally available NHS resources, schemes are being subsidized through national and regional capital budgets. PFI schemes have thus failed to deliver within the

---

[6] Despite the introduction of this bias against public procurement, the Dartford trust notes that the public sector option 'is cheaper in cash terms during the early years of the project by £1.7 million per annum. However, this is primarily caused by a requirement for the investment to be repaid over 25 years under PFI compared with the 40-year depreciation policy in the Public Sector Comparator [and because] the PSC ignores risk adjustment and is bound to be understated.' The trust concludes 'This affordability comparison, therefore, is misleading', a judgement it would be difficult to argue with.

[7] In this context, it is worth noting that government Interest Bearing Debt principal is recovered over 25 years, not over the lifetime of the assets.

affordability limits originally set for them, and those limits have been relaxed to accommodate them.

There is no reason to believe that these problems will disappear as the volume of PFI investment increases. Although current government policy seems to be to keep hospital beds open, the current wave of major investment in the NHS—'the largest new hospital building programme in the history of the NHS' (GB Department of Health, 1997)—is fundamentally dependent on the downsizing of the NHS, its facilities and its workforce. The implications for patient care and the goals and values of the NHS are very serious indeed.

Other countries intending to adopt NHS market models and macro-policy instruments such as resource accounting and the private finance initiative would do well to learn from the case study of the UK NHS before embarking on the same route.

References

Calderdale Healthcare NHS Trust. *Bid for a new hospital in Halifax.* May 1997

Centre for Mental Health Services Development, King's College London, *Future configuration of mental health services in Calderdale: Final report.* October 1997

Dartford and Gravesham NHS Trust, *New Acute General Hospital: Addendum to the Full Business Case.* 1998, pp 48–49

Dartford and Gravesham NHS Trust *Full Business Case.* 1996, p 31

Financial Times. NHS set for extra hospital beds. *Financial Times,* 8 June 1998

Gaffney D, Pollock AM. Can the NHS afford the PFI? London: British Medical Association Health Policy and Evaluation Unit, 1997

GB Department of Health. Local authority personal social services statistics 1995: statistical bulletin 1995/21. London: Government Statistical Services, 1995 (Crown Copyright)

GB Department of Health. Local authority personal social services. Community Care: detailed statistics on local authority personal social services for adults: England 1995; government statistical services, Department of Health, 1996

GB Department of Health. Press release 97/151. Alan Milburn announces primary care act pilots: patients to get one-stop shop community health service. 1 July 1997

GB Department of Health *Statistical Bulletin: NHS hospital activity statistics 1996-7*

GB House of Commons *Treasury Committee Sixth Report: The Private Finance Initiative (HoC 1995-6)* (HMSO 1996) pp 4–5

GB HM Treasury. *Financial Statement and Budget Report.* London: The Stationery Office, 1996. House of Commons paper HC90

GB HM Treasury, *Appraisal and Evaluation in Central Government: The Green Book* London: HM Treasury, 1997, p 84

Harrington C, Pollock AM. Decentralisation and privatisation of long-term care in the UK and USA. *Lancet,* 1998; **351**:1805–1808

Henwood M. Through a Glass Darkly. London: King's Fund, 1991

Mayston D. NHS capital charging, PFI contracts and value for money in healthcare (forthcoming)

National Health Service and Community Care Act 1990. London: HM Stationery Office [http://www.hmso.gov.uk/acts/summary.01990019.htm]

Newchurch and Company. *UK Health Care after the White Papers. PFI Futures: Capital Investment after the White Paper*. London: Newchurch and Company, 1997

Pollock AM. The NHS goes private. *Lancet*, 1995a; **346**: 683–684

Pollock AM. Where should health services go: local authorities versus the NHS? *British Medical Journal*, 1995b; **310**: 1580–1584

Pollock A, Gaffney D. Capital charges: a tax on the NHS. *British Medical Journal*, 1998; **317**: 157–158

Pollock AM, Dunnigan M, Gaffney D, Macfarlane A, Majeed FA. What happens when the private sector plans hospital services for the NHS: three case studies under the private finance initiative. *British Medical Journal*, 1997; **314**:1266–1271

Shaoul J. Charging for capital in the NHS trusts: to improve efficiency? *Management Accounting Research*, 1998; **9**: 95–112

South Manchester University Hospitals NHS Trust *Summary of the full business case for the reconfiguration of hospital services in South Manchester.* 1997

Webster C. *The Health Services since the War. Volume 1: Problems of Health Care: the National Health Service before 1957*. London: HM Stationery Office, 1988

Worcester Royal Infirmary NHS Trust. *Outline Business Case*, 1996, p 51

12
Designing and implementing successful health reforms: the role of research and research institutions

Somsak Chunharas and David Harrison

Health Systems Research Institute, Thailand and Health Systems Trust, South Africa

Health reforms in different parts of the world

The term 'health reform' has permeated the vocabularies of health sectors and health authorities in various parts of the world, although it is defined and even interpreted differently. Health reform concerns in Western countries have centred on cost containment, coping with increasing and changing demands for service provision, and simultaneously ensuring adequate financing for new and more sophisticated services. On the other hand, the major focus of reform in many developing countries has been to define new roles for government in service provision, aiming in the first instance not at cost containment, but rather at better use of limited resources to benefit the population as a whole.

The envisaged final products of health reform might be the creation of new organizations, the establishment of new relationships between existing organizations, new methods of work, or new performance tools—with or without significant structural changes. Reform may also involve changes in the basic values and attitudes towards health and health care among all concerned. It is no overstatement to say that, unless there are efforts to move beyond technical models and methodologies, efforts at health reform may not achieve their intended consequences. We risk inventing new tools or organizations that fail to have any real impact on health care provision, let alone the quality of people's lives. The essential characteristics of health reform should involve change in the structure and relationships of various institutions and stakeholders, including their attitudes and practices, and not only in the forms (rules, regulations, criteria, etc.) and mechanisms (organizations, channels, etc.) through which they interact.

An alternative term currently used for the worldwide efforts to improve health sectors is 'health system development'. This term has been used for quite some time and most often by the World Health Organization. It implies a somewhat different understanding of the process of change. 'Health reform' suggests that there is something that needs to be tackled with speed in order to fix things that have gone wrong. Once they are fixed, better health or more rational spending for health would be restored or achieved. 'Health system development', on the other hand, suggests that the system needs to be changed or improved continuously, rather than a once-off effort at health reform. Conceptually, the terms are not mutually exclusive. Present health systems are the outcomes of cumulative historical events, and what was deemed acceptable or appropriate in the past may not necessarily be so today. There may be a need for fundamental changes in design; however, the rapidly changing macro-environment of the present day leaves no room for complacency once we think we have reformed the system. On the contrary, it is always wise to keep a close eye on the results of the change and subsequent dynamics. Thus 'health reform' (with its connotation of fundamental change) and 'health systems development' (implying continuous monitoring and incremental change) are twin instruments that need to be applied by those wishing to ensure health for the mass of the population.

Health reform requires change, and change requires knowledge. It is always arguable whether specific changes are affected by knowledge: many changes take place with limited use of external information or knowledge, but rather based mainly on the decision-maker's own experiences, ideas or preferences. When expected changes do not occur, it may be due to a lack of information or knowledge, or it may stem from a lack of determination to take action, or even management deficiencies which thwart the ability to bring about the desirable changes.

The World Development Report 1993 (World Bank, 1993) called for attention to reappraise and redesign how countries invest for health. Many new concepts and criteria as well as methodologies were introduced to guide decisions on resource allocation. This certainly brought out very clearly the need for more information and knowledge to help decision makers evaluate these new approaches. The World Health Organization has produced an agenda for research, aimed at guiding countries to undertake important research in pursuit of health system development and health sector reform (Janovsky, 1996). The Report on Investing for Health Research and Development has identified research strategies for improving health on a global scale. Although it was not aimed exclusively at health reform, it pinpointed health policy development as one of the four major research components (WHO Ad Hoc Committee on Health Research, 1996). Included among the areas for international focus are health care financing, decentralization, quality of health services, private/public mix in health care, needs assessment and priority setting for health.

At the country level, the goal of health reform and the need for research vary from one country to another, depending on many factors, including political concerns and commitment, the strength of the research communities, interests of the public at large, and those of health professionals and service providers in both the public and private sectors. In addition, there are many other potential actors such as pharmaceutical companies and private health insurers. The macro socio-economic and political environment also determines how much reform can be anticipated, and the extent to which research guides decisions. In Thailand, national policies stipulated in the periodic five-year health development plans did not clearly articulate the need for health reform, until the recent eighth five-year plan (1997-2001) (Thailand Ministry of Public Health, 1981; 1986; 1992; 1996). Neither were policy changes initiated by governments. Attempts to bring about health reform seemed to be concentrated more among technical staff in the ministry of public health and academics in universities (Green, 1997). With the establishment of the Health Systems Research Institute in 1992 as a national institute to promote research for continuous health system development, health reform efforts in Thailand have become very much driven by research (Thailand Health Systems Research Institute, 1994; 1998). At the same time, certain issues for reform are also being pursued by the ministry of public health directly through legislative effort (Thailand Ministry of Public Health, 1997). In the Philippines, political factors were the main driving force behind the devolution of the health sector (Reodica, 1997). However, research efforts in the form of intensive monitoring have been launched to monitor and support local government units to offset undesirable outcomes (Perez, 1997). The reform of the national health service in the United Kingdom was also made with little input from the research communities (Hunter and Stockford, 1997). In the United States, many reform options were proposed by groups of researchers and academicians to influence the reform initiative led by Hillary Clinton, (Blendon *et al*, 1992) but political action proved impossible.

Research and decision making in health reform

Reason suggests that all decisions should be based on a thorough assessment of available relevant information, and there are illustrations which support this belief (WHO, 1991). Whether this is generally the case with health reform is a matter worth exploring. In health reform, crucial decisions need to be made with regard to three major questions:

- where the reform should be made;
- its objectives and
- how it can be carried out.

The identification of problems and shortcomings often occurs through a variety of means, and not necessarily through research. Research studies and information systems in many countries have pointed out defects, but decision-makers have been reluctant to act, indifferent or even sceptical of the information received. In conventional models of scientific research leading to change, the knowledge generated by one researcher is taken up by other scientists who carry out further studies until a product, generally a technology, is generated. We may call this a 'technological model' of research as an agent of change. In an alternative model, research leads to better understanding on a particular subject or issue, which enables people informed through this research to modify the relationship with their environment and/or the people with whom they work. This may be called a 'behavioural model', as research is expected to create behavioural changes directly, not through the production of technologies. Regrettably, this highly desirable situation is rare.

In health reform, research may be expected to adhere more closely to the 'behavioural model'. But it may also adopt the 'technological model' by producing certain 'tools' or ' blue prints' for creating and better managing the health system. However, for research to be useful for health reform efforts, it is important that the stakeholders—especially researchers and decision-makers—understand the nature of the interaction between information and decision-making and the complex interplay of various groups in the health systems (Goodman *et al*, 1992).

A number of observations help define the relationship between information and decision-making.

First, information makes sense only to the receptive. Information generated by research normally consists of facts or figures, or even ideas and recommendations generated as a result of such facts. 'Facts' do not necessarily mean the same thing to all people, and some facts are meaningful only to some people. In addition, ideas and recommendations may be proposed by researchers, and understood but not accepted by the target audience. For research findings to be useful, the target audience needs to be receptive—and in many cases they have to be 'primed' to be receptive. This means that ideas and recommendations have to be made relevant and communicated well, taking into account the concepts and values of the target audience. This does not imply manipulation, but rather a packaging of information in a manner which is sensitive to the audience's concerns and understandings. In this way, key messages emerging from research stand a better chance of serious consideration.

Second, mere facts are not enough. Researchers often believe that figures will speak for themselves, but this is usually a misconception—especially for complex subjects like health systems reform. Being able to turn the figures into understandable messages is key to making the target audience properly informed.

Third, interaction is important. Researchers are used to practising impartiality, but attempts at objective distance may be interpreted as indifference. Academic fear of losing neutrality may lead them to avoid interaction with the audience. Consequently, their research efforts could be rendered futile. The 'technological' model does not readily lend itself to the work of health reform, where the 'behavioural' model is more suitable. The latter can be considered comparable to the incrementalist approach to policy change (Walt, 1996). Given the interactive nature of policy processes, health system researchers rarely have the luxury of the objective distance afforded researchers in some other medical disciplines, but also need to guard against being driven by their own presuppositions:

> If researchers and analysts really want to have a direct impact on policy—one that goes beyond the diffuse enlightenment function—they may need to abandon the posture of the neutral technician and embrace the more actively committed role of the advocate. At the very least, policy projects should recognise that much of what they are about is persuasion and argumentation, and not simply the kind of self-confined academic research effort that has inspired the (self-centred) utilisation question (Porter, 1995).

This enhanced, more proactive role for researchers means treading a fine line in the policy process. But researchers will soon discover that much of their legitimacy in this new role stems from the validity and merit of their work. Equally important is a sensitivity to others' ideas and perceptions in interactions, so that crucial messages can be successfully conveyed, and further work based on a consensus of issues that require further clarification.

Fourth, there is always more than one group that needs to be informed, and they need to be able to interpret the message from their perspective. Health is the concern of all in society. Even in countries where government plays a major role in managing and controlling the health care delivery system, it is important to keep in mind that the general population still need to be properly informed—especially on health reform where the government has a dominant role, they tend to be seen as the prime target audience for research studies. However, other groups of stake-holders are also influential, either in advocating for or campaigning against reform efforts, and are thus important groups to be considered in the dissemination and discussion of research results. Related to this is the need to formulate research questions which are of relevance and concern to these interest groups, and not to focus narrowly on what is of relevance only to governments or politicians. Core messages may need to be packaged in different ways to inform different interest groups.

Finally, the complex language of health systems and health reform and that of researchers is often alienating to decision-makers and other interest groups. The study and analysis of health systems inevitably involves a diversity of concepts and employs a number of different academic disciplines. But this complex integration of the terminologies of economists, theories of social scientists, jargon of epidemiologists, techniques of management experts and so on needs to be minimized when communicating research results aimed at influencing reform decisions. The need for crisp and clear messages derived from research work cannot be overemphasized. Complex language is not only an obstacle to effective communication with policy makers, but is also a hindrance to comprehensive, interdisciplinary approaches to research. Moreover, unnecessarily complex language inhibits effective communication with non-technical people, and also creates barriers among technocrats. The need for a medium, a person or a mechanism that can integrate and communicate with the various disciplines, at the same time understanding the non-technical people, is therefore crucial for the successful integration of research into the reform efforts.

Key actors in research for health reform

Many groups of people assume different roles in the interplay between research and health reform. We can categorize them as three major groups: funders, researchers, and users of research. They adopt different roles and make their contribution at different stages from research planning to research utilization. Their relationship along the process may change from one stage to another, and it is useful to understand who they are and what are their characteristics.

1. Funders of research

These normally determine what research is to be carried out, although many rely, in turn, on researchers to submit their proposals and plans, and limit their task to selecting the best among proposals submitted by researchers. In the light of the expectation that research should contribute to health reform, it is certainly far from adequate for research funders to adopt one or other of the two extremes: either defining priority agendas and areas for research on their own; or waiting for proposals to come from researchers. A focus on research that feeds into reform implies changing roles and practices in research management, as a more participatory approach will be crucial for funding agencies wanting to support research that will be useful and relevant.

Funding of research for health reform can come from either national or international sources. In developing countries where health research funds are limited, it is usually the case that international sources play a major role. However, even where national sources of funds for health research are available, it is not necessarily the case that research for health reform will be identified as a priority. This depends very much on how the national budget for research is allocated. In

many instances, the process of allocation is supervised or directions set by
ministries dealing with science and technology which perpetuates funding bias
towards technologies, rather than health system development.

2. Researchers

In many countries, researchers working on issues of health reform are based in
universities. The influence of university-based research on health reform varies
from country to country, depending on the background and roles of universities in
various settings. In most cases, universities are hampered by their separation from
the mainstream of the health system, and thus may not have the proper
understanding of the functioning of the health system. Moreover, the careers of
university staff are evaluated on their general academic performance, and not
usually on the contribution of their academic work to the improvement of society.
(Given the nature of academic work, the difficulties of evaluation based on
academic criteria is acknowledged.) This system of merit assessment could also be
due to the fact that the university structure is usually discipline-based, and requires
intensive management either from within, or by funding agencies to ensure that
universities can be mobilized to make a concerted contribution to health systems
improvement.

Arguably, those working in the health services delivery system, and not
academics, are best acquainted with the system, are not limited to the interests of a
particular discipline, and thus make better researchers for health reform. A further
argument is that research for health reform is meant to be change-oriented, and
change through research will not happen easily unless those in the system are
involved. The first argument implies a shift in emphasis in flows of research
funding from academics to those in the health service. The same conclusion does
not necessarily hold for the latter argument, in that it does not automatically follow
that those in the health system have to work as researchers. Involvement in
research efforts can take many forms, and there are different ways in which their
limited time may be more productively used than participating in the core research
team. Whatever the precise arrangements, it is clear that researchers working in the
field of health reform will have to abandon or at least modify conventional ways of
working.

First, they will have to be ready to align their work with priority research
agendas and not just stay with their own initiatives and ideas. Second, researchers
must be ready to involve many other people in the process of research
implementation instead of working in isolation and waiting until the final results
are obtained before discussing with others! Third, they might have to be prepared
to modify their research plan, if necessary and if not conflicting with the goals and
quality of research work. Fourth, the management norms and evaluation criteria for
academic performance may need to be modified in order that universities may be
effectively involved in research for health reform. The organizational structure may
need to be changed as well. Some units may need to be created to help in

mobilizing researchers from various disciplines to work together. Whether this means a unit created by universities, by agencies outside universities or by research funding agencies is a matter that needs to be assessed and decided on independently by each country, taking into account the unique contexts of their academic institutions and relationships with other partners.

3. Users of research

In health reform, those who need to change, those who want changes to happen and those who can help catalyse changes are all potential users of research results. In the first instance, this certainly implies a wide range of possible contact points for disseminating research results. A common misconception is that health reform can happen only with high political commitment and concern, and therefore politicians or top level administrators are regarded as the most crucial users of research. In more democratic societies, the concerns of the public are articulated through a range of often powerful interest groups. By interacting only with health authorities or the policy level, researchers may miss the opportunity for their results to be properly considered or used, as they will be judged solely by those in power who may have different agendas and concerns. In many instances, it may in fact be those in power who resist change, and at whom change needs to be directed. Influential policy actors operating within civil society include the media, lobbyists and non-government organizations. The private sector plays a significant role in many health systems, and needs to be included in interaction and information exchange. In the United States, increasingly sophisticated lobbyists in the health system use their significant informational base and analytical capacity to entrench policies or resist change (Ginzberg 1991). Continuing interaction should help reduce the polarization between the public and private health sectors.

But the role of potential users of research results should go beyond utilization of available information, to participation in determining or identifying priority research agendas for reform. It is generally not a very easy task to involve the general public at those two crucial stages of research. Sometimes, on their own, researchers or even ministries of health attempt to establish 'representative fora' through meetings, mail surveys or other channels. Often, the consequence is a fairly contrived wish-list of needs, little different from any that could be drawn up independently. Recognition of and interaction with organizations of civil society who already have an established role as the 'voice of the people' may generate a more specific and manageable research agenda. These organizations include parliamentary committees on health, the media and NGOs. The crux of the issue is to ensure that as many user groups as possible have the opportunity to shape the research agenda, rather than it being the domain of a limited few who may have particular interest in retaining the *status quo*.

The contribution of these three major groups of active players and the roles they play in ensuring that research will be useful for health reform are summarized in Table 12.1.

Table 12.1 Possible participation/roles of different groups in the process of research for health reforms

Actors/ Functions	Setting research agendas/ questions	Carrying out research	Making use of research
Users			
Health authorities	++++[1]	+++	++++
General public	++	++	+++
Other groups (media, NGOs, lobby groups, parliamentarians)	++	++	+++
Researchers			
Universities	++++	++++	+++
Those in service delivery systems	++++	++++	+++
Funders			
National			
– general health research	+++	++	++
– health system research	++++	+++	++++
International	++++	++	++

[1] indicates degree of involvement

Mechanisms to generate information for health reform

In order to guide decisions for health reform through research, many countries and international organizations have established various types of mechanism to generate essential information. It has become apparent that, no matter how much international effort and interest are put into this area, a positive impact on the country health systems will not be achieved unless there are active country-initiated efforts. The model supporting these efforts may vary from one country to another, but essentially takes one or a combination of the following forms.

1. A research project approach

This seems to be the most common form in many countries, and is usually promoted through various international programmes or organizations which fund research for health reform at the country level. Commonly, it is also due to the lack of a dedicated country mechanism to organize research for health reform. Examples of international programmes that support research projects for reform include the International Health Policy Program (IHPP) (IHPP, 1998), and the International Clearing House for Health Systems Reform Initiatives (ICHHSRI) (ICHHSRI, 1997). Sometimes the relationship between the international efforts and the country is better established and more formalized, and takes the form of a special project or unit at the country level (see 5 below). This allows for a more continuous and integrated approach rather than an *ad hoc* research project based solely on competition for funds from international programmes or organizations.

The advantage of this first mechanism is that it is easy to create research projects for health reform, as the international programmes act to ensure that issues of reform of relevance and interest to them are addressed. The disadvantage is that it is based mainly on competition and the judgement rests purely in the hands of international experts rather than countries. The criteria for selection may differ between the two.

2. A research programme approach

This may differ from the project approach in two important respects. First, it allows for multiple questions and issues to be asked at the same time through multiple projects rather than through a single project (that may address a number of questions, but be more limited in scope). Second, the programme approach means that the research work will be more continuous rather than a once-off effort dictated in duration by project funding. The programme approach might be a result of international funding or be supported from the national budget—or a combination of both. Competitive grant practices may run contrary to the need for continuity enshrined in the programme approach, even though they may support multiple projects at the same time and not necessarily a single project in addressing a particular reform question (Zhan, 1995).

3. Existing research promoting mechanism

These include Medical Research Councils (MRC) or an Essential National Health Research (ENHR) mechanism. In many countries, such mechanisms already exist, and may be expected to play a more active role in promoting research for health reform, although long-established history and practices may hamper transformation (WHO, 1997). Special efforts may be needed to reorient such bodies to carry out the new roles effectively. The Council on Health Research and Development (COHRED) has promoted and supported countries to establish a national mechanism to promote essential national health research. Although the focus of

ENHR is not purely on health system development and reform but also includes relevant biomedical research (COHRED, 1990), many of the ENHR mechanisms in countries work to promote and create relevant research for health reform. Such mechanisms usually derive the bulk of their funding from national sources.

4. Research promoting mechanism dedicated to health systems change

This allows a more continuous or even long-term approach. Adoption of this approach is consistent with the interpretation that health reform is not a cross-sectional, once-off effort that takes place only when called for, but rather a process that evolves over time, with research inputs as an integral part of the process. Note that this mechanism is slightly different from the use of existing and more general-purpose health research-promoting mechanisms (see 3 above). This distinction is based on the argument that research for health reform needs special emphasis, separate from the more conventional research promotion for biomedical research. Combining the two may dilute the emphasis on research for health reform, which is usually less established. Moreover, such research promotion may also require management approaches different from the conventional 'technological' model. Examples of mechanisms include the Health Systems Trust (HST) in South Africa (Health Systems Trust, 1995), the Health Systems Research Institute (HSRI) in Thailand (Thai Government, 1992), the plan to establish a health policy and system research unit in the University of Singapore (Phua Kai Hong, personal communication, February 1997) and the creation of a self-financed health policy research unit in Hong Kong (Geoffrey Liu, personal communication, February 1997).

Common to both this and the mechanism outlined in 3 is the ability to define the needs for research in countries and interact with different sources of funds to create relevant and continuous research work. This characteristic suggests that they may be the most desirable working models for supporting health systems development, although acceptance of this requires changes of attitude and practices from the various partners, both national and international.

5. MOH special research units for health reform

In certain cases, the need for concerted research support for health reform is perceived by ministries of health who respond by creating special units for such purposes. The unit might carry out only a few research projects, or many projects over a long period under different and changing macro-environments. However, creating the special unit usually implies the relatively temporary nature of such an undertaking. It may be phased out due to changing financial, political or technical constraints although, compared to the project or programme approach which might be created outside the ministry, there is a better chance for it to be integrated into the system or to provide needed information. One of the significant limitations of a unit based within the ministry of health is the potential for its monitoring role to be constrained, particularly in terms of progress towards equity in health care provision.

Whether units have a comparative advantage in guaranteeing a more continuous research input into health reform is not clear and depends very much on the factors motivating the creation of mechanisms. The Local Government Assistance and Monitoring Services (LGAMS) that works to monitor and facilitate decentralization and health in the Philippines could be taken as an example of such a unit created by the ministry of health. The Health Care Reform Project in Thailand supported by the European Union is a combination of the programme and the unit approach (Thai Government, 1997).

These various approaches are not mutually exclusive but can actually be related or combined (Figure 12.1). It is, however, useful to bear in mind that certain examples in some countries may take the form of a project or programme approach which is quite temporary in nature and can be heavily influenced by the agendas of funding agencies which have little knowledge of country situations.

Research management and health reform

The need for proper management to ensure that research contributes to health reform cannot be overemphasized. Management is the key to successes in many other business and undertakings (Drucker, 1992) but many research communities still see research as best left to individual initiatives and imagination, avoiding influence from those intimately involved with the issues. On the other hand, funding agencies, national or international, generally believe in a competitive model for granting research funding, and restrict their management to ensuring that the competition will be as fair as possible, based often only on academic criteria. Researchers limit their roles to proposing the projects most attractive to the funding agencies and then carrying out the research work as best they can. This leaves several gaps in leadership and direction that need to be filled and call for more intensive management. The most crucial goal of such management may be to ensure that all involved are reoriented and shift their thinking from the conventional practices of research management which focus on supporting the most interesting ideas, to supporting those most related to the needs for reform. Table 12.2) lists some of the concepts and practices that may need to be addressed.

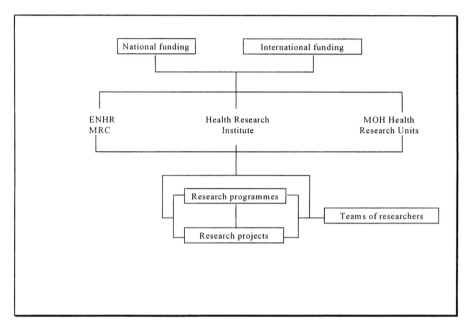

Figure 12.1 Relationship between funding sources, research promoting mechanisms and research programmes and projects

1. Change orientation

Research for reform is change oriented and not curiosity driven. Ensuring that this common understanding exists is not easy, and often needs to be tackled case by case. In many of the planning processes of research for reform, it is useful to start by analysing the intended end points or changes anticipate, and then to work backwards to see which questions still need to be addressed in reaching those end points. Starting from the end helps to provide focus and substance for research, and conducted properly, the research should still help to confirm, modify or even dispute the end point. This argument does not trivialize the importance of research which aims to provide a better understanding of the situation, causal factors and actors. However, it is far from adequate to focus research only on issues of context, as research input is required for many other aspects leading towards reform (Figure 12.2).

Table 12.2 Comparison of conventional research funding management with decision-linked research management

Stages of research	Setting the research questions	Soliciting best proposal	Carrying out the research	Ensuring good quality	Dissemination
Active players					
Conventional	Funding agencies	Funder + researcher (proposal + defend)	Researcher (funding agencies monitor)	– Funder – researchers	– Researchers – publishers – funder
Decision-linked research	– Users – funder – researcher	– Funder – researcher – users	– Researchers – funder – users	– Funder – users – researchers	– Funder – researcher – users
Objectives (or focus)					
Conventional	– interesting to the funder – relevance – change?	–technical soundness (methodologic-ally)	– the best data quality	–data analysis quality –generaliza-bility	–to international scientific community
Decision-linked research	Change-oriented	–addressing the question – timing	– timeliness – focus on the content/question	– practical application – useful recom-mendations	– utilization by relevant stakeholders

2. User involvement

Being change-oriented also implies that research managers need to involve those who are expected to bring about those changes in the process of research. In conventional management related to research utilization, the emphasis is on ensuring the research results are easily understood by the users, for example through training researchers in how best to present results (Smitasiri, 1997). In an area as complex as health reform, it is simplistic to expect that such a practice would translate into better use of research results. Involvement of research users before the very first step of research planning and identification of research questions all the way to the process of monitoring research progress and modification of research plans has been a lesson learnt by different countries (Munishi, 1995; Okello, 1995). In other words, research may have greatest value when it is regarded as an integral part of a bigger policy initiative, in which researchers may not even have a major role in initiation or leadership.

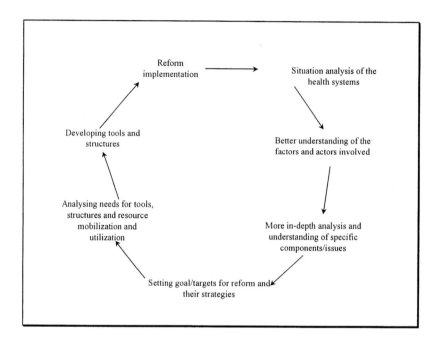

Figure 12.2 Different sets of research questions and their contribution to the reform process

3. Going beyond the facts and findings of research work

Conventionally, research work is regarded as completed when the findings have been made and accepted as scientifically sound. For reform purposes, those findings need to be converted into recommendations that are meaningful to various groups of research users. Studies on existing and comparable practices will be useful to suggest possible future action, but researchers may be required to do further analysis on possible financial or resource implications of applying such practices. They may also be asked to come up with workable models or even manuals that would make implementation possible. Often, this activity is left to agencies implementing the reform and is not regarded as the work of research teams. But for those who are anxious to ensure that research is useful and relevant to reform efforts, creative ways of education and communication will certainly constitute part of their management undertakings. This requirement on the research management unit will vary from one country to another, depending on how effective the implementing agencies are in making use of technical information. In addition, a proactive and creative research management unit may help to guide decisions for reform by limiting its role not only to research work, but also supporting syntheses based on the compilation and review of various types of data or relevant research studies.

4. Being mindful of the policy process and the politics involved

Health reform is political in nature. It is easy to expect researchers to keep their distance from politics, but it may be more productive to make them aware of and acquainted with the policy process involved in anticipated reform. Most researchers cannot be expected to handle complex policy processes. Thus, research for health reform requires management practices and management mechanisms different from conventional research work. Understanding the policy process and the politics involved will enable the research management unit to help the researchers identify proper entry points for their research agendas, involve those who need to be involved, avoid biased views and influences, and finally adjust the overall management plan to the changing macro or micro political environment.

5. Effective dissemination of research findings

Making results of research work known to those concerned is a crucial step in research management for change. Effective communication requires thorough consideration and detailed planning at various stages of research dissemination. First, there is a need to make the findings meaningful and understandable. This involves further synthesis and interpretation as mentioned in 3 above. It also means analysing each of the various groups of potential research users and trying to convert the messages so they can be understood by these various groups from the perspective of their own concerns and context. The forms needed to disseminate information to these many groups also vary. Researchers like to organize dissemination workshops with policy makers but usually find that few show up or busy themselves with something else. Policy briefs constitute another form by which researchers attempt to reach policy makers. Reaching the general public often involves dissemination through the media or large meetings that allow broad-based participation, though the costs are often prohibitive. In many cases, disseminating information through the media is often the most effective way to reach politicians. However, this interaction with the media depends on the socio-political environment and is not necessarily always as effective as might be expected.

Effective research dissemination needs to be planned and budgeted for by management. Conventional research funding confines support to publishing research reports. In order to formulate more meaningful messages for various groups of people we need those who know how to convert technical messages into understandable terms. The Health Systems Trust in South Africa has established partnerships with two national newspapers, whose journalists help them convert messages for the general public as well as politicians. Besides lengthy and technical reports, the IHPP has produced short summary reports aiming specifically at decision-makers. In some cases the efforts to disseminate research findings to potential users are extensive and time-consuming. On several occasions, research briefs on the reform of the Civil Servant Medical Benefit Scheme in Thailand had to go through the director-general of each of the responsible departments, and then to the permanent secretary of the finance ministry, and then to the secretary-general of the civil service office, and then to the deputy minister of finance and finally to the media. Yet despite this process, the recommendations of the research were not effectively adopted by those concerned, and also not well received by the civil servants who were affected by the reform.

6. Different criteria to evaluate the quality of research work

Critical evaluation of research work—from proposal review to the final judgement on the value and quality of research work—contributes significantly to the planning and formulation of research proposals and their outcome. Being change-oriented, and evidence of appropriate user involvement are important criteria in the evaluation of research proposals or research results. The emphasis on sound methodologies should not be lost, but should be assessed together with the need to ensure that relevant data is being collected and meaningful information generated. Adhering only to methodologies, data analysis techniques or research design based on theoretical concerns may omit key concerns, and thus be unacceptable or oversimplified. In addition, sophisticated analytical techniques are not necessarily preferable to carefully designed data gathering and simple tabulation for descriptive purposes.

The criterion of judging whether research will produce new knowledge or not (and thus justifies support) should be applied with discrimination. Knowledge that is well established elsewhere might need to be reassessed or studied in a different context. On the other hand, existing data or studies might suffice to guide certain decisions and need not be repeated. Unswerving dedication to representativeness, careful case-control study design and elimination of confounding factors may need to be traded off with the reality that circumstances may render such practices next to impossible—and the only way to take the various confounding factors into consideration is in the discussion of results and their implications. International publishability is another criterion which may conflict with the need to design a study which is country-specific and decision-relevant.

7. Fuzzy logic rather than rock logic

Managing research for health reform means the ability to incorporate different viewpoints and come up with the one that best represents the concerns of all parties, rather than adhering only to one set of standards or needs. This does not imply compromise at all costs, but rather being able to create dialogue whereby all parties can be heard and given due consideration. The outcome of this dialogue may help enrich, clarify or modify the implications of research findings, keeping in mind the final goal of the research undertaken and reform objectives. It certainly requires managers who have a strong technical background, knowledge of the realities of the system and most importantly, sensitivity to differences of opinion and potential areas of convergence.

Institutionalizing research management for health reform

If health reform is perceived necessarily as an ongoing process rather than a once-off undertaking, studies into health systems need to be carried out on a continuous basis and the need to institutionalize research management for health reform is indisputable. It is clear from many experiences that when reforms are called for, there is often no time for studies and whatever information is available will be used to guide the reform process. Since research for health reform requires solid understanding of the health system, the need for continuing dialogue between various groups of stakeholders, and the imperative of moving beyond the publication of research findings, it is clear that a mechanism to carry out all these functions would be beneficial to the system as a whole. A basic model for effecting this is suggested in Figure 12.3. The focal point for research management serves many functions, from ensuring a relevant research agenda to proper use of research results. The main strategies employed are participatory rather than self-executing, integrating rather than polarizing, and interactive rather than isolating. In attempting to institutionalize research management for health reforms, certain crucial questions need to be addressed.

1. Where should this research management unit be?

A unit situated appropriately to promote and manage the generation of relevant and useful research for health reform should be able to understand the system, yet remain impartial. It should also possess enough potential for sustained financing (see 2 below). The ministry of health, as the national health authority, is normally expected to carry out such functions. In certain cases—actually the norm in most developing countries—the ministries of health also work as service providers and health programme executing agents. This makes the ministry far from being impartial, and may therefore prevent it from being able to see the needs for reform clearly, even when they are compelling. A mechanism which is not part of the ministry of health in this case is therefore desirable. Whether this should be an NGO or part of government machinery that has a more general function of

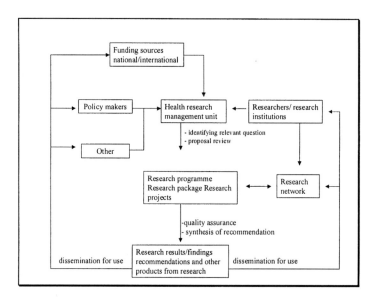

Figure 12.3 Research management in research for health reform

evaluating system performance and promoting relevant research studies will depend on each country's situation. The case of HSRI in Thailand, created as a semi-governmental agency but overseen by the ministry of public health and receiving its budget from the government through the ministry of public health, is an example of such a mechanism. It was created in response not to a specific need for health reform, but rather to the need for a mechanism to generate research and information that would guide the Thai health system in a rapidly changing environment. In practice, its major research agendas are oriented towards the need to guide many aspects of the reform efforts of the country. The Health System Trust in South Africa, created through international support to best serve national interests and concerns to reconstruct the health service system after the apartheid regime, is another good example. It was established as a non-governmental organization with no direct line-of-command relationship with the ministry of health, neither through its governance nor financing, but has contributed significantly to meeting the information needs of the ministry of health. The Foundation for ENHR in the Philippines is a private sector foundation with links to the ministry of health of the Philippines (Neufeld *et al*, 1997). Advantages and disadvantages of these comparable models could be learnt by many other countries contemplating similar mechanisms.

2. Financing for the mechanism

Financing for research is limited especially in developing countries. Dependence on international sources is common. It is important to ensure that funds available to support research for health reform allows for dialogue and development processes, taking into consideration the need to involve various stakeholders along the way. Such funding cannot be provided on a project-by-project basis, judged mainly on technical merit and on a competitive basis. In addition, there is a need for funds to support the work of the management unit. In most cases, especially with international sources, funds might be available to support individual projects but not the management mechanism. Countries may be reluctant to support the management mechanism for fear of it becoming redundant or unable to mobilize additional funds, as most international funding agencies prefer to work directly with individual research groups. Governments may also be concerned about establishing units with a greater degree of autonomy, especially those tasked with evaluating a political hot potato such as health reform! If funding comes from international sources, the provision of blocks of funds for a period of time may allow for management roles to be delegated to reliable national institutions or mechanisms. The experiences of the National Epidemiology Board of Thailand (1990) supported by the Rockefeller Foundation and the South African HST supported by the Kaiser Family Foundation may serve as interesting examples.

With regard to national funding, it is worth mentioning that the conditions attached to the funds will affect the efficiency of such management units. Provision of a block grant to an autonomous management system independent from bureaucratic rules and regulations is crucial. Moreover, the provision of a government budget to support research projects through such a management mechanism will both increase the effectiveness of strategies of mobilization and interaction, and act as a lever for raising money from other funding sources.

3. Research management capacity

One major barrier to institutionalizing research management for health reform is the need for competent managers. This requires a person who understands the health system as well as research concepts and methodologies. S/he also needs to be managerially competent and well oriented to policy processes. It may not be easy to find people ready made with such competencies and orientation, and even more difficult to find those prepared to deal with such diverse areas (Thai Health Systems Research Institute, 1997). Conventional research managers focusing only on technical concerns can learn to pay attention to other aspects, if they realize and agree that research for health reform is change-oriented and not merely productive of new facts or new theories or explanations. The prevailing model of research management based mainly on the belief that research requires individual innovation and that there should be minimal interference with the ideas or work of researchers may hinder attempts to establish research management capacity for the purpose of health reform.

4. Networking and partnership building

One of the important components for successful institutionalization is the creation of networks and institutional linkages with those in the field of research for health reform, both nationally and internationally. Linkage with international funding mechanisms is important to consolidate the limited national expertise and capacity in this field and thus facilitate the management process. Networking of national actors includes networks of researchers that might be grouped according to reform areas or disciplines or institutions. It also involves networking with decision-makers through some established mechanism rather than through *ad hoc* interactions. Linking with the media helps to convey messages to the public at large. Wherever feasible, public involvement through consumer advocacy groups or other types of community groups or organs of civil society is also desirable. International institutes and groups with technical expertise relevant to the needs for reform in countries can also act as a stabilizing factor in the institutionalization effort. Creating networks and partnerships of various kinds help to ensure that the institutionalization efforts will create a dynamic mechanism for knowledge-based health reform (Task Force on Health Research for Development, 1991).

5. Research careers and academicians

Most research capacity in countries is in universities, and research for health reform will not be firmly established without strengthening the capacity and concern of universities in these areas. There is a need to restructure or re-create incentive systems, especially career paths so that university researchers can benefit from research work that contributes to health reform—and not just limit their contribution to those topics that are more theoretical or technical in nature. Without such career structures, the involvement of researchers from universities will be *ad hoc* and dependent upon individual and personal interests, without the momentum for long-term development of the health system.

International mechanisms and research for health reform

It is undeniable that many of the research efforts in countries related to health reform, especially developing countries, are the result of international organizations working with researchers at the country level. It is customary for international organizations, in these cases, to deal with academics in universities rather than with national authorities, as they believe that academicians are less biased in looking at the system and needs for reform. They also believe that academicians in universities have a good grasp of research methodologies. This leads to the practice of soliciting research projects from countries which will then be judged on a competitive basis using multiple criteria set by the international mechanism. Certain international programmes such as IHPP, wanting to ensure that researchers do have a link with the system, mandate that each project submitted by researchers carry with them a policy adviser. Others may require that certain methodologies be employed (Bobadilla and Conley, 1995). Many set the priority issues or areas under which funding will be made available, believing that these are the areas that need to be explored even though not yet perceived by countries. Some agencies adopt a more open policy, mandating only very broad policy directions and objectives rather than specific agendas or methodologies, or even managerial processes and structures such as the National Epidemiology Board approach of the Rockefeller Foundation. A number of issues related to the practices of international mechanisms in supporting health research for reform need to be reviewed to ensure that international efforts really promote and support national efforts.

1. What are the preconditions that need to be set in order for an international mechanism to support research efforts for health reform at the country level? Should support be based on area of interest, either research agenda or methodologies, determined by the supporting international organizations? Could such requirements be made in a more interactive way?

2. Calling for proposals from research institutions at the country level should be weighed against the need to strengthen national mechanisms that will manage research for health reform. In those countries where such mechanisms exist, the international mechanism should be encouraged to work with them as much as possible rather than trying to directly solicit and support research projects on a vertical basis. This will not only strengthen the national mechanism but also ensure a better chance of the research being considered or further developed by the parties concerned.

3. In the effort to promote or support countries to carry out research for health reform, it might be better for international mechanisms to aim at strengthening both national mechanisms for managing research for health reform, and units responsible for health policy development, rather than aiming only at directly

supporting individual research teams. Research work by individual research teams might contribute to the wealth of knowledge accumulated by international agencies but may be of little use to countries.

Conclusion

This paper has sought to address the question of how we can work to ensure that research becomes an integral and useful component of the reform process. Leaving health research management to conventional models of researcher-initiated and technically-oriented research funding will not bring about the anticipated impact on health reform. A different planning process is required, based on an interactive working model which does not leave the task of identifying relevant research questions in the hands of researchers alone. It also does not end with producing research findings by researchers and then passing them on to whichever users are deemed relevant. The need to go beyond findings to formulate meaningful messages, design workable models, or refocus efforts into the development of relevant tools for reforms, are a few examples where researchers might be required to work in paradigms beyond conventional research. This implies the need for a mechanism at the country level to carry out many co-ordinating and facilitating roles. Existing mechanisms to fund health research such as medical research councils might need to be reviewed with the new roles and practices in mind. How such a mechanism should or could be established depends very much on the stage of development and the concern of countries, taking into consideration the overall political and economic environment, concerns of the general public, and the academic and technical capacity in health research. The Health Systems Research Institute of Thailand and the Health Systems Trust of South Africa are illustrations of two country mechanisms dedicated to support of research for health reform which have proved quite effective.

International agencies and mechanisms play a great role in creating awareness of the need for reform, as well as in promoting and mobilizing research communities in countries. Deficiencies in their funding practices need to be rectified, bearing in mind the need for interaction and dialogue to make research efforts useful to countries. Typical vertical funding practices dealing directly with individual researchers or research teams rather than with existing national mechanisms that facilitate the linking of research with the reform process should be avoided. There is a need for international organizations to help build up such managerial units and capacity wherever necessary, rather than continuing the practice of separately supporting national research teams on a competitive basis using the criteria set mainly by the international funding mechanism. This implies a different way of working with countries where health reforms are needed.

This new approach is not without its pitfalls, which need to be recognized in order to be avoided. The first is that the national mechanism may be construed as a way of concentrating control of research for health reform in the hands of a few national people. Second, there may be anxiety about shrinking the diversity of funding sources available for health systems research. Third, there may be concerns that innovation is undermined through the removal of competition for international research funds. These are legitimate concerns. But in fact, the very success of any national mechanism rests in it being able to avoid these pitfalls. It has to be seen to be participatory in outlook, reaching out to groups and constituencies previously overlooked. It needs to be able to mobilize funds, not only for itself, but for research groups who will actually do the work. It also needs to encourage and support in-country researchers to seek funding independently. Finally, it will have to continue to motivate for funding from both national and international funding sources based on its ability to deliver the goods. If it fails to achieve this, it will rapidly lose legitimacy and funding. If it succeeds, it can be a powerful force for health systems development.

References

Blendon RJ, Edwards JN, Hyams AL. Making the critical choices. *Journal of the American Medical Association*,1992; **267**: 2509–2520

Bobadilla JL, Conley P. Designing and implementing packages of essential health services. *Journal of International Development*, 1995; **7**: 543–554

Commission on Health Research for Development. *Health Research: Essential Link to Equity in Development.* New York: Oxford University Press, 1990

Drucker PF. *Managing for the Future.* New York: Butterworth-Heineman, 1992

Ginzberg E (ed) Health Services Research: Key to Health Policy. A Report from The Foundation for Health Services Research. Harvard University Press, Cambridge Massachusetts, 1991

Goodman RA, Remington PL, Howard RJ. Communicating information for action. *Mortality and Morbidity Weekly Report*, 1992; **41** suppl: 143–147

Green A. Health Sector reform: policy formulation and implementation: country report on Thailand. Leeds: Nuffield Institute for Health, 1997

Health Systems Trust. *Health Systems Trust: Annual Report* 1994. Durban: Health Systems Trust, 1995

Hunter DJ, Stockford D. Health care reform in the United Kingdom. In: Nitayarumphong S (ed) *Health Care Reform: at the Frontier of Research and Policy Decisions.* Nonthaburi, Thailand: Office of Health Care Reform. Ministry of Public Health, 1997: pp71–99

International Clearing House of Health Systems Reform Initiatives. www.insp.mx/ichri/index.htm/, April 1997

International Health Policies Program. www.health.org/afronts/ihpl.htm, 1998

Janovsky K (ed) *Health Policy and Systems Development: an Agenda for Research.* Geneva: World Health Organization, 1996 (WHO/SHS/NHP/96.1)

Munishi G. Paper on impact of research on policy. Workshop paper on International Health Policy Program, sixth meeting of participants, 2-7 October 1995, Beijing, 1995

National Epidemiology Board of Thailand. Chunharas S, Choprapawon CH (eds) *The National Epidemiology Board of Thailand: the first four years(1987 1990).* Bangkok: The National Epidemiology Board of Thailand, 1990

Neufeld V, Dlamini QQ, Tan-Torres T, Pruzanski M. *The Next Step: an Interim Assessment of ENHR and COHRED.* Geneva: Council on Health Research for Development(COHRED), 1997

Okello DO. IHPP Supported project in Uganda: attempts made to reach the findings of phase I research project results to policy makers. Workshop paper on International Health Policy Program, sixth meeting of participants, 2–7 October 1995, Beijing, 1995

Perez JA. *Operationalizing equity: the Philippiness: decenterized health care system.* Department of Health. Local Government Assistance & Monitoring Service. Presentation made to the travelling seminar on the attainability and affordability of equity in health care provision, 29 June 1997 Manila, Philippine, 1997 (unpublished)

Porter RW. *Knowledge Utilisation and the Process of Policy Formulation: Toward a Framework for Africa.* Washington DC: Support for Analysis and Research in Africa (SARA), 1995

Reodica, N. *The Philippine health systems and transformation process of the past decade.* Paper presented to the travelling seminar on the attainability and affordability of equity in health care provision, 29 June 1997 Manila, Philippine, 1997 (unpublished)

Smitasiri, S. A report. Workshop on policy communication 1–3 March 1997, Regent Cha-Am. Bangkok: National Health Foundation, 1997

Task Force on Health Research for Development. *Essential National Health Research. A Strategy for Action in Health and Human Development.* Geneva: Task Force on Health Research for Development, 1991

Thai Government. *Health Care Reform Project.* Nonthaburi: Office of Health Care Reform Project, 1997

Thai Government Gazette. Health Systems Research Institute Act B.E. 2535(A.D.1992). Vol. 109, Part 45

Thailand Health Systems Research Institute. Health Systems Research Institute Plan (1993-1996). Health Systems Research Institute, 1994

Thailand Health Systems Research Institute. Health Systems Research Management Guideline (in Thai). Nonthaburi: Health Systems Research, 1997

Thailand Health Systems Research Institute. Health Systems Research: an agenda for health reform. Bangkok: HSRI Publishing Project, Health Systems Research Institute, 1998

Thailand Ministry of Public Health. *The National Health Development Plan in the 5th National Economic and Social Development Plan.* Bangkok: Thailand Ministry of Public Health, Health Planning Division, 1981

Thailand Ministry of Public Health. *The National Health Development Plan in the 6th National Economic and Social Development Plan.* Bangkok: Thailand Ministry of Public Health, Health Planning Division, 1986

Thailand Ministry of Public Health. *The National Health Development Plan in the 7th National Economic and Social Development Plan.* Bangkok: Thailand Ministry of Public Health, Health Planning Division, 1992

Thailand Ministry of Public Health. *The National Health Development Plan in the 8th National Economic and Social Development Plan.* Bangkok: Thailand Ministry of Public Health, Health Planning Division, 1996

Thailand Ministry of Public Health and Parliamentary Health Committee. (Draft) National Health Insurance Act B.E, 1997

Walt G. Policy analysis: an approach. In: Janovsky K (ed) *Health Policy and Systems Development: an Agenda for Research.* Geneva: World Health Organization, 1996, pp 225–241 (WHO/SHS/NHP/96.1)

World Bank. *World Development Report 1993: Investing in Health.* New York: Oxford University Press, 1993

World Health Organization. *From research to decision making: case study on the use of health systems research.* Programme on Health Systems Research and Development. World Health Organization, 1991

World Health Organization. *Tenth meeting of the directors of medical research councils or analogous bodies and concerned research foci in The Relevant Ministries. Report to the Regional Director, Bandung, Indonesia, 21–25 October 1996.* New Delhi: World Health Organization Regional Office for South East Asia, 1997

World Health Organization Ad Hoc Committee on Health Research Relating to Future Intervention Options. Investing in Health Research and Development. Geneva: World Health Organization, 1996 (WHO/TDR/GET/96.1)

Zhan Shao Kang. Financing of health services in Poor Rural China. Workshop paper on International Health Policy Program, sixth meeting of participants, 2–7 October 1995, Beijing, 1995

13
Implementing successful health care reforms: minding the process

Josep Figueras, Richard B. Saltman*, Tom Rathwell**, Gill Walt***

*World Health Organization Regional Office for Europe, Copenhagen; *The Rollins School of Public Health, Emory University, Atlanta, USA;** School of Health Services Administration, Dalhousie University, Halifax, Canada; ***London School of Hygiene & Tropical Medicine, UK*

Over the last decade, governments in Europe and elsewhere have been reviewing the suitability of their patterns of finance, organization and delivery of health care services. In many instances this has led to setting in motion health care reform programmes. There have been substantial difficulties in implementing reforms, however. These difficulties often have less to do with the content of the reform programmes, but rather reflect insufficient attention to the process of implementation. A variety of factors including the economic, political and social environment within which the reforms take place, as well as the support—or lack of it—of key actors such as the medical profession, can be more important in determining the success of reforms than the actual content of the reform programme itself (Walt and Gilson, 1994). The significance of these factors increases in the current climate of cross-fertilization of reform ideas between countries. Reform models are sometimes transferred across national boundaries and incorporated in reform programmes in receiving countries without adequate regard to political, cultural and social differences.

The reform literature and debate in general have paid relatively little attention to the problems of reform implementation and to strategies for dealing with them. This lack of emphasis has served to open a gap between research and the decisions that policy makers actually confront. While analysts have focused considerable research effort on developing sophisticated organizational and financial strategies, policy makers have been struggling to introduce minimal, less sophisticated change in their health care systems.

Recently, research efforts have begun to focus on the context and process of health care reform. This research applies social and political science techniques to analyse the influences that affect the process of reform implementation in the health field. Work has concentrated predominantly on highlighting the complexities of reform implementation, however, placing less emphasis on the implications for design and implementation of future reform.

This chapter views reform from the perspective of policy makers, planners and implementers who are given the task of managing reform implementation, sometimes amidst difficult political and economic circumstances over which they have little or no influence, and frequently without the support of key stakeholders. The chapter is structured as a series of issues for managing the reform process, drawn from experience to date with the implementation of health reforms mainly in the European region[1] and including the countries of Central and Eastern Europe (CEE) and the Commonwealth of Independent States (CIS). The chapter focuses particularly on the more complicated aspects of implementation and suggests potential strategies to deal with them.

Understanding the nature of reform

In trying to diagnose the difficulties in reform implementation, one needs first to have a clear understanding of the notion of 'reform' itself. This concept tends to be used and interpreted in several different ways. If the political value attributed to reform is high, policy makers may seek to magnify small changes and call them 'reform' (Figueras *et al*, 1997). In some cases there is what can be termed 'cosmetic reform' when change takes place only at terminological and superficial levels. For instance, following the widespread dissemination of the internal market model of health care reform into Eastern Europe, several countries begun to use terms such as 'purchaser provider split' and 'contracting' as labels for what largely remain their traditional health system arrangements. In contrast, if the political value of reform is low, policy makers may deny the existence of 'reform' while in fact seeking to undertake relatively radical changes in the health care system.

Kroneman and van der Zee (1997) attribute the problems in understanding and measuring reform to the 'fuzzy' nature of reforms. They argue that the main cause for fuzziness is the gradual introduction of reforms, a process which can be

---

[1] Examples are primarily based on the evidence collected and generated by the European Observatory on Health Care Systems, notably the Health Care Systems in Transition (HiT) profiles (now available for 35 European countries) and the results of a recent study on reforms in the European Region collected in two publications (World Health Organization, 1997; Saltman *et al*, 1998). A literature review of recent publications on reform implementation has also been employed.

disrupted at any point in time. Also, in some cases no clear starting point can be distinguished and the formal date of implementation, sometimes marked by the passing of the law, may not indicate the real commencement of reform.

Given different understandings of reform, it is important that, at the outset, implementers examine the specific nature of the reform process in their own setting. Table 13.1 outlines dimensions along which to consider a definition of health sector reform. The approach adopted in this chapter defines reform as a purposive process involving sustained and profound structural change, top down, led by national, regional or local governments, and seeking to achieve a series of explicit policy objectives (Saltman and Figueras, 1997).

Table 13.1 Key dimensions for a definitional framework of health sector reform

- Structural vs. evolutionary change
- Change in policy objectives followed by institutional change vs. redefinition of policies alone
- Purposive vs. haphazard change
- Sustained and long-term vs. one-off change
- Top-down vs. bottom-up
- Politically led vs. non-politically led

Source: Figueras *et al*, 1997

Managing external influences: the role of values, culture and society

The international character of the health reform process can be attributed to the interaction of separate but related activities. One is the seemingly independent genesis of reform activities in a number of countries, driven by a confluence of domestic or domestically-felt pressures (e.g. demographic, technological and economic). A second element is the rapid transference of certain basic reform notions across national boundaries: for example, the concept of creating a contract relationship inside publicly operated health systems, between purchasers and what then become independently managed provider institutions. This involves the application of innovative solutions to what are essentially similar structural dilemmas. International organizations sometimes contribute to this phenomenon of rapid transfer of reform ideas through their project development and consultation activities, particularly when these are linked to international loan requirements. Some observers, however, question the cultural, social and, particularly, the technical appropriateness of some of this activity (Collins *et al*, 1994). Countries with very different health sector traditions and expectations, and, in CEE/CIS countries, with a dearth of managerial capacity, are sometimes being lured down a perilous path into adopting structural arrangements that they have neither the societal interest nor the organizational capacity to sustain.

From the perspective of those implementing reforms, several basic strategies have emerged in response to international transference. Ideas which are useful but not entirely culturally appropriate have typically been substantially adapted before introduction. National policy makers have also found it effective consciously to develop techniques to 'manage the donors' (e.g. to steer international agencies toward a more appropriate mix of reform activities). Both responses, however, require national policy makers to generate a clear set of health sector objectives, and then to implement those policy objectives consistently. This has proved difficult to achieve in some CEE/CIS countries undergoing economic transition. However, unless health sector reform strategies are capable of rooting themselves in national cultural 'soil', they are not likely to produce the expected outcomes nor to be sustainable over the medium to long term.

Achieving reform sustainability under macroeconomic constraints

Macro-economic constraints constitute both a main stimulus for health care reform as well as a primary obstacle to its implementation. A number of reforms have been triggered by concern about increasing cost pressures within a context of macro-economic recession. In the same way, a central constraint in implementing reform is the relative strength and resilience of the national economy. This is true for both western and eastern Europe. In western Europe, macro-economic policy increasingly reflects intense concern about national competitiveness in a period of regionalization and globalization of industrial production and trade. For the member states of the European Union, the Maastricht criteria for admission to the forthcoming European Monetary Union are also having a powerful effect on macro-economic policy. Both concerns have led economic policy makers to call for sharp reductions in public sector spending, particularly for human services such as health care (Kanavos, 1997).

Macro-economic pressures are even more acute in CEE/CIS countries than in western Europe. The element in common across the board in CEE/CIS countries has been the deep recession in all countries, following the demise of communist governments. In CEE countries, although several years of negative economic growth have now been replaced by improvements in overall gross domestic product, only in Poland and Slovenia have current levels of production returned to their 1989 levels. In CIS countries, economic productivity in 1997 was estimated to be barely more than half what it was in 1989 (EBRD, 1998). This severe economic situation has led to a significant decline in the financial resources officially available for the health services, with considerable implications for health care provision in these countries (Goldstein et al, 1996; Kanavos, 1997; McKee et al, 1998). In some CIS countries the financial cuts (of up to 50% of the health care budget) have slowed down or stalled the implementation of desired health care reform, as well as creating a substantial flow of informal payments.

Not surprisingly, economic retrenchment and decreasing health budgets affect the scale of reform and the extent of implementation. But the issue for implementers is whether financial constraints preclude the introduction of reform entirely. To the extent that many reform strategies aim at containing costs and/or generating savings, reform should improve rather than worsen at least the long-term financial sustainability of the health care system. Introducing reforms under these circumstances, however, involves at least three dilemmas. First, organizational reforms such as hospital contracting require substantial additional investment in management training and information systems to put them in place (Saltman and Figueras, 1997). Second, efficiency increases tend to appear in the form of increases in productivity rather than in actual savings. Even when the latter occur, the effects are not likely to be felt in the short run. Finally, in reforms aimed at reducing services such as the closure of hospitals, the extent of savings generated should not be overestimated (Edwards *et al*, 1998) and should be balanced against redundancy and social costs.

These dilemmas do not inexorably lead to the conclusion that reform is not possible, given existing financial constraints. Rather, the main obstacle may be unrealistic expectations about the likely benefits of reform, both from decision-makers and the population at large. In many CIS countries, market-style reforms have been expected to increase quality while maintaining universality despite reduced financial resources. The reality often has not matched these expectations. There are nonetheless strategies that national policy makers can adopt. One is to acknowledge up front the full financial implications of the reforms proposed. Often this means that implementers will need to shift the focus of reform towards less 'glamorous' but more affordable health care areas such as the strengthening of primary health care. A second strategy is to accept that the programmes of reform initially may need to be less ambitious, maintaining current structures and concentrating on marginal priority shifts between areas. Third, policy makers need to recognize that resource scarcity does not imply that existing patterns of provision and treatment are necessarily appropriate. For instance the health services in many CIS countries, while enduring enormous financial pressures, still maintain expensive human-resource-intensive services and treatments, inherited from the former Soviet Union, which in many cases are of dubious effectiveness. Finally, in some countries the financial constraints in the public health care system co-exist with considerable informal or 'under-the-table' payments (Delcheva *et al*, 1997) which reflect the inability of fiscal systems to reach the informal economy. Implementers might consider increasing resources in the public sector by formalizing 'under the table payments' while still maintaining existing structures of solidarity. Even when their implementation may require additional financial resources, these strategies offer a realistic and affordable approach to reform within macro-economic constraints.

Ensuring political will

A significant factor affecting reform implementation is what is frequently referred to as political will. It is influenced either by (explicit or implicit) opposition to reform or by political instability, and frequently constitutes a central obstacle. In some cases, the lack of political willingness to implement reform is not surprising. The nature of health care reform, as a highly complex process which requires major changes from the status quo and whose benefits are only felt in the long term (Walt, 1998), clashes with the short-term nature of political agendas, a problem which can be made worse by weak coalition governments and political instability.

The slowness in introducing health sector reform in many CEE countries is in considerable part a function of political instability. Frequent political changes—not only of governments and ministers but also of high-level officials within the relevant Ministries—have led to multiple reform proposals often leading to overall inaction (Rathwell, 1998). By contrast, political stability and strong political will can sometimes achieve reform implementation even in unfavourable circumstances. Two examples of this are New Zealand and the UK. The governments in these countries exerted their politically stable majority to introduce major health sector reforms in a relatively short period of time and in spite of prevailing opposition (Rathwell, 1998).

The issue faced by implementers is how to raise political commitment to reform and/or to ensure reform stability amidst political change. While there are no obvious answers, four sets of strategies may assist implementers in increasing political willingness to reform. First, implementers may use a number of epidemiological, economic and social science techniques to assess the problems of the health care system and thus to demonstrate the need for reform and its expected benefits. In particular, the use of comparative analysis techniques, showing the situation of a particular country within a broader international context, may spur politicians into considering change. Second, the use of demonstration or pilot sites to highlight the impact of specific reform strategies seems to be a particularly effective way to gain political willingness for more widespread change. However, as discussed below, this approach is not without problems. Third, implementers can increase reform sustainability by decentralizing implementation to a technocratic project office, to lower levels within the public sector, to NGOs, or to other key health service actors. In pluralistic or decentralized countries, reform implementation typically is less affected by periods of political instability. Lastly, one can try to ensure at the outset a wide consensus for reform between (and within) political parties, and with other key stakeholders. While this is often difficult to achieve, it is nonetheless a good way to ensure reform success. Key actors can constitute a substantial support to reform as well as impede reform altogether, even when there is substantial political will. The role of other key actors in reform implementation is discussed in the next section.

Mapping actors' agendas and setting strategic alliances

The nature and role of various central health sector actors have been well known for many years, both in the social science literature generally as well as in specifically health system focused assessments. A classic observation about physicians, for example, was made by Aneurin Bevan in 1948, when he noted that the best way to convince British doctors to support the nascent National Health Service was to 'stuff their mouths with gold'. Similarly at an institutional level, there are numerous examples of various hospital strategies to defeat political efforts to close redundant facilities. Recent studies of health reform have also provided clear maps for the interests and strategies of key actors (Reich, 1993; Gonzalez, 1995; Walt, 1998).

Where recent efforts have been less adequate is in the development of suitable strategies by which to steer these divergent interests into policy coalitions capable of designing, implementing, and sustaining sector-wide change. As national policy makers in western Europe know well, and as policy makers in CEE/CIS countries are rapidly discovering, a critical element in bringing the various actors together is to develop a policy champion. While ministries of health sometimes see themselves in this role, it typically is important to have one or more health sector actors who feel that their basic interests are also aligned with a proposed reform. Thus national policy makers often find themselves in the role not only of designing reforms, but of adjusting those reforms to facilitate the recruitment of one or more health sector interest groups to serve as their champions. These champions typically concentrate their efforts on coalition building among other health system actors. Through this process, national policy makers can help limit the likelihood that a strong opponent of the reforms will emerge to forge a negative coalition against the proposed changes. Policy makers should note that it can be difficult to recruit champions since they run the risk of drawing criticism or worse from vested interests who hope to prevent change.

Steering the process

Prior sections have reviewed strategies that can accommodate the context of reform implementation and the actors involved in this process. This section addresses the design and management of the implementation process itself (i.e. the stages or steps required to introduce change). Inadequate planning and management of this process has helped account for numerous reform failures. Yet it is this aspect which is mostly under the control of implementers and thus depends on their own ability to design and manage the process appropriately.

Helpful techniques here include setting explicit reform objectives; establishing a management structure and allocating responsibility; assessing available financial, technical and managerial resources; using mechanisms such as legislative and financial incentive tools,and putting in place appropriate information and monitoring systems. Overall, the effectiveness of these organizational management techniques in the health sector reform field is uncontroversial. Three of these strategies, however, deserve further discussion here.

Explicitness of reform objectives

A number of analysts believe that aims and objectives must be clear and easily understood to give a sense of direction and facilitate social consensus. However, policy makers sometimes argue that keeping the actual goals implicit and conducting the debate at a symbolic level may speed the initial process. In certain circumstances keeping the objectives deliberately vague may be the only way of ensuring, if not co-operation and support, at least limited opposition to changes, or of protecting hidden agendas (e.g. protecting jobs). Whether or not the objectives are ultimately expressed in clear and unambiguous language, or defined in ways open to different interpretation, will depend on whether the government has a strong mandate and is confident that it can carry through reform even in the face of opposition (Saltman and Figueras, 1997).

Establishment of management structures and allocation of responsibility for implementation

There is no single approach to ensure effective implementation. European countries differ in the structural, organizational and managerial arrangements introduced to run the reform process. A great deal will depend on aspects such as the decision-making structure and the distribution of authority between central and local levels. A key feature of many reforms is decentralization, the devolvement to certain groups of responsibility for activities and tasks previously undertaken by the government and its agencies. For example, countries as diverse as Britain, Germany and the Russian Federation did not establish formal mechanisms for implementation, relying instead on a combination of legislation and professional group support (often secured with specific incentives) to achieve their objectives. Other countries such as Turkey have taken a different approach, establishing a small unit specifically for implementation. This approach can work well, as long as the body responsible for managing the process retains political support and has access to adequate managerial, financial and legislative resources.

Development of enabling legislation

The development of enabling legislation is central to implementation, yet there is considerable uncertainty as to how best to support the process of change. There is wide variation among countries in the significance and usefulness of legislation for implementation. Health system reform in Northern Europe often relies on legislative legitimacy for implementation. In Germany, for instance, the implementation of reform has relied on a series of cost containment acts (Schwartz *et al*, 1997). Reform underpinned by regulation has been easier to implement than reform based on negotiation. In contrast, in other countries particularly in the South and Eastern parts of Europe, having legislation in place does not necessarily generate subsequent implementation. In parts of the CIS, legislation can act as a formulaic expression of official values to which no one subscribes in practice. Thus agreeing the laws does not imply that these are sufficient to steer the reform process or even that they will be implemented. Moreover, events frequently develop faster than the legislative cycle is able to respond.

New legislation is not always essential for health sector reform. In some instances, particularly at the outset of the reform process, it may be more effective to implement change through pushing the limits of existing legislation and/or through passing inconspicuous ministerial or royal decrees. This approach has been recently used by countries as diverse as Chile and Portugal. Nevertheless, in the medium-term, the lack of legislation can constitute a major block for health sector reform. The failure to enact required legislation due to political uncertainty resulting from short-term coalition governments has been a major obstacle to reform implementation in several CEE countries.

A central question for implementers is what type of legislation best facilitates reform implementation. Over-elaborate laws and regulations can slow down and restrict implementation. It may be best to rely on basic framework legislation establishing the broad principles of reform and allowing for flexible implementation. This type of legislation is particularly appropriate when there is substantial uncertainty as to the impact of the proposed reform and/or when the pace of change is likely to be swift. Ultimately, however, while legislation is important, it needs to be accompanied by other implementation measures: of itself, it will not produce the desired outcomes.

One aspect of steering the process of reform which has been the subject of some controversy is the timing and pacing of reform. This is dealt with separately in the next section.

Setting the time and pace of change

The timing of reform and the speed of change are important determinants of implementation success. Choosing the most appropriate time to reform, such as when there are appropriate or specific political, social or economic circumstances that favour change, is an important factor in successful implementation. A new government may have the legitimacy to execute policies denied to previous governments. Also, times of wide political and social transformation offer historical windows for introducing change (Saltman and Figueras, 1997). This window of opportunity is amply illustrated in many CEE/CIS countries, where the breakdown of the old communist regime has led to wide-ranging economic, social and political reforms. Similarly, the introduction of National Health Services in Spain, Portugal and Greece in the early 1980s took place at the end of long periods of totalitarian rule and followed the approval of new democratic constitutions that established health as a social right (Figueras *et al*, 1994). Chinitz also highlights the importance of timing when he refers to the 'end of history' (Fukuyama, 1989) to describe the changes in Israel's health policy in 1994 when, after reform proposals had been blocked for decades, policy subsystems had changed enough to make reform implementation possible (Chinitz, 1995).

These windows of opportunity favour the introduction of radical change. Yet the likelihood of achieving a rapid pace of reform depends on other factors discussed above, such as political will and stability, the macro-economic situation, the configuration of governance structures, and the degree of support from key stakeholders. Rapid 'big bang' reforms involving the top-down introduction of a grand plan, as in the Czech Republic, New Zealand and the United Kingdom, have been effective in bringing about change in a short time (Klein, 1995). In contrast to this 'big bang' approach to health system reform, changes in Finland, Germany, the Netherlands, Spain and Sweden have been more incremental.

There is a considerable debate about the relative merits of swift and radical reform compared with more incremental approaches (Maynard, 1994; Chinitz, 1995; Klein, 1995; Saltman and Figueras, 1997; Rathwell, 1998). In practice, however, the extent to which implementers can choose the pace of change is a somewhat rhetorical issue. In nations such as the Scandinavian countries, Germany and the Netherlands, with decentralized or pluralistic arrangements in the health sector with a system of 'checks and balances' overseeing the actions of the executive, the introduction of swift radical health reform is more difficult unless wide social consensus has already been achieved among major social actors. In the same way, the incrementalist nature of health reforms in CEE/CIS countries such as Bulgaria, Poland, Romania or Russia is more by default than by design, and is explained by contextual factors including political instability and macro-economic constraints. Lastly, both radical 'big bang' and incrementalism are relative concepts which are subject to different interpretations by observers. For instance, there has been some discussion as to whether health care reforms in the UK have been incremental or 'big bang'.

The question faced by implementers is whether, when (and if) contextual circumstances are appropriate, they should launch into radical 'big bang' reform. Available evidence to date indicates that a rapid pace of change is difficult to sustain. If 'big bang' reform is to be successful in the long term, it requires two prerequisites: first, a degree of technical 'certainty' as regards the reform model to be introduced; and, second, a broad social consensus behind that chosen model. Both prerequisites are often difficult to achieve. In the UK, experience with implementation of the (previously untested) internal market reforms, the lack of social consensus and the recent change of government have all contributed to a softening of some market strategies, encouraging a more moderate position that relies on contestability, long-term relationships and collaboration between purchasers and providers (Ham, 1996; GB Department of Health, 1997). Similarly, in the Czech Republic some of the fee-for-service schemes introduced at the outset of the reform led to a cost explosion and have subsequently been modified (Goldstein *et al*, 1996; Struk and Marshall, 1996).

A more incremental approach, whereby change is tested locally before being extended to the country as a whole, may be more effective (Borren and Maynard, 1994). This approach yields more evidence about the effectiveness of different approaches, allowing better decision-making. In the long run, an incremental approach may lead to more socially sustainable policies than the wholesale changes introduced in 'big bang' reforms. Sweden provides an example of the advantages of locally tested reforms, with major organizational changes being first introduced by individual county councils (Anell, 1995).

A local testing or incremental approach, however, also can have a number of drawbacks. A slow pace of reform allows key groups of stakeholders to organize before change is introduced, building up resistance. This can be seen in the reform process in the Netherlands, where the slow implementation of the Dekker proposals allowed time for a wave of mergers between health insurance companies and among some larger hospitals, in order to protect their market share if the proposals became policy (Groenewegen, 1994).

Another drawback of incremental approaches reflects the difficulties of generalizing the results of pilot experiences. Several countries in Europe, such as Kazakhstan, Poland, Portugal, Romania, Russia, Spain and Sweden, have put in place pilot projects to test various reform strategies. While pilots generate valuable evidence for future reform design and implementation, decision-makers frequently encounter obstacles when attempting to extend pilot experiences nationwide.

Three issues are of particular relevance. First, the human resources participating in pilot projects often are not representative of those available in the country as a whole. In many cases, these are self-selected groups who are motivated to embrace new ideas and whose baseline performance is well above national average. This factor may have played a significant role in explaining the positive results obtained by the first wave of GP fundholders in the UK (Glennerster *et al*, 1995). Second, pilot projects tend to be well funded and bring with them a strong infrastructure and financial incentives for the participating personnel. Often these conditions cannot be replicated when the experience is extended to the whole country. Lastly, pilots often benefit from a 'Hawthorne effect' caused by the interest generated by these experiences as well as by the evaluation mechanisms put into place.

Ultimately, the best implementation approach in each country will depend on its particular social, cultural and economic characteristics. However, there seems to be a consensus about the need to build flexibility into the implementation process. Policy makers should be able to modify the course of reform in the light of the evidence collected about its impact (Saltman and Figueras, 1997). One strategy is to combine an incremental approach to the overall reform programme with a series of small 'bangs' to put in place particular reform strategies, particularly in areas where there is both organizational certainty and social consensus.

Building institutional, human and management capacity

The success of reform implementation depends to a great extent on the existing institutional, human and management capacity (see Bennett, this volume). Many reform strategies such as the introduction of provider markets require sophisticated information systems as well as substantial technical and managerial skills which are lacking in a number of countries, particularly in the eastern part of the European region. The absence of these preconditions helps explain the minimal progress achieved when versions of provider-market reforms have been adopted in CEE/CIS countries.

A related factor in determining reform success is the extent to which there is institutional capacity, particularly in the public sector, to steer the reform process. The decentralization of State functions, together with the advent of market mechanisms in health care, has highlighted the need to increase the capacity of the State for governance, monitoring and regulating these new organizational relationships (Saltman and Figueras, 1997). A key factor in the failure of reforms in a number of CEE/CIS countries is the lack of capacity of the Ministry of Health to adopt new regulatory and information functions (Kokko et al, 1998; Figueras and Marshall, forthcoming). One contributory factor has been the rapid turnover of public sector personnel, with some of the best people migrating to better paying jobs in the private sector or with international organizations. In several CEE/CIS countries, the decentralization of authority to health insurance agencies or/and to regional and local level has left health ministries with accountability for implementation but with little authority and/or mechanisms to drive reforms.

Implementers can utilize a number of strategies to address the lack of technical and institutional capacity. In the first instance, implementers need to review available technical and managerial resources in the light of the requirements to implement desired reforms. When available resources are inadequate or insufficient, implementers may need to modify the pace of implementation to adapt to the existing capacity. At the same time, there will be a need to plan for the required skill mix of personnel by putting in place appropriate training programmes. At the outset these programmes need to be aimed at retraining existing human resources. Countries such as the Czech Republic or Hungary, which appear to have been more successful in this process, have involved interest groups such as the medical profession in building capacity and worked with external agencies in obtaining support to train and retrain their human resources. Finally, at the centre of strategies to build capacity to implement reform, there is a need for programmes of institutional strengthening and governance aimed at public bodies and in particular Ministries of Health charged with the responsibility to implement, regulate and monitor health care reform.

Concluding remarks

This chapter adds to the evidence that 'minding the implementation process' is essential if reforms are to be successful. However, the evidence reviewed also shows that implementation is not an exact science. There is no agreed set of strategies that can be applied in all countries and circumstances and which, if followed faithfully, will lead to success.

The chapter identifies a number of key issues in managing the reform process across Europe, and reviews a number of strategies that have met with success at least in some countries. First, the chapter highlights the need for implementers to recognize contextual factors, in particular the effects of macro-economic constraints and the important role of culture and values in adapting external influences. Some pragmatic strategies are suggested to deal with these contextual factors. Second, implementers can use a number of strategies to ensure the support of key actors, amongst whom the politicians themselves are particularly important stakeholders. Indeed, strategies to strengthen political will are central to reform implementation. Third, the chapter shows the range of available strategies to steer the process of change and to set the time and pace of change. Lastly, a key precondition for the implementation strategies reviewed is the availability of sufficient institutional, technical and managerial capacity. In this respect the establishment of training programmes should parallel the development of appropriate reform programmes.

References

Anell A. Implementing planned markets in health care: the Swedish case. In: Saltman RB, von Otter C (eds) *Implementing planned markets in health care: balancing social and economic responsibilities.* Buckingham: Open University Press, 1995, pp 209–226

Borren P, Maynard A. The market reform of the New Zealand health care system: searching for the Holy Grail in the Antipodes. *Health Policy,* 1994; 27:233–252

Chinitz D. Israel's health policy breakthrough: the politics of reform and the reform of politics. *Journal of Health Politics, Policy and Law,* 1995; **20**: 909–932

Collins C, Green A, Hunter D. International transfers of national health service reforms: problems and issues. *The Lancet,* 1994; **344**: 248-250

Delcheva E, Balabanova B, McKee M. Under-the-counter payments for health care: evidence from Bulgaria. *Health Policy,* 1997; **42**: 89–100

Edwards N, Hensher M, Werneke U. Changing hospital systems. In: Saltman RB, Figueras J, Sakellarides C (eds) *Critical challenges for health care reform in Europe.* Buckingham: Open University Press, 1998

European Bank for Reconstruction and Development. *Transition report: Infrastructures and savings.* London: European Bank for Reconstruction and Development, 1998

Figueras J, Mossialos E, McKee M, Sassi F. Health care systems in Southern Europe: is there a Mediterranean paradigm? *International Journal of Health Sciences,* 1994; 5:135–146

Figueras J, Saltman RB, Mossialos E. *Challenges in evaluating health sector reform: An overview*. London: London School of Economics and Political Science, 1997

Figueras J, Marshall T. Health reform trends in the European Region: balancing the role of the state and market. In: Alvarez-Dardet C (ed) *European Public Health*. London: Global Healthcare Communications Group, forthcoming

Fukuyama F. The End of History. *The National Interest*, 1989; Summer:3–35

Glennerster H, Matsaganis M, Owens P, Hancock S. *Implementing GP fundholding: wild card or winning hand?* Buckingham: Open University Press, 1995

Goldstein E, Preker AS, Adeyi O, Chellaraj G. *Trends in Health Status, Services and Finance: The Transition in Central and Eastern Europe*. Volume 1. World Bank Technical Paper No.341. Washington, DC: World Bank, 1996

Gonzalez AEA. *La dimension politica en los procesos de reforma del sistema de salud*. Mexico, D. F.: Fundacion Mexicana para la Salud, 1995

Great Britain Department of Health. *The new NHS: Modern, dependable*. London: The Stationery Office, 1997

Groenewegen PP. The shadow of the future: institutional change in health care. *Health Affairs*, 1994; **13**:137–148

Ham C. Contestability: a middle path for health care. *British Medical Journal*,1996; **312**: 70–71

Kanavos P. Health expenditures in CEE: friend or foe? In: Saltman R, Figueras J (eds) *European health care reform: analysis of current strategies*. Copenhagen: World Health Organization Regional Office for Europe, 1997

Klein R. Big bang health care reform - does it work? The case of Britain's 1991 National Health Service reforms. *Milbank Quarterly*, 1995; **73**:299–337

Kokko S, Hava P, Ortun V, Leppo K. The role of the State in health care reform. In: Saltman RB, Figueras J, Sakellarides C (eds) *Critical challenges for health care reform in Europe*. Buckingham: Open University Press, 1998

Kroneman MW, van der Zee J. Health Policy as a fuzzy concept: methodological problems encountered when evaluating health policy reforms in an international prespective.*Health Policy*, 1997; **40**:139–155

Maynard A. Can competition enhance efficiency in health care? Lessons from the reform of the UK national health service. *Social Science and Medicine*, 1994; **39**:1433–1445

McKee M, Figueras J, Chenet L. Health sector reform in the former soviet republics of Central Asia. *International Journal of Health Planning and Management*, 1998; **13**: 131–147

Rathwell T. Implementing health care reform: A review of current experience. In: Saltman RB, Figueras J, Sakellarides C (eds) *Critical challenges for health care reform in Europe*. Buckingham: Open University Press, 1998

Reich MR. *Political mapping of health policy*. Boston: Harvard University Press, 1993

Saltman R, Figueras J (eds) *European health care reform: Analysis of current strategies*. Copenhagen: World Health Organization Regional Office for Europe, 1997

Saltman RB, Figueras J, Sakellarides C (eds) *Critical Challenges for Health Care Reform in Europe*. Buckingham: Open University Press, 1998

Schwartz FW, Busse R. Germany. In: Ham C (ed) *Health Care Reform: learning from International Experience*. Buckingham: Open University Press, 1997, pp 104–118

Struk P, Marshall T. *Health care systems in transition: Czech Republic*. Copenhagen: WHO Regional Office for Europe, 1996

Walt G, Gilson L. Reforming the health sector in developing countries: the central role of policy analysis. *Health Policy and Planning*, 1994; **9**: 353–370

Walt G. Implementing health care reform: A framework for discussion. In: Saltman RB, Figueras J, Sakellarides C (eds). *Critical challenges for health care reform in Europe.* Buckingham: Open University Press, 1998

14
Rethinking health sector reform: personal reflections

Anne Mills

London School of Hygiene & Tropical Medicine, UK

The preceding chapters testify to the worldwide interest in reshaping health systems, and indicate the extent to which there is a global terminology—even though each country may make different decisions on which changes to introduce, influenced by its own particular historical inheritance, current institutions and structures, and political and economic pressures.

A key feature of this volume is the inclusion of papers addressing the experiences and concerns of countries at all levels of development, from some of the richest to some of the poorest. From this unusual interaction came much of the richness of the discussions, and valuable questioning of the assumptions of researchers and commentators whose analyses are inevitably bounded by the experiences of the countries they know best.

This final chapter seeks to draw on the fervour and depth of debate at the Forum and reflect on key points that emerged from the interaction of ideas from very different countries and regions.

Fundamental forces

All sessions at the Forum, even those more focused on the technical content of reforms, highlighted that reform is fundamentally about who gains and who loses, and the power that different groups have to impede or encourage reform. The chapter by Evans makes this point very powerfully, and highlights that the conventional tools of economics tend to obscure issues of the distribution of gains and losses. Yet such forces can ultimately dictate whether or not reforms succeed:

for example in the US, opposition from the health professions and insurers undermined the Clinton proposals. However, it should not be assumed—as for example is often the case in the UK—that the medical profession is necessarily always reactionary, and opposed to change. In some middle-income countries, for example, the medical profession has supported the introduction of compulsory insurance. In countries where purchasing power limits the size of the private market and doctors are not in short supply, the medical profession may see insurance as a secure source of income and thus in its own interests, even though it implies greater dependence on an external paymaster.

At the country level, the categorization of different interest groups is very similar—the medical profession with sub-groups within it, private insurer and provider groups, politicians, labour unions etc. In developed countries, it is frequently argued that the number and size of competing groups makes fundamental reform almost impossible to achieve. However, it is by no means clear that the same conclusion holds true across all countries in the world or at all times within a given country. The balance of power between, for example, the state, the medical profession and labour interests may vary greatly. For example, the medical profession may be more fragmented; labour interests less well organized; and consumer special interest groups (such as the elderly) non-existent. To date, political scientists have been most active in studying the North American health system; they should encourage their colleagues in low- and middle-income countries to analyse similarly their own health systems. We may then be in a better position to understand the influences on health policy, and the scope for change in different settings.

Underlying Evans' theme that health reform is in essence about distribution is the fundamental accounting identity which, over all individuals in society, links total expenditure on health goods and services, total revenues raised to pay for those services, and total incomes earned from the provision of services. This immediately highlights a key difference between rich countries and poorer ones, which is that for the latter group this identity does not hold true at the country level because of the often very substantial flows of resources from outside. For example, in some of the poorest countries up to 50% of ministry of health recurrent funds may originate from outside the country. The importance of this flow of funds in this context is that it fundamentally changes the balance of power in the health system. It is likely both to weaken the power of some internal groups, and to strengthen the power of those who can leverage external resources. At the same time it clearly gives external funders, especially where there are a few large ones, considerable potential to influence country reforms (Pavignani et al, 1998).

These influences help to explain the arguments over models or blueprints of reforms. On the one hand commentators, notably Marmor in this volume, emphasize that employing the term 'health reform' misleadingly suggests common diagnoses and remedies, argue that a search for the best model is wishful thinking, and condemn much of the rhetoric about worldwide health reform. In practice, country-specific circumstances dictate both what is desirable and what is feasible.

From a North American or European perspective, such arguments appear eminently reasonable. However, the reality of poorer countries is that models tried in richer countries are suggested to them as offering possibly useful lessons. Influences flow through external technical experts and through the training received by local analysts and decision-makers in developed country universities. There has not as yet been any concerted effort to build capacity in countries to formulate their own health policy and systems thinking, so they are all the more vulnerable to ideas imported from outside.

The power of words

Bringing together a large group from a very wide-ranging set of countries highlighted both the commonality of the language we use to describe health reform and some fundamental differences in interpretation and terminology. There appear to be regional differences in whether we talk about health care reform, health sector reform, health system reform, or just health reform. While we could argue about the particular nuances that any one of these implies, it is clear that in general the last two are distinguished by their much broader consideration of health, as opposed to the narrower concerns implied by the term 'health care reform'. In a school of public health, it is important to remind ourselves that medical care, although it may preoccupy the bulk of reformers' time, is only one element in a strategy to improve population health.

Marmor warns us not to be deceived by the fashionable terms used to describe particular reform components. He highlighted 'managed competition' and 'health maintenance organizations' as being particular examples of the way in which terms can be used, as in advertising slogans, to convey desirable images which are actually quite at odds with the phenomena being described. To this list could be added 'sophisticated payment systems'. Such systems are frequently being recommended, and involve combining several payment approaches together rather than just employing fee-for-service, or capitation, or case-based payment alone. However, the chapter by Scheffler makes clear their accompanying disadvantage: very substantial management costs.

Controversy

A particularly valuable contribution of the Forum was to highlight controversy. Published descriptions of reforms may gloss over controversies, or even be written largely by partisans of the reforms. In addition global myths can develop about particular country reforms, where certain countries are held up as good examples to the outside world even though those within the country see all the imperfections.

Two particular types of controversy were evident. One was whether to interpret a particular country's reforms as a success or failure. For example, in the case of UK reforms, the Forum exposed the fundamental debates that have persisted over the internal market reforms. Commentators differed over whether the internal market had ever existed. If it did, has it stopped existing? Was it a fundamental change or not? Has it had a fundamental effect or not? The chapter by Mays in this volume both sheds light on these questions, and highlights the many methodological difficulties that countries face in trying to evaluate reforms.

The second type of controversy was whether or not any of the principles of managed markets were desirable, and especially those reforms that opened up insurers and providers to competition. My opening paper identified this as a key issue, and expressed some scepticism about the value and relevance of these principles in low-income countries; the papers from North America by Evans and Scheffler portrayed very different views of the desirability of North American trends; and the papers by Frenk and McPake clearly saw value in incorporating elements of competition within systems of financing and provision, especially in the context of Latin America, and in redefining the role of the state to reduce its involvement in direct provision and increase it in the area of regulation and standard setting. However, the chapter by Bennett highlights the nature of the capacities required by states if they are to fulfil these roles effectively. These debates merge into issues of the relative roles of public and private sectors, and again considerable controversy was apparent, not least in relation to the private finance initiative in the UK described in the chapter by Pollock. Some commentators saw the state as essentially failing in its responsibilities especially in the provision of care, and wanted to see a much greater role played by private sector providers and autonomous public ones. Others, such as Evans and Gilson, emphasized the vital role of the state in setting public policy and addressing inequalities.

Lack of knowledge

The papers in this volume emphasize that different ways of funding and organizing health systems have fundamental implications for the health care provided and for the health status of the population. Some hints of what these might be emerged during the Forum. For example Martin McKee, in his remarks on the paper by Evans, commented that antibiotic resistance was highest in countries in Europe with more fragmented health systems; and the chapter by Yepes suggests that the Colombian reforms have adversely affected the performance of the public health function of disease surveillance and control. Yet in general, this book highlights that it is not yet possible to predict the effects of reforms, nor easily judge their effects after they have been implemented. One of the discussants, Alex Preker, listed some key unknowns:

- where should the boundary be placed between public and private, and what determines where the boundary should be placed?
- what are the implications of moving towards a greater private sector role in the health system?
- to what extent should the institutions of the health system be under political as opposed to administrative control?
- what should the balance be between centralization and decentralization?
- should health systems be single-payer or multi-payer: i.e should there be a single public insurer or many?
- how should health system performance be measured? Can we identify 'tracer conditions' (for example the extent to which benefits have accrued to priority population groups) that might provide insight into the impact of reforms?

A particularly large gap, and a challenge thrown out by a number of speakers, was to improve knowledge of specific public policies which can be implemented to improve the health of the most disadvantaged. Key themes which emerged from the Forum were those of universality and solidarity, but how these principles can be applied in the context of poor countries requires much more thought and experimentation.

Gains in knowledge

Nonetheless, it was apparent that there have been substantial gains in knowledge over the last decade, and that we are able to engage in a much higher level of debate than was the case some years ago. One key feature was the engagement of a number of disciplinary perspectives. It has often been said that health sector reforms have been driven by economists; however the Forum demonstrated that even if this had been the case, it was no longer so. Discussion drew widely on the contributions of many disciplines, and there was a notable presence of political science.

Another key feature resulted from the interaction of researchers and decision-makers both at the Forum and as reflected in the content of the papers. Several speakers addressed how research and policy might best interact. Somsak Chunharas' chapter emphasizes the importance, from the perspective of countries where much research funding is external, of managing research for health reform, to ensure that it is relevant to countries and communicated to decision makers in appropriate ways and using a variety of channels. Josep Figueras' chapter emphasizes how the ways in which decision-makers go about implementing reforms have a vital influence on whether or not change actually happens.

The Forum also heard some of the latest evidence on the impact of reforms, notably in the case of the UK and Colombia. While this may not be definitive—at least in the case of Colombia where the new system is being phased in gradually—it begins to enable us to highlight key aspects of the content and processes of reform that appear influential in influencing reform impact. While there were a number of common themes, one notable one was the importance of the general public. There has been a tendency for reforms to have been driven either by technocrats or politicians, with little involvement of the general public. Yet benefits for the general public—which substantially depend on how they respond to reforms—are a major endpoint of reforms. The lack of attention given to consulting and involving the general public is thus not only strange but perverse. Where reforms involve giving people choice of insurer, as in Colombia, or choice of provider, as in the Thai social insurance scheme, careful thought needs to be given to how to make that choice as informed as possible.

And finally, the Forum provided many rich examples of the practical issues of implementing reforms. It is easy for researchers to get carried away by controversies over grand designs, but decision makers are concerned about much more practical and pragmatic issues, especially where government capacity is limited. These are also important areas where research can help countries to implement successful reforms.

References

Pavignani E, Walt G, Gilson L, Howe G (1998). *Managing external resources in the health sector.* Final report to the Department of International Development, London School of Hygiene & Tropical Medicine.